LF

ELDERCARE

ELDERCARE
A Practical Guide to Clinical Geriatrics

Editors

Mary O'Hara-Devereaux, F.N.P., PH.D.
Director of Research, Foundation for Comprehensive Health Services
Sebastopol, California
Co-Director, Family Nurse Practitioner and Physician's Assistant Program
Department of Family Practice, School of Medicine
University of California at Davis
Sacramento, California

Len Hughes Andrus, M.D.
President, Foundation for Comprehensive Health Services
Sebastopol, California
Professor, Department of Family Practice
School of Medicine
University of California at Davis
Sacramento, California

Cynthia D. Scott, M.P.H.
Education Specialist
Foundation for Comprehensive Health Services
Sebastopol, California
Coordinator of Geriatric Education
The Aging Health Policy Center
Department of Social and Behavioral Sciences
University of California at San Francisco

Technical Editor

Mary I. Gary
Research Associate/Editor
Foundation for Comprehensive Health Services
Sebastopol, California
Family Nurse Practitioner and Physician's Assistant Program
Department of Family Practice, School of Medicine
University of California at Davis
Sacramento, California

Grune & Stratton
A Subsidiary of Harcourt Brace Jovanovich, Publishers
New York   London   Toronto   Sydney   San Francisco

Library of Congress Cataloging in Publication Data
Main entry under title:

Eldercare: a practical guide to clinical geriatrics.

Bibliography:
Includes indexes.
1. Geriatrics. 2. Gerontology. I. O'Hara-
Devereaux, Mary. II. Andrus, Len Hughes.
III. Scott, Cynthia D. [DNLM: 1. Geriatrics.
WT 100 E37]
RC952.E46   618.97   80–39592
ISBN 0–8089–1285–2

Grune & Stratton, Inc.
111 Fifth Avenue
New York, New York 10003

Distributed in the United Kingdom by
Academic Press Inc. (London) Ltd.
24/28 Oval Road, London NW 1

Library of Congress Catalog Number 80–39592
International Standard Book Number 0–8089–1285–2

Printed in the United States of America

ERRATA

Page 64 should read as follows:

cord becomes more than a communication system. When properly utilized, it sets the stage for the team approach.

Comprehensive Patient-Centered Care

The comprehensive approach to eldercare addresses the totality of the patient's existence, the problems, and the needs; health care is only part of the picture. In addition to the patient's physical and emotional status and daily activities, other factors must be considered, such as the patient's physical environment. Getting old usually means an increasingly solitary experience and, for many, a time of institutionalization. Older people are also much more vulnerable to the dangers in our society of crime and abuse. Loneliness, despair, and paranoia are understandable byproducts. To counter these depressing forces and prevent the patient from assuming the cloak of invalidism, it is important to play into personal strengths, utilize expectations positively, and foster self-responsibility.

Fortunately, most older patients with chronic illnesses are able to take care of themselves to a great extent. The majority of older people are at home and have friends and family involved in their care. Only 5 percent of elders are in institutions.

Our goal is to help the older patient assume responsibility whenever possible for his or her own care. This means the patient must become involved in the identification and definition of his or her problems and needs. Ideally, the needs of the patient and the problem list are developed by the primary health care team under the leadership of the physician, and a plan for each problem is established. Depending on the nature and complexity of the problems, responsibility for sharing care is assigned to various team members. Through regular, as well as informal and impromptu, conferences, the progress is evaluated and the problem list updated. The patient and others involved should be informed in such a way that they will understand the patient's health status including the symptoms of each problem and the potential complications. Such information should be conveyed in an honest, simple, and easily understood manner, avoiding frightening language or scare techniques, and expressing optimism and reassurance whenever possible.

Clear instructions need to be given on recommended activities, nutrition, preventive measures, and both medications and possible side effects. Instructions should be in writing for the patient and others involved in the patient's care. Patients in general, but particularly elders under the tension and confusion of the clinical setting, have difficulty remembering directions. A well-organized, written regimen that is typed in large print gives the patient a visual and conceptual framework for regularity and compliance with therapeutic programs.

The key to patient-oriented care is *patient education and the education of family, friends, and others involved in the patient's care.* Doctors frequently do not have the time or inclination for proper patient education, while other team members can handle this function well. Managing chronic illness by utilizing the primary health care team, the patient's family, and community resources in a comprehensive patient-centered approach leads to better and more humanistic patient care and is professionally stimulating, rewarding, as well as personally satisfying.

REFERENCES

1. Weed LL: Medical Records, Medical Education and Patient Care, The Problem Oriented Record as a Basic Tool. Cleveland, Ohio, The Press of Case Western Reserve University, 1969

On page 93, the last two lines of the first column should read:

The hypochondriacal preoccupation is often a socially acceptable emotional crutch that may be

Dedicated to my mother, Kathleen O'Hara-Devereaux, who encouraged me to always reach for my highest aims; to my grandmother, Anna O. Devereaux, who had a great capacity for love and family; and to my grandmother, Sarah O'Hara, who taught me to seek adventure and see the humor of life.

Mary O'Hara-Devereaux, F.N.P., Ph.D.

Dedicated to Leonard Milo Andrus, M.D., my 85-year-old father, who always had a special way with older patients, and to my mother, who always had a special way with him.

Len Hughes Andrus, M.D.

Dedicated to the grandpersons in my life: Amos and Fern Hoff and Hazel Abbe, who inspired strength and commitment in the lives they touched.

Cynthia D. Scott, M.P.H.

Dedicated to my father, Fred P. Roessel, Ph.D., whose altruistic philosophy and dedication to education greatly enhanced the lives of his children, grandchildren, and his many students; and to my mother, Emma I. Roessel, who taught me the value of patience and perseverance.

Mary Gary

Contents

SECTION 3. COMMUNITY AND MEDICAL RESOURCES

Acknowledgments

The original concept for this book evolved out of our education and service activities in primary care, in which it became increasingly apparent that the care of elders was an important and neglected area. Although not directly supporting the preparation of this volume, the Division of Nursing, DHEW (Grant 7D24 NU00056), did support our efforts to develop and implement in primary care a geriatrics curriculum for our Family Nurse Practitioner students, Department of Family Practice, University of California at Davis. The undergraduate, graduate, and continuing education curriculums that resulted have been utilized and studied by family nurse practitioners, as well as by physicians, physician's assistants, nurses, social workers, and others over the last four years.

In addition to the editors' positions with the University of California, all are members of the Foundation for Comprehensive Health Services, a nonprofit organization founded by Len Hughes Andrus, M.D. The Foundation is devoted to activities in the research and development of new approaches to the delivery of basic health services, emphasizing work in underserved areas and with underserved populations. The Foundation's activities in geriatrics provided a solid basis for our ideas and philosophy of eldercare. A DHEW research and development grant (90-A-160) from the Administration on Aging to the Foundation helped establish a private-team practice model consisting of a physician, family nurse practitioner, medical social workers, and clinical pharmacist. This grant provided support for our advocacy of the sociomedical team model for delivering health care to elders.

For several years, the W. K. Kellogg and the Robert Wood Johnson Foundations supported our activities in primary care education and team training. The California Health Manpower Policy Commission also supported our work over the last several years. The philosophy of copractice (with physicians, family nurse practitioners, and physician's assistants) and the role of geriatrics in primary care developed through these efforts.

Our gratitude extends to many people: first, to our coauthors who share our philosophy and commitment to improving eldercare. Warm thanks to our colleagues in the Family Nurse Practitioner and Physician's Assistant Program and our graduates who worked closely with us to develop our geriatric education and service approach. Special thanks to David Daehler, M.D., and Peggy Davis, M.S.W., for their valuable assistance with Chapter 5, "Caring for Elders." We extend a special acknowledgment to Mary Gary, who did the major editorial work and who worked tirelessly and enthusiastically to complete the volume on target. We wish to thank Mora Chartrand and Marilyn Rigby for their typing assistance, Ollie Butler for her administrative support, and our families and friends, who were cheerful and supportive while we completed our work. A special thanks to Leona and Charlie Judson, who kept the home fires burning.

The original drawings in Chapter 15 were developed by David Daehler, M.D. from concepts in Williams Flexion Exercises, also utilizing ideas from professional association with Ralph Soto-Hall, M.D. and Rene Cailliet, M.D.

Foreword

It is now appreciated that proper care of people in their elder years will do a great deal to extend their lifespans and increase the quality of their lives. I feel that *Eldercare: A Practical Guide to Clinical Geriatrics* will be helpful to all health care professionals involved with older people. It will also be a useful resource to many older people who would like to make the most of their later years and for their families to read for their own guidance. I am 85 years old and am enjoying a most productive period by following the principles laid down in this book. It should be a very valuable book for the whole field of gerontology.

RUSSELL V. LEE, M.D.
Founder and Consultant
Palo Alto Medical Clinic
Palo Alto, CA

Preface

In many ways elders are the forgotten members of our society. Our social policies and programs do not support or serve them well. This is also true for our health care system. Our specialized medical care system has fragmented care for those most in need of a comprehensive and personal approach.

It is our belief that the most comprehensive, personal, and economical way to deliver services to elders is by a primary health care team. With their appropriate bright attitude, knowledge, and skills, the members of this team can effectively deliver 90 percent of the care needed.

Eldercare provides the primary care clinician with a diagnostic and therapeutic approach to the most common clinical problems in geriatrics. The first section of this book discusses normal aging processes and ethical considerations as a way to provide a perspective and context for delivering health services. It is our opinion that clinicians cannot effectively care for elders without understanding the social and political realities of aging.

In Section 2, we elected to present several chapters on the clinical problems confronting elders, chapters which have been written by primary care physicians, nurse practitioners, or physician assistants and coauthored by specialists in this particular field of geriatrics. The team approach to preparing the book reflects our commitment to the philosophy of copractice as a model of care. We have tried to make this section practical and an easy-to-use reference guide for a wide spectrum of health care professionals dealing with elders.

This section is meant not to be an exhaustive clinical review but rather to focus on common problems and to provide practical hints—a "how-to" approach. There is an overview of each system, of the incidence of problems in primary care, and a short review of uncommon problems. The emphasis is on diagnosis and treatment of common problems, again emphasizing the practical approach. We have attempted to maintain a sensitivity to elders, as well as to those near and dear to them, and to assume a philosophy of caring without assuming total responsibility for elders. It is hoped that this approach both encourages elders to use their own individual resources and promotes family and community involvement in eldercare. We tried to imply that health care for elders is best accomplished through a team approach.

Also included in this section is a chapter on alternative therapies, which provides information to clinicians on some of the new and effective therapies.

The third section focuses on community resources and alternatives to institutionalization. Coordination and cooperation with these professionals and programs are cornerstones of good health care.

The ongoing theme throughout the book is that the quality of the lives of elders should be made as meaningful and active as possible. It is hoped that health care providers can make a contribution to the health of older persons by increasing and promoting self-care and prevention.

MARY O'HARA-DEVEREAUX, F.N.P., PH.D.
LEN HUGHES ANDRUS, M.D.
CYNTHIA D. SCOTT, M.P.H.

Contributors

Len Hughes Andrus, M.D.
Professor, Department of Family Practice
School of Medicine
University of California at Davis
President, Foundation for Comprehensive Health
    Services
Sebastopol, California

Georgia Barrow, Ph.D.
Instructor
Department of Behavioral Sciences
Santa Rosa Junior College
Santa Rosa, California

Rodney S. W. Basler, M.D.
Consultant in Dermatology
University of Nebraska
Lincoln, Nebraska
President, American Dermatologic Health
    Association

James Bennett, D.D.S., M.S.
Professor and Director
General Dental Residency Program
University of Oregon Health Sciences Center
Portland, Oregon

Andre Calin, M.D., M.R.C.P.
Assistant Professor of Medicine
Stanford University
Director, Department of Rheumatology
VA Hospital
Palo Alto, California

James W. Cooper, Ph.D., F.C.P.
Associate Professor and Head
Department of Pharmacy Practice
School of Pharmacy
Assistant Clinical Professor
Medical College of Georgia
University of Georgia
Associate Director, Pharmacy Services
Athens Convalescent Center
Athens, Georgia

Howard Creamer, Ph.D.
Associate Professor
Chairman, Department of Microbiology
School of Dentistry
University Oregon Health Sciences Center
Portland, Oregon

James L. Creighton
Stress Management Consultant
Saratogo, California

Donat P. Cyr, M.D.
Former Chief of Hematology Section
Department of Internal Medicine
Lahey Clinic
Boston, Massachusetts

David Daehler, M.D.
Clinical Assistant Professor
Department of Family Practice
School of Medicine
University of California at Davis
Medical Director
River City Family Medical Group
Sacramento, California

John Dervin, M.D.
Clinical Assistant Professor
Division of Family and Community Medicine
University of California at San Francisco
Associate Director
Family Practice Residency Program
Community Hospital of Sonoma County
Santa Rosa, California

Patricia Dervin, R.N., M.S.
Research Analyst
Foundation for Comprehensive Health Services
Sebastopol, California

Ken Dychtwald, Ph.D.
Director
Association for Humanistic Gerontology
Berkeley, California

Carroll Estes, Ph.D.
Professor of Sociology
Director, Aging Health Policy Center
School of Nursing
University of California at San Francisco
San Francisco, California

Donna J. Fontana-Smith, R.D.H.
Coordinator of Nursing Home Dental Group
Geriatrics Dental Group
Portland, Oregon

Virginia Fowkes, F.N.P., M.H.S.
Lecturer, Division of Family Medicine
Director, Primary Care Associate Program
Stanford University School of Medicine
Stanford, California

William C. Fowkes, Jr., M.D.
Associate Professor and Chief
Division of Family Medicine
Stanford University School of Medicine
Stanford, California

Martha Holstein, M.A.
Deputy Director, Western Gerontological Society
San Francisco, California

Roger Jacobs, Ph.D.
Post-Doctoral Fellow
Department of Obstetrics and Gynecology
Columbia University
College of Physicians and Surgeons
New York, New York

Darlene Jelinek, R.N., F.N.P.
Instructor
Department of Family, Community, and
  Emergency Medicine
University of New Mexico School of Medicine
Albuquerque, New Mexico

Jean Johnson, M.S.N., N.P.
Director of the Adult and Geriatric Nurse
  Practitioner Program
Department of Health Care Sciences
George Washington University
Washington, D.C.

Albert R. Jonsen, Ph.D.
Professor of Ethics and Medicine
School of Medicine
Health Policy Program
University of California at San Francisco
San Francisco, California

Leona Judson, F.N.P., M.H.S.
Clinical Faculty Division

Family Nurse Practitioner and Physician's
  Assistant Program
Department of Family Practice
University of California at Davis
Occidental Area Health Center
Occidental, California

Jack Kleh, M.D.
Medical Director
Gerontological Treatment Center
Associate Clinical Professor
School of Medicine
George Washington University
Washington, D.C.

Philip R. Lee, M.D.
Professor of Social Medicine
Director, Health Policy Program
School of Medicine
University of California at San Francisco
San Francisco, California

Glen A. Lillington, M.D., F.R.C.P.(C), F.A.C.P.
Professor and Chief
Section of Pulmonary Medicine
Department of Internal Medicine
School of Medicine
University of California at Davis
Sacramento, California

Parveen Malik, M.D.
Assistant Director
San Joaquin County Family Practice Residency
  Program
University of California at Davis
French Camp, California

Jack McAninch, M.D.
Associate Professor, School of Medicine
University of California at San Francisco
Chief of Urology
San Francisco General Hospital
San Francisco, California

Jan McCann, F.N.P., M.H.S.
Lecturer, Family Nurse Practitioner and
  Physician's Assistant Program
Department of Family Practice
School of Medicine
University of California at Davis
Sacramento, California

Henry S. Metz, M.D.
Chairman, Department of Ophthalmology
University of Rochester Medical Center
Rochester, New York

Clark H. Millikan, M.D.
Professor
Department of Neurology
University of Utah Medical Center
Salt Lake City, Utah

Walter Morgan, M.D.
Assistant Clinical Professor
Department of Family Practice
Medical Director, Family Nurse Practitioner
and Physician's Assistant Program
School of Medicine
University of California at Davis
Sacramento, California

Thomas Novotny, M.D.
Clinical Faculty
Division of Family Medicine
School of Medicine
University of California at San Francisco
Russian River Health Center
Guerneville, California

Mary O'Hara-Devereaux, F.N.P., Ph.D.
Co-Director, Family Nurse Practitioner and
Physician's Assistant Program
Department of Family Practice
School of Medicine
University of California at Davis
Director of Research, Foundation for
Comprehensive Health Services
Sebastopol, California

Gibbe H. Parsons, M.D.
Assistant Professor
Department of Internal Medicine
Pulmonary Section, School of Medicine
University of California at Davis
Sacramento, California

L. Gregory Pawlson, M.D., M.P.H.
Director of the Center for Aging Studies
and Services
Department of Health Care Services
George Washington University
Washington, D.C.

Michael Podlone, M.D.
Clinical Assistant Professor
Department of Medicine
Medical Director
Primary Care Associate Program
Stanford University
Palo Alto, California

Jack Rodnick, M.D.
Assistant Professor and Vice Chairman

Division of Family Medicine
School of Medicine
University of California at San Francisco
Associate Director
Family Practice Program
Community Hospital of Sonoma County
Santa Rosa, California

JoAnne Rolando, R.N.
Geriatric Nurse Practitioner Program
University of Utah
Salt Lake City, Utah

Robert J. Ruben, M.D.
Professor and Chairman
Department of Otolaryngology
Albert Einstein College of Medicine
Montefiore Hospital and Medical Center
Bronx, New York

John Santos, Ph.D.
Professor of Psychology
Director in Gerontological Education
Research and Services
University of Notre Dame
Notre Dame, Indiana

Marvin Schuster, M.D.
Professor, School of Medicine
Johns Hopkins University
Chief, Gastroenterology
Baltimore City Hospital
Baltimore, Maryland

Cynthia D. Scott, M.P.H.
Coordinator of Geriatric Education
The Aging Health Policy Center
Department of Social and Behavioral Sciences
University of California at San Francisco
Education Specialist
Foundation for Comprehensive Health Services
Sebastopol, California

Joseph C. Scott, Jr., M.D.
Professor and Chairman
Department of Obstetrics and Gynecology
University of Nebraska Medical Center
Omaha, Nebraska

Nancy D. Sullivan, F.N.P., M.S.
Lecturer, Family Nurse Practitioner and
Physician's Assistant Program
Department of Family Practice
School of Medicine
University of California at Davis
Sacramento, California

David N. Sundwall, M.D.
Assistant Professor
Department of Family and Community Medicine
University of Utah
Salt Lake City, Utah

Dennis A. Taisch, M.D.†
Clinical Instructor
Department of Ophthalmology
Pacific Medical Center
San Francisco, California
Attending Physician
Highland General Hospital
Oakland, California

Elizabeth A. Taisch, F.N.P., M.H.S.
Lecturer, Department of Family Practice
School of Medicine
University of California at Davis
Sacramento, California

Corinne Thomas, F.N.P., M.H.S.
Private Family Practice
Instructor, College of the Redwoods
Fortuna, California

George W. Thorn, M.D.
Professor in Chief, Emeritus
Peter Bent Brigham Hospital
Hersey Professor of the Theory and Practice
of Physic, Emeritus
Harvard Medical School
Boston, Massachusetts

James A. Thorson, Ed.D.
Associate Professor and Director
Gerontology Program
University of Nebraska at Omaha
Omaha, Nebraska

Judy Thorson, R.N., M.Ed.
Coordinator of Staff Development

Division of Nursing Service
University of Nebraska Medical Center
Omaha, Nebraska

JoAnn Trolinger, F.N.P., M.H.S.
Lecturer, Family Nurse Practitioner and
Physician's Assistant Program
Department of Family Practice
School of Medicine
University of California at Davis
Sacramento, California

Berthold E. Umland, M.D.
Assistant Professor
Department of Family, Community, and
Emergency Medicine
Medical Director, Family Practice Clinic
University of New Mexico School of Medicine
Albuquerque, New Mexico

Betty Walraven, F.N.P., M.H.S.
Clinical Faculty
Family Nurse Practitioner and Physician's
Assistant Program
Department of Family Practice
School of Medicine
University of California at Davis
Sacramento, California

William M. Whelihan, Ph.D.
Chief Clinical Research Psychologist
Philadelphia Geriatric Center
Philadelphia, Pennsylvania

Lynda White, P.A., M.H.S.
Lecturer, Family Nurse Practitioner and
Physician's Assistant Program
Department of Family Practice
School of Medicine
University of California at Davis
Sacramento, California

Section 1
THE AGING PROCESS

1

Aging in America

Carroll L. Estes, Ph.D.
Philip R. Lee, M.D.

FACTS AND FALLACIES ABOUT THE AGED

Older people are becoming more and more important in the United States. One reason is the sheer increase in their number in recent years. In 1940 there were 9.0 million aged (6.8 percent of the population); by 1965, the year that Medicare and Medicaid were enacted, the number had doubled to 18.5 million aged (9.5 percent of the population). There are now more than 22.5 million aged and it is estimated that in the year 2000, 31.8 million Americans (10.5 percent of the population) will be aged 65 or older.[1]

The growing importance of the aged and their role in American society make it imperative for health professionals who work with elderly people to understand that the major problems faced by the aged are socially constructed as a result of society's conception of aging and the aged. What we know about aging and the aged, as well as what is done for them, are products of our conceptions of aging.

The quality of life of the aged—their incomes and opportunities, their participation in community affairs, their personal levels of gratification, and indeed even their health—are largely determined by social forces. Individual differences in inherited social and economic status, in marital status, and in racial and ethnic origins influence the lives of the aged, but the major determinants of the standards of living enjoyed or endured by older people are national social and economic policies, political decisions at all levels of government, the power of organized interest groups, and the policies of business and industry. Of particular importance are income and opportunities for employment.

In this era when so much attention is directed to the role of the individual, including the role of taking responsibility for one's own health, it is essential to recognize how these broader social forces and conditions create the context within which the individual exercises choice. For example, the lives and opportunities of the wealthy farmer and the migrant worker, the slum landlord and slum housing tenant, and the middle-class white and the poor black are immensely different. In addition, society places special limits on individual choices of the aged because of the social conception of aging and the aged.

THE SOCIAL CONSTRUCTION OF REALITY CONCERNING OLDER PERSONS IN THE UNITED STATES

It is not easy to apply generalizations about the social construction of reality concerning older persons in the United States because there are so many different people from so many different backgrounds and cultures living in such a variety of different places, and under so many different conditions. There are, however, dominant views that affect virtually all of their lives.

As examined in *The Aging Enterprise*,[2] the perception of the aged in the United States is:

1. That they are themselves, a special problem. Old age is in itself perceived as a problem.
2. Old age is special and different: it is characterized by special needs requiring special programs. This has led to separatism of the aged via public policies.

3. Old age with its concomitant social problems is seen as resolvable by the application of services at the individual level. This concept of need as met through services has justified inadequate income maintenance, employment, and retirement policies, because the dominant conception is that services, not income or employment, can solve "the problem."

4. The services strategy that has been adopted preserves and reinforces the existing social class structure. Three classes of the aged are entitled to some type of government program: the middle- and upper-class (nonpoor) aged; the newly poor in old age (the deserving poor); and the aged who have always been poor (the underserving poor).[3] The nonpoor aged have the resources to permit access to public and private services without the necessity of government intervention. They also receive a disproportionate share of the benefits of the largest federal programs for the aged (e.g., Social Security, Medicare, and retirement tax credits). Most services policies tend to favor the newly poor in old age, largely because they are thought of as both deserving and deprived. Services have been designed largely to assist the recently deprived aged to maintain their lifestyles, rather than to provide the more crucial life-support services (e.g., income) needed by the poor aged. The aged who have been life-long poor are assisted largely through inadequate income-maintenance policies, such as Supplemental Security Income (SSI), and through Medicaid which is highly variable from state to state.

5. Old age is commonly perceived as characterized by inevitable physical decline, presumably occurring with chronological aging. The biomedical model of aging and its decremental-decline concepts have gained wide acceptance, particularly with society's increasing tendency to conceptualize social problems as medical in origin and to look to medicine for solutions.

6. The problems of old age in our society are characterized as having reached crisis proportions, as evidenced in testimony on Social Security, Medicare, Medicaid, and the Older Americans Act. Such crisis definitions fuel the activities of interest groups and promote their demands for an ever-increasing supply of resources to fund the respective services with which they promise to solve the problem. The result is a wasteful patchwork of often contradictory solutions, none of which is capable of ameliorating the defined problems in the long run.[4]

7. Older people are seen as unproductive and dependent, as a burden on society and also somehow to blame. They are accused of not saving enough, of living too long, of using too many health services, and of contributing to the spiraling costs of government programs including the costs of Medicare and Medicaid.

8. Given the social construction of reality about the problems of old age in America, the perception is that it is impossible to redistribute resources to older people in order to alter their status. Rather, it is only possible (and with great sacrifice of other generations) to hold older people in place, despite the fact that social policies, such as forced retirement, create new dependency for the middle-class old and exacerbate the dependency of those who are poor prior to old age.

THE NEEDS OF THE AGED

Older people are dependent on public policies and programs because of their relatively low economic status, their burden of illness and disability, and their need for a wide range of health and social services.

THE ECONOMIC STATUS OF OLDER PEOPLE

Inadequate retirement income is the most serious problem facing older Americans. A host of income and poverty statistics testify to this fact. The problem was summed up by the Select Committee on Aging, United States House of Representatives[5]:

Although persons above 65 constitute little more than one-tenth of the population, they account for 29 percent of all persons in America receiving an income below $3200. Currently the median income of all families headed by a person 65 or over is 43.1 percent lower than the median income for all families; the income of individuals 65 or older is 33.4 percent lower than the median income for all individuals.

Although the number of aged living in poverty declined from 5.5 million in 1959 to 3.2 million in 1977, there has been virtually no reduction in the number of elderly living in poverty during the 1970s. The economic status of millions of the nation's elderly has a negative impact on their health status, and it severely limits their access to needed medical care.

THE BURDEN OF CHRONIC ILLNESS AND DISABILITY

Although it is difficult to be precise about the numbers and kinds of persons needing medical and social services, the chronically ill and disabled utilize these services far more than those who do not suffer with such problems. Among the elderly in 1970, five percent were residents of institutions, and millions suffer from chronic illness and disability.[1] In 1975, almost half of noninstitutionalized elderly were limited in their activities because of chronic conditions, including 17 percent who were unable to carry on their major activity. Activity limitation is far more common (56 percent) for those 75 years of age and over, in contrast to those 65–74 years of age (42 percent).[1] It is also more common among the poor. Those aged 65 and over who are poor had 46.6 days of limited activity per year, compared with 31.2 for the nonpoor aged.[6]

The problems of those aged 75 and older are of particular importance, because this group bears a high burden of illness and disability. They are often poor and without family or other social support systems.[2] Indeed, half of the residents of long-term care facilities are aged 80 or older; the great majority (68 percent) have family incomes of less than $3,000 annually, almost half are widowed, divorced, or never married.[7]

Previously, we summarized the impact of chronic illness on the elderly as follows[8]:

The impact of this illness burden on the quality of life of the aged is enormous. Over 1 million are in nursing homes, over 3.8 million are unable to carry on their normal activities, and at least 11 million are limited in their activities. The problems increase with advancing age. Illness and disability are cited as the major reason that those 65 and over are unable to work. Not only do illness and disability restrict the earning capacity of the aged, but the costs of medical care drive many to a state of impoverishment. Poor health is a significant factor in accentuating and deepening the poverty of the aged; in turn, their poverty contributes to their poor health and disability. High medical care costs for the aged reflect their growing numbers, their disproportionate burden of illness, the increasing percentage who are 75 years old and older, and the devastating effect of price inflation during the past 15 years.

THE MEDICAL CARE NEEDS OF THE AGED AND THEIR USE OF HEALTH SERVICES

The added burden of chronic illness and disability among the aged is also reflected in data on the use of health services. In 1975 the aged saw physicians 50 percent more often than did those under 65, and they had twice as many hospital stays per capita and remained in the hospital almost twice as long as younger persons. Still, over 80 percent reported no hospitalization during the year, and over 13 percent did not consult a physician. Wide variation existed in the utilization of medical care by the aged with particular chronic conditions. For example, only 43 percent of the elderly reported to have arthritis had seen a physician about this condition during the year, while 80 percent of the aged with diabetes mellitus, hypertension, and heart disease had done so.[1]

THE IMPACT OF RISING MEDICAL CARE COSTS ON THE AGED

The cost of health care is rising in all industrial societies, and the percentage of the Gross National Product allocated to health services in more developed countries has essentially doubled in recent decades.[9] Older people are particularly concerned about the rapid and continued increase in the cost of medical care, because it is imposing an increasing financial burden on them. In the decade from 1966–1976, per capita health expenditures for the elderly rose from $455–1521 annually.[10] Although the most rapid increase was in hospital and physician services (Table 1-1) that are covered in part by Medicare, direct out-of-pocket costs rose rapidly because of the cost of prescription drugs, payment of physician fees not covered by Medicare, Medicare (Part B) premiums, Medicare copayments and deductibles, private health insurance premiums, and long term care services. [In 1966, direct out-of-pocket costs for medical care for the aged were $237 annually. In 1976, they had risen to $404 annually (Table 1-2). In aggregate terms direct out-of-pocket expenditures for medical care rose from $4.38 billion in 1960 to $8.71 billion in 1975.][11] The cost of prescription drugs presents a special problem for the aged. Although the elderly comprise only about 10 percent of the population, they bear

Table 1-1
Per Capita Health Expenditures for the Elderly, 1966 and 1976

Type of Expenditure	1966	1976
Total	$ 455	$ 1521
Hospital care	178	689
Physician's services	90	256
Dentist's services	13	32
Other professional services	12	23
Drugs and drug sundries	62	121
Eyeglasses and appliances	15	19
Nursing home care	68	351
Other health services	7	31

US Senate Special Committee on Aging: Developments in Aging: 1977. Report No. 95–771, part 1. Washington DC: US Government Printing Office, 1978.

the cost of roughly 25 percent of all out-of-hospital drug expenditures–expenses that most older people must meet by out-of-pocket spending.[12] In 1975, the average drug bill for the elderly was more than four times the average drug expense for individuals under 19 years of age and almost two and one-half times the bill for persons aged 19–64.[13]

Current health expenditure data reveal that drugs represent one of the largest out-of-pocket medical expenses for the aged. In 1976, per capita drug expenditures for the elderly were $121 annually. More important than the per capita expenditure is the fact that because of their burden of illness and disability, 10 percent of the aged account for more than 40 percent of all prescription drug charges for the aged.[14] In addition to the problem of direct cost to the aged, it has been suggested that improving access of the aged to appropriate drug use—especially out-of-hospital—can minimize more costly physician visits and hospitalization, as well as limit needless illness and disability.[12]

It was hoped at the time of Medicare's enactment that private health insurance would respond and fill the gaps and permit a better distribution of the costs of care. This hope has not been realized. Private health insurance pays for only about 5.4 percent of the costs of personal health care for the aged. Since 1966, private health insurance has never met more than 5.9 percent of the annual costs of health care for the aged.[11] This does not appear to be a viable alternative for the aged to meet the costs imposed by Medicare's gaps.

Although Medicare and Medicaid are vitally important to the aged in providing access to needed medical care and in providing financial protection for millions against the high costs of medical care,

Table 1-2
Medical Care Expenditures, 1966 and 1976

		Directly Out-of-Pocket	Third-party Payments			
	Total		Total	Government	Private Health Insurance	Philanthropy and Industry
Amount:						
Under 65:						
1966	$ 154	$ 79	$ 75	$ 30	$ 42	$ 3
1976	438	153	285	127	151	7
Over 65:						
1966	466	237	209	133	71	5
1976	1521	404	1117	1030	81	6
Distribution: (Percent)						
Under 65:						
1966	100.0	51.1	48.9	19.4	27.3	2.2
1976	100.0	34.9	65.1	29.0	34.5	1.7
Over 65:						
1966	100.0	53.2	46.8	29.8	15.9	1.1
1976	100.0	26.5	73.5	67.7	5.4	.4

Gornick M: Ten years of Medicare: Impact on the covered population. Social Security Bulletin 39:16, 1976 (table 17); and Gibson RM, Mueller MS, Fisher CR: Age differences in health care spending, fiscal year 1976. Social Security Bulletin 40:5, 1977 (table 2).

both programs have serious gaps that are creating increasing problems for the aged. The rising out-of-pocket costs for physicians' services and prescription drugs, the very limited coverage for long-term care services, and the present method of reimbursing hospitals and physicians are contributing to the rapid increase in the cost of care and services.

In 1977, Medicare expenditures totalled $20.77 billion, and the Medicaid total, including federal, state, and local government expenditures, was $16.25 billion. Of the Medicaid total, we estimate that approximately $6.2 billion was spent on health services for the aged.[12,15] Although these expenditures are large and of vital importance to the aged, it is the gaps, particularly in Medicare and Medicaid, that are of particular concern to older people.

Medicaid, as the welfare component of federally authorized health care, is a state-administered program of medical assistance for the aged poor and other low-income families.[16] A major limitation in the Medicaid program is the existence of wide state variations in coverage, in terms of both services offered and program eligibility. States have the discretion to limit coverage to the categorically needy (excluding the "medically needy" option) and to provide only six basic services out of a possible 23 services. The problems of elderly poor have been described in a recent staff report of the House Select Committee on Aging which stressed the lack of uniformity among Medicaid programs[5] and the limited range of services provided in many states[5] as particularly serious deficiencies. As fiscal limitations extend themselves at state and local levels, even the bare minimum eligibility and scope of services standards are likely to be reduced.

PUBLIC POLICIES AND THE AGED

For the past 40 years, the United States has been moving gradually toward a national aging policy. Federal policies and programs designed to serve the elderly directly or indirectly that are key elements of national aging policy include[17]:

- Income maintenance
- Employment and volunteer service
- Housing
- Health care
- Social service programs
- Transportation
- Training and research programs

The elderly may benefit from these programs because of their age, because they are poor, or because they are designated as a beneficiary (of a program such as Social Security). They may also benefit because they live in a community served by a particular program or because they have a special problem, such as unemployment. Although the full range of these programs is of importance to the aged, we will address only those that bear primarily on the medical and long-term care needs of the aged.

MEDICAL CARE FOR THE AGED—THE GROWING ROLE OF GOVERNMENT

Medical care is one of the nation's largest industries in terms of employment and expenditures. The role of government is of major importance in regulating and financing medical care, in supporting the research that lies behind many of the advances in medical care, in supporting the education and training of health professionals who provide the care, and in adopting policies that permit expansion and modernization of hospitals and other health care facilities. The enactment of the Social Security Amendments of 1965, which included Medicare and Medicaid, was the turning point in terms of the role of government in planning, financing, and the regulating health care. In 1977, 40 percent of all costs of personal health care was paid by government (federal, state, and local) funds; 30 percent was paid directly out-of-pocket by individuals and their families; 25 percent was paid through private health insurance, while charitable contributions and services provided by industry directly to employees accounted for an additional 2 percent.[15] With increased third-party payments, both public and private, costs have been rising rapidly, an increasing percentage of which is devoted to hospital and nursing home care, particularly for the aged.[18]

The decade from 1966–1976 was one of dramatic change in health care for the aged. The total amount of money spent on medical care for the aged rose from $8.6 billion annually in fiscal year 1966 to $34.9 billion in fiscal year 1976. Inflation accounted for the bulk of this increase (50 percent), increased services for 36 percent, and the increase in the number of aged for 14 percent.[1] The rapid increase in the cost of medical care has imposed a special burden on government funds because of the expanded role of the federal and state governments in financing medical care for the aged.[15]

Health care for the aged involves not only the expenditure of large sums of money, including public money. It also represents an area of great complexity because of the nature of the health care system. In perhaps no other sector of the economy is there such a mixture of public and private financing and delivery of services. Physicians, pharmacists, and dentists are generally in private practice, which is a profit-making enterprise. By contrast, most hospitals are either nonprofit community hospitals or public institutions. Nursing homes, on the other hand, are almost entirely profit-making institutions, even though almost 50 percent of their income is derived from government funds.

PUBLIC POLICIES AND LONG-TERM CARE

A number of major programs established during the past 20 years have had a major impact on long-term care services. These include Medicare, Medicaid, Title XX (social services) of the Social Security Act, Supplemental Security Income, and the Older Americans Act. Medical care programs have dominated the picture.

Medical Care

The enactment of Medicare and Medicaid as Titles XVIII and XIX of the Social Security Act ushered in the current era of long-term care policy. Long-term care was to be predominantly a health service, reimbursed through medical care programs. Medicare and Medicaid differed, however, in eligibility, benefits, financing, and administration. The limitations of the Medicare Program, particularly in relation to nursing home care and home delivered services, were to result in Medicaid's becoming the primary vehicle for the payment of long-term care services.

There are marked differences between benefits for Medicare and Medicaid. Medicare provides up to 100 days of skilled nursing home care per benefit period; these days must be preceded by at least three days of hospitalization. In fiscal year 1977, Medicare expenditures for nursing homes paid for by Medicare was 24 days, which was considerably

shorter than the median stay paid for by sources other than Medicare. Medicare expenditures actually represented only about nine percent of federal spending for nursing home care in fiscal 1977, and long-term care represented only two percent of total Medicare expenditures.[19]

Medicaid, by contrast, paid a total of $6.4 billion in federal and state funds for nursing home care in fiscal 1977, representing more than 50 percent of all public and private expenditures for such care and almost 38 percent of total Medicaid expenditures.[20] These services were provided primarily in skilled nursing facilities (SNF) and intermediate care facilities (ICF). Although ICF care is an optional benefit, it is paid for in every participating state. In 19 states nursing homes account for the bulk of Medicaid expenditures.[19] Below the level of ICF care is domiciliary or custodial care for which Supplemental Security Income payments to elderly beneficiaries are the main source of payment.

Home-health services are authorized under both Medicare and Medicaid, but together these programs provide minimal funding for noninstitutional service. Medicare is the primary source of payment for home-health services. It provides coverage for home-health visits when they are preceded by a hospital inpatient stay of at least three days (Part A) and when they are ordered by a physician for patients who have not been hospitalized (Part B). In both cases, visits are limited to 100 visits per calendar year. Both require that patients be homebound and in need of skilled care, and the services must be ordered by a physician. In 1977, Medicare expenditures for home-health services were $433 million, while Medicaid expenditures were only about $82 million for home-health services.

Long-term care expenditures, particularly for SNF and ICF care, constitute an increasing share of total Medicaid costs. From 1969, when ICF care was first paid for under the Old Age Assistance Program, to 1976, the total of SNF and ICF Medicaid expenditures rose from $1.386 billion to $5.380 billion, or from 31.8 percent of expenditures to 37.7 percent. In 1974, SNF/ICF expenditures exceeded Medicaid inpatient hospital care expenditures for the first time. In 1976, SNF/ICF expenditures exceeded inpatient Medicaid expenditures by more than $1.2 billion.[20]

State discretionary policy is particularly important in relation to long-term care services because state officials have a number of options related to eligibility, scope and duration of benefits, reimbursement, standards of care, and utilization review. The result is a wide disparity among states in terms of long-term care services provided. In fiscal year 1976, for example, state-level Medicaid expenditures for long-term care ranged from 66.6 percent of total Medicaid expenditures in Wyoming to only 19.3 percent in the District of Columbia.[20]

Social Support and Social Services

Families, friends, voluntary associations, churches, and other institutions provide most of the social support systems and social services needed by the aged. This is particularly true of those in the upper and middle classes, who are not rendered poor by retirement and inadequate private pensions and Social Security retirement benefits.

The Older Americans Act, enacted in 1965 but significantly modified in the 1970s, was originally designed to support the development of community services to meet the needs of all of the aged. Two programs—area planning and social services (Title III) and nutrition (Title VII prior to 1978)—are of potential importance in filling gaps in the continuum of long-term care services. This potential has not been realized, because appropriations for Title III programs (now including nutrition) have been severely limited in relation to the needs, and most states have spent less than 25 percent of these funds on long-term care services.

A far larger program, Title XX (social services) of the Social Security Act, has been of limited benefit to the aged. Title XX was enacted in 1974 as part of the new federalism strategy. It consolidated previous social service programs, set limits on federal matching, and restricted eligibility to the poor. On average, less than 10 percent of Title XX funds are expended on services for the aged.[2] The potential exists for funding of services for the aged if the ceilings on federal matching and income eligibility restrictions are lifted.

Housing

Housing is another key area of public policy that affects the elderly and is of particular importance with respect to long-term care. Millions of elderly live in substandard housing that is deteriorating or dilapidated and scarcely habitable. Such housing may lack inside toilet, hot water, and adequate heat. Physical conditions are often deplorable, and costs are often prohibitive for the elderly on fixed incomes. Housing represents the single most signifi-

cant expenditure for the elderly, accounting for almost 29 percent of their total budget.

Ninety-five percent of the elderly reside in a community. Over 50 percent of those living in a community live with a spouse (11.4 million), and an additional 27 percent live alone (6 million). Still, many are in need of housing assistance.[21] Obtaining adequate, affordable housing is a major problem. Many elderly homeowners face high costs for utilities, maintenance, and property taxes. The aged who rent homes or apartments face particularly difficult problems because of rising costs.

The federal Department of Housing and Urban Development offers assistance to elderly individuals and couples through a variety of authorities, particularly Sections 8, 202, and 236 of the Housing and Community Development Act. Although 25–30 percent of the nation's elderly live in substandard housing, only a tiny minority—probably less than five percent—benefit from these federal programs.[8] Public housing policies provide adequate authority to meet the housing needs of the elderly, particularly those who need or desire congregate housing. Funding for these programs, however, remains far below that required to meet even the minimum needs of the elderly.

Income

The most important federal programs for the aged are those providing income and financial support. Social Security has become increasingly important as the mainstay of retirement income for the vast majority of the nation's elderly. This has been particularly important because of the mandatory retirement policies of government, business, and industry, and because of the inadequacy of private pensions. Almost 16 million retired workers received Social Security retirement benefits in 1977, and without it 60 percent of elderly families would be poor.[8,22] Even with Social Security benefits, over 4.9 million aged (30.6 percent) are poor or near poor by government standards. The number is reduced to 3.9 million (24.4 percent) when other government programs, such as SSI and Food Stamps, are added. Although these figures appear impressive, the relative financial status of the aged, compared with the financial status of those under 65, has changed very little in 25 years.[23]

The SSI program is important in long term-care because it is a source of income for the aged poor and because of its relationship to Medicaid eligibility and domiciliary care. The law provides automatic Medicaid eligibility for SSI beneficiaries (aged, blind, and disabled) unless states adopt more stringent standards based on their 1972 Medicaid eligibility. The law also permits states to provide additional payments to SSI beneficiaries to cover the costs of congregate housing or domiciliary care. Because states vary in their coverage of institutional settings (both the types and numbers of categories) and in the levels of supplementation, SSI policies may affect Medicaid caseloads and expenditures as well as the development of particular segments of long-term care services.

State Discretionary Policy

A key factor affecting long-term care services is the discretion permitted state and local officials in the major federal–state programs (Medicaid, Title XX, SSI, Older Americans Act) that relate to long-term care. The development of new federalism policies in the 1970s gave a strong boost to the role of the states in domestic social programs, including those affecting long-term care. The new federalism strategy was designed to both decentralize program control to state and local government and limit federal involvement in social programs, including those related to long-term care services.[2]

New federalism has made it more difficult to define the appropriate roles for federal, state, and local governments within long-term care. The problem has been made even more complex by the emergence of fiscal crisis conditions at various levels of government and the "taxpayer revolts" that have followed. These changes in fiscal conditions can be expected to produce new state and local strategies for shifting fiscal responsibilities within programs created or redesigned within the new federalism strategy. State-level attempts are likely to be made to shift more of the costs to the federal government (e.g., federalize Medicaid) while returning administrative control to the state or local government. The federal government, on the other hand, is expected to attempt to shift an increasing share of the cost burden to states and localities.

The Policy Process and Interest-Group Influence

Important elements in the failure of domestic social programs, particularly those affecting medical care and long-term services are: (1) the role and influence American political processes accord special interests, and (2) the fact that ambiguous legislative mandates permit and encourage special-interest influence in all processes of implementation.[2] Some have argued that competition of multiple special interests automatically results in policies and priorities that are in the national interest. We do not agree. We find the observations of David Broder, one of America's most distinguished political reporters, far more accurate. Broder observed that "There is no 'free market' in the political influence game. Some interests are far more powerful than others, so powerful that they can almost rig the game to assure a favorable outcome to themselves."[24] The dominance of special interests and interest group bargaining in determining social policies has had important consequences for the aged and for long-term care policies.

The decentralization of responsibility, with broad discretion in program implementation provided to state and local officials, has meant that choices concerning program priorities, service emphasis, and eligibility occur in the less visible implementation processes rather than in the more visible (and more publicly accountable) legislative processes. This permits the interest groups to exert their influence at every step of the implementation process, and it tends to hide the facts of power from those over whom it is exercised. Further, it provides opportunities for the powerful to dramatize and build on the problem as they define it, expanding the problem definition and its magnitude without having to demonstrate performance.[25]

The Aging Enterprise

Formulation of the problem of aging in America is such that policy prescriptions tend to fall into services strategies, with power largely in the hands of service providers. Such policies provide reimbursement for providers but fail to alter the dependency status of the aged, because there are no programs either for continued employment or for adequate retirement incomes. The policies that have emerged also have the core characteristic of being largely separatist in nature; that is, separating the aged from other groups in society based on their special need. As a consequence of this problem formulation and policy prescription, an "aging enterprise" has been created to serve the aged. The "aging enterprise" includes the congeries of programs, industries, and professionals that serve the aged in one capacity or another.[2] The major components are physicians; hospitals; the Social Security Administration; the Administration on Aging; the Health Care Financing Administration; state health and welfare agencies; state and area agencies on aging; Congressional committees on health care financing; aging, pharmaceutical, and medical equipment and supply companies; and the nursing home and insurance industries. As a result, the dominant influence on policies affecting the aged, including long-term care policies, is the "aging enterprise" and not the aged. Provider interests, rather than consumer interests, dominate the policy process.

The results of the current policy emphasis on medical and institutional care as the primary means of meeting the needs of the elderly for long-term care services have been: (1) a failure to deal with the basic income, housing, and nonmedical social support needs of the aged that might prevent, delay, or reduce the need for medical services; (2) high costs, which have had a major impact on public expenditures for medical care at the state and federal levels, thereby limiting the availability of funds for other needs; and (3) gross inequities among states in eligibility for services and in the scope and duration of services provided.

CREATING A CONTINUUM OF EFFORT

Responsibility for the pursuit of health and for care of the ill is a cooperative venture involving government, the health professions, business and industry, voluntary health organizations, mutual aid and self-help groups, families, and individuals. The health of the aged, no less than that of the young and middle aged, is dependent on how well the various groups work together toward agreed-upon goals. Although emphasis has been placed on the role of medicine and the role of government in medical care and long-term care, it is individuals and families who are primarily responsible for health promotion and who treat from two-thirds to three-quarters of all episodes of illness and injury in the United States. The aged, perhaps because of their frequency of symptoms, are very much a part of this self-care system.

Self-care is not only a common practice; it is the universal first option in health care. In fact, self-care encompasses a wide range of activities, including:

- Health maintenance
- Disease prevention
- Self-diagnosis, self-medication, and self-treatment
- Patient participation in professional care

At an individual level, choices relating to health revolve around efforts to remove personal or behavioral barriers to health: smoking, drinking, reckless driving, physical inactivity, improper diet, and poor sanitary or hygiene habits. These issues are variously labeled as lifestyle problems, behavioral problems, and individual problems. They are individual problems, however, only if the individual alone can solve them. In most cases, individuals need help in solving these problems that stem from social, economic, and cultural conditions and not solely from the behavior of the individual. Individuals need information and skills; they need protection from environmental hazards; they need incentives and resources in order to alter their behavior. Most of all, they need the freedom to act in what they consider to be their own best interest.

At a governmental level, policy choices revolve around attempts to remove social and environmental barriers to health, such as poverty, unemployment, lack of educational opportunities, poor nutrition, environmental and occupational hazards, and unequal access to health care. In an ideal sense, government should be involved in doing for individuals only what they cannot do for themselves.

Practicing health professionals, particularly primary care physicians, sit at midpoint on this continuum. Once an individual decides to seek advice for a health problem, the threshold is crossed into the health care system. It is then the primary physician or doctor of first contact who deals with the symptoms, diseases, and associated problems that the individual decides require skilled professional management.

Physicians and other primary care practitioners cannot, however, limit their activities to care of the sick. They must carefully examine the role of medicine and its emphasis on disease, acute care, modern hospitals, and advanced technology, as well as on professional and financial rewards for nonprimary care practitioners.

Why has medicine accorded a low priorty for primary care and long-term care services needed by the aged and disabled? Why does medicine give lower status to professionals who provide primary care and work in long-term care institutions?

Medicine's views of its function have a profound impact on the views and actions of society. Medical care generally is equated with improved health and well being. More and more resources are being invested in its development. The number of social and behavioral disorders that are included within the jurisdiction of medicine and its practitioners is increasing, lending support to the claim that the American society is being medicalized.[26] As a result of the policies that flow from this perspective, aging is being medicalized with disastrous consequences for the aged.

MEDICINE'S VALUES AND THE PROSPECTS FOR THE FUTURE

Policies affecting medical and long-term care services reflect the values of the medical profession and the profession's influence on public policy. Medicare emphasizes acute care, particularly hospital care. The systems of reimbursing physicians and hospitals have had a major impact on rising medical care costs, and they are increaseingly pricing the aged out of the mainstream of medical care. Medicaid policies, because the poor are accorded a low priority, have been left largely in the hands of the states, thus creating great inequities in access to and the quality of services available across the states.

Long-term care has been medicalized, because this was the only avenue open to support the development of needed services. In the process, however, long-term care has been accorded a low priority because physicians and hospitals find it less prestigious and economically rewarding than acute care. Institutional care (hospitals and nursing homes) has been emphasized at the expense of community and home care services. Nursing homes have been required to perform multiple functions— custodial care, acute illness care, rehabilitation, chronic care, and terminal care—without the resources to perform these tasks. Alternative policies for income maintenance and housing have not been adequately considered because the medical model has been so dominant and so costly.

Efforts to improve long-term care services via professionalization, medicalization, regulation, or the introduction of alternatives to nursing homes will not touch the basic problems of the aged. None of these developments will alter either their status or condition. If the current development of services under long-term care strategies continues, they will emphasize screening, assessment, and coordination.

These new long-term care services will remain marginal in their capacity either to improve the lives of the aged or to reduce the escalation of economic cost, for they are likely to provide little in the way of needed social support or home help; nor are they likely to alter current health reimbursement policies. Further, these policies continue to treat problems of the aged as independent of social and economic origins, while positing solutions involving the consumption of largely acute-care services. Both health and social services policies and programs emerge essentially as consequences of interest-group politics. The most disadvantaged aged and the poor of all ages are left to the discretionary policy choices across the states, resulting in great disparities in eligibility and services.

What is called for is a major reexamination of federal and federal–state policies that affect the needs of the aged, particularly the current emphasis on the services strategy. Of major importance are income maintenance, housing, medical care, and social services policies. A basic question that must be asked is whether or not particular long-term care goals and priorities should be in some sense national, rather than state or local. A systematic examination of the many state policies affecting the delivery of long-term care services for the aged and medical care for the poor is required in order to determine what the current national policies are and to define the alternatives and options. The goals of such studies should be to distinguish those responsibilities that are logically state and local in nature from those that are so significant in impact that they require definitive national policy.

National policies should be geared to: (1) supporting the individual in the community with an adequate income; (2) promoting the right to employment and decent housing; and (3) providing access to good medical care and community-based, long-term care services while providing adequate protection against the rising costs of medical care, food, and energy. The burden should not be borne entirely by federal funds, but the federal government does have a responsibility to remove the gross inequities in services and eligibility created by the great variation across the states in Medicaid, social services, and income supplementation programs for the aged. It also has the obligation to assure income support above the poverty level for everyone. Continuing down the path of incrementalism, interest-group politics, and the medicalization of long-term care will not serve the aged, nor will it serve the needs of society.

REFERENCES

1. Kovar MG: Elderly people: The population 65 years and over, in National Center for Health Statistics, Health: United States, 1976–1977. Washington, DC, US Government Printing Office, 1977

2. Estes CL: The Aging Enterprise. San Francisco, Jossey-Bass, 1979

3. Nelson G: Perspectives on social need and social services for the aged. School of Social Welfare, University of California, Berkeley, 1978 (unpublished)

4. Edelman M: Political Language: Words That Succeed and Policies That Fail. New York, Academic Press, 1977

5. US House of Representatives, Select Committee on Aging: Poverty Among America's Aged. Washington, DC, US Government Printing Office, 1978

6. Butler L, Newacheck P, Harper P, et al: Income and Illness. Health Policy Program, University of California, San Francisco, 1979 (unpublished)

7. Joe T, Meltzer J: Policies and Strategies for Long-Term Care. San Francisco, Health Policy Program, University of California, 1976

8. Lee PR, Estes CL: Eighty federal programs for the elderly, in Estes CL: The Aging Enterprise. San Francisco, Jossey-Bass, 1979

9. Shanas E, Maddox GL: Aging, health, and the organization of health resources, in Binstock RH, Shanas E (eds): Handbook Of Aging and the Social Sciences. New York, Van Nostrand Reinhold, 1976

10. Paringer L, Bluck J, Feder J, et al: Health Status and Use of Medical Services: Evidence on the Poor, the Black, and the Rural Elderly. Washington, DC, Urban Institute, 1979, p 3

11. US House of Representatives, Select Committee on Aging, Subcommittee on Health and Long-Term Care: Medicare Gaps and Limitations. Washington, DC, US Government Printing Office, 1977a

12. Silverman M, Lydecker M: Drug Coverage Under National Health Insurance: Proceedings of the National Conference. Hyattsville, Md., National Center for Health Services Research, 1978, p 12

13. Mueller MS, Gibson RM: National health expenditures fiscal year 1975. Soc Secur Bull 39:19, 1976

14. Lennox K: Expanding Health Benefits for the Elderly, vol 2: Prescription Drugs. Washington, DC, Urban Institute, 1979, p 9

15. Gibson RM, Fisher CR: Age differences in health care spending, fiscal year 1977. Soc Secur Bull 42:8, 1978

16. Davis K, Schoen C: Health and the War on Poverty: A Ten-Year Approach. Washington, DC, Brookings, 1978

17. US House of Representatives, Select Committee on Aging: Fragmentation of Services for the Elderly. Washington, DC, US Government Printing Office, 1977b

18. Gibson RM: National health expenditures, 1978. Health Financ Rev 1:1–36, 1979

19. Weissert WG: Long term care: An overview in US Department of Health, Education, and Welfare: Health—United States 1978. Washington, DC, 1978, p 96

20. US Department of Health, Education, and Welfare, Health Care Financing Administration: Data on the Medicaid Program: Eligibility, Services, Expenditures. Fiscal Years 1966–1976. Washington, DC, The Institute for Medical Management, 1977

21. Scanlon W, DiFederico E, Stassen M: Long-Term Care: Current Experience and a Framework for Analysis. Washington, DC, Urban Institute, p 73

22. Ball RM: Social Security Today and Tomorrow. New York, Columbia University Press, 1978

23. Clark RB, Kreps J, Spangler J: Economics of aging. J Econom Lit 16:919–962, 1978

24. Broder D: The Party's Over: The Failure of Politics in America. New York, Harper & Row, 1972

25. Estes CL, Noble M: Paperwork and the Older Americans Act. Problems in Implementing Accountability. Washington, DC, US Government Printing Office, 1978

26. Fox RC: The medicalization and demedicalization of American society. Daedalus 106:9, 1977

2

Ethical Considerations in Eldercare

John Dervin, M.D.
Patricia Dervin, R.N., M.S.
Albert R. Jonsen, Ph.D.

From an ethical viewpoint there are a wide range of issues of concern in the care of the elderly. This chapter focuses on the issue of decision making about the use of medical interventions: *who will decide—with what risks and for which outcomes—which medical interventions will or will not be used?* The term medical interventions is used to refer to not only the heroic treatment of common or uncommon disease but also the routine measures used for the common serious illnesses of the seventh, eighth, and ninth decades of life. Because the elderly are more vulnerable to the untoward effects of medical interventions, this issue of *who will decide* is central in their care.

As a practical strategy to guide decision making about the use of medical interventions, the clinician uses feedback from the patient to gauge the fit of the medical intervention to the patient's need. Based on patient feedback, medical interventions are then modified, retained, or eliminated. For the elderly patient who is dying, the problems involved in decision making are made more complex when clinicians do not consider the issues involved until it is too late for the patient to help with feedback and decision making. Without patient feedback, how will the clinician know if the decisions that were made were in the patient's best interest? *How will the dead testify as to the fit of their dying?*

In this chapter, the question of *who will decide* is explored from the following considerations: ethical, professional, sociological, and those of the patient. The first part of the chapter, Decision Making: Considerations Involved, responds to this question by building a foundation for practice based on the

values of respect for the person and honesty in human relations. The second part of the chapter, Decision Making: Working Towards Resolutions, discusses means by which the clinician can implement these values into clinical practice.

Throughout this chapter, decision making is discussed in the context of the care of the dying because decision making about how to live while dying is the most pressing and inevitable concern in eldercare. However, as the principles discussed are fundamental in health care, they can be applied to other ethical problems surrounding decision making about the use of medical interventions encountered in clinical practice.

DECISION MAKING: CONSIDERATIONS INVOLVED

Ethical Considerations

The primary care clinician will probably become frustrated in reviewing the medical ethics literature for an answer when confronted with ethical dilemnas in everyday practice. Ethics offer the primary care clinician opinions that need to be judged as more or less reasonable, more or less plausible. In this respect, ethical opinions are like clinical opinions. While there may be agreement as to the general principles involved, the working options as to what to do are strongly influenced by the nuances of a particular patient's situation and personal opinion. When there is significant divergence of opinion about options, a difficult judgment must be made.

This judgment is not easily reached by following any methodological straight line. Rather, the judgment is made by testing the opinion in the fire of debate, challenging its assumptions, drawing out its implications, questioning its terms, and measuring its fit to a range of practical problems.

Despite the debates, however, primary care clinicians must make decisions, as well as implement and defend them. It is useful for the clinician, then, to recall that all ethical positions try to answer the question of what kinds of acts are right? What is the moral thing to do? In answering this question, there are two basic values that transcend time and culture:

The first of these is respect for the individual. In its ultimate form it is respect for human life, including a concern for others, a caring and compassion. In its broader form it is taken to mean respect for the human person. Aspects of this respect include the rights of the individual, freedom of choice, and freedom to act within the context of the rights of others.

The second value is a basic honesty in human relations . . . all ethical systems include a condemnation of deception, dishonesty, and trickery. If there were not a minimal level of honesty in a society, a basic trust in others, the social order would collapse.[1]

These basic human values, *respect for the individual and basic honesty in human relations,* form the guiding themes for this chapter. The work for the clinician in making an ethical decision is to take these values, to understand their meaning and apply them to the resolution of the particular moral problem encountered in daily practice.

In eldercare, these values may come into conflict with other factors and be debated under such issues as mercy killing, truth telling, patient autonomy, and when to terminate life-support systems. How these values and the professional injunctions "do no harm" and "to prolong life" may appear to come into conflict in the clinical setting is the subject of the next section.

Professional Considerations

THE CLASSICAL INJUNCTIONS

Traditionally, the clinician has been directed in decision making by guidelines or rules that have been a trademark, such as the Hippocratic Oath and the Florence Nightingale Pledge. All of these guidelines agree that the clinician's loyalty is to the patient. Two precepts, accepted as bedrock ethical principles by health professions, which underscore

this loyalty are to prolong life and to "do no harm." As these precepts are used to interpret the clinician's moral duty, they deserve special comment.

The precept "do no harm" had its origin in ancient times, and though it is commonly thought to be in the Hippocratic Oath, it actually appears in Epidemics: "As to diseases make a habit of two things—to help, or at least to 'do no harm.[2]'" The origin is clear. What is less clear is the meaning.

The most commonly accepted meaning of "do no harm" stresses due care on the part of the physician. Several other interpretations of do no harm are possible: that medicine is a moral enterprise, that the risk–benefit ratio of a medical undertaking must be considered, and that the precept serves not so much as a minimal morality of practice but as a warning to practice with humility. The latter is important because: "When persons possess great powers and yield them on behalf of others, they sometimes fail to see the harm done as they ply their beneficial craft."[3]

Under the precept, "do no harm," some clinicians may see themselves as sanctioned to practice in ways that might conflict with the values of their patients. Such clinicians invoke "do no harm" as a justification for unilateral decision making. For instance, some consider it permissible to withhold the truth in those instances in which they perceive it will "harm" the patient. When the clinician decides the truth may be harmful to the patient, the clinician often decides for the patient, or informs the patient in such a manner that the patient's decision is directed by the professional. This misuse of the precept "do no harm" to justify manipulation of information is unacceptable clinical practice.

It is not clear whether the precept "to prolong life" had its origin in ancient times. The actual practice of medicine in greco-roman times valued the right of individuals to freely dispose of their lives. Suicide was considered honorable and physicians of the time frequently rendered assistance. Abortion was practiced, and active euthanasia (mercy killing) was commonplace. While the Hippocratic writings prohibit abortions and assistance in suicide, they are neutral towards the issue of euthanasia. What seems clear is that in ancient times a physician " . . . who prolonged or attempted to prolong the life of a man who could not ultimately recover his health was viewed as acting unethically."[4]

The ethical basis for modern practice became established from 1100–1500 A.D. Important factors in this development were the cultural influence of the doctrines of the Catholic Church, the development of medical guilds with codes, and the establishment of medical education in university settings. In the Christian Era, physicians became more likely to refuse to perform abortions or to assist in suicide. By the tenth through the sixteenth centuries, suicide, abortion, and euthanasia were forbidden.

In the seventeenth century, Francis Bacon wrote that medicine has three tasks: to preserve health, to cure diseases, and to prolong life. However, he chastises physicians for their practices which prolong dying: "but the physicians contrariwise do make a kind of scruple and religion to stay with the patient after the disease is deplored; whereas in my judgment they ought both to inquire the skill and to give the attendances, for the facilitating and assuaging of the pains and agonies of death."[5] Not finding cures for incurable diseases, futile cure-seeking for patients when the situation is hopeless, not finding and applying means to make death less unpleasant—these problems unresolved in history are of equal or even greater importance today.

PROGNOSIS

Decision making in all medical diagnosis and treatment depends on the professional's access to scientific facts and his or her ability to predict the future based on these facts—the facility of prognosis. On the basis of prognosis, the clinician is able to inform the patient of the various options and outcomes of the patient's condition. While knowledge of what *can* be done for a patient's condition is within the professional realm, the decision about what *ought* to be done goes beyond scientific expertise and into the realm of moral judgment.

Today, because of its increased sophistication, prognosis is valued as a guide in decision making in a number of areas with ethical importance. For example, the adoption of the Harvard Criteria for determination of brain death is founded on prognosis. Unreceptivity and unresponsiveness, no movements or breathing, no reflexes, and a flat EEG have been accepted as clinical criteria for brain death precisely because the prognosis for recovery from such a state is without precedent.[6] In these situations the Harvard criteria serve as a guideline for not instituting or for discontinuing recovery oriented medical interventions. In the case of the severely burned patient, in whom prognosis for survival is nil, approaches have been instituted making full application of technology an option dependent on the patient's desires.[7] In the situation of

cardiopulmonary resuscitation, where prognosis for survival is extremely unlikely, a team of emergency care professionals has defined guidelines for not instituting or for discontinuing advanced life-support measures.[8] These examples illustrate that when *death* is the inevitable outcome, prognosis has simplified decision making about when and when not to use medical interventions. Prognosis has also simplified decision making about using medical interventions in those conditions where an *unimpaired* level of existence is likely to result from medical interventions (e.g., treatment of hemorrhagic shock, or coma from drug overdose).

In other areas of medicine prognosis cannot simplify decision making because prognosis alone cannot resolve the moral issue of *who will decide*. The care of the severely brain-injured and fresh-water drowning victims who have undergone cardiac arrest are cases in point. These situations are characterized by certainty of poor prognosis but differ in that death is not the only outcome. Instead there is a range of outcomes: severe impairment, a vegetative state, or death. In these patient situations, application of medical interventions without reference to the patient's values is standard practice by many clinicians.

A number of reasons are given by clinicians for treating these patient situations differently from those situations in which death or an unimpaired existence is the inevitable outcome:

- We can't be really sure our diagnosis and prognosis are accurate.
- Even if our reasoning is correct, perhaps this case will be an exception.
- What if in the course of treatment we come up with a new cure for the problem?

All of these assertions masquerade as reasonable doubts. In reality they only ask a more fundamental question: can we ever be sure of anything, particularly in the future? What degree of certainty is required for judgment? In any human endeavor there is always some degree of uncertainty. The tragedy in these patient situations is that medical interventions are unquestioningly applied under the guise of uncertainty about prognosis.

The issue that focuses decision making in patient situations where the prognosis is for severely impaired level of existence, a vegetative state, or death is this: is a severely impaired level of existence or vegetative state better than, worse than, or equal to death? From this flows the question of who will decide what quality of life is to be valued? That is, *who will decide, with what risks and for which outcomes— which interventions will or will not be used?* Particularly for the elderly because they are less resilient to injury, disease, and the untoward effects of medical interventions, this issue is central in their care.

Prognosis, therefore, in situations where death or an unimpaired level of existence is the outcome, has simplified decision making. The problem area remaining concerns those patient situations in which there are a range of possible outcomes—severe impairment, a vegetative state, or death. In these situations, clinicians often practice differently. While some clinicians control decision making and the use of medical interventions to allow death to come, others control decision making and interventions so that a severely impaired level of existence or vegetative state is the patient's outcome. What is important here and illustrates the limitations of reliance on the clinician as sole decision maker is the clinician's subsequent unilateral handling of the situation according to how the clinician perceives the benefits of the various prognoses. The decision, however, of an inevitably severely impaired existence or vegetative state as compared to allowing death to come is certainly one that belongs rightfully to the patient. This decision should be made by the patient with due care and thoughtful guidance from his or her primary care clinician. This decision should necessarily be made well in advance of any critical event or deterioration.

Sociological Considerations

This section discusses how *who knows what* about a given patient situation explains what happens in that situation. It presents how the professional often controls who knows what by the ways in which patient access to information is managed. Since *who knows what* principally determines *who will decide*, the values of respect for the person and basic honesty in human relations are essential in patient–professional relationships.

AWARENESS CONTEXTS

Social scientists explain what goes on around a patient from the viewpoint of a phenomenon known as the awareness context. It is important for clinicians to understand awareness contexts because *who knows what* surrounds and affects interaction in health care. In the case of a dying patient, the awareness context means "who, in the dying situa-tion, knows what about the probabilities of death for the patient."[9]

Four general types of awareness contexts are used to explain the common interactions surrounding a dying patient. (For the sake of simplicity in the following listing, two interactants are assumed, the patient and the clinician.)

1. *Open awareness:* the clinician and the patient know that he or she is dying and acknowledge it in their actions.
2. *Closed awareness:* the patient does not recognize impending death even though the clinicians have the information.
3. *Suspicion awareness:* the patient does not know, but only suspects with varying degrees of certainty, that the clinician believes the patient to be dying.
4. *Pretense awareness:* the patient and clinician both know that the patient is dying, but pretend otherwise.[9]

Knowledge of which awareness context is operating is important: as each context has its own consequences, outcomes from the context are predictable. The point here is not an ethical one— which of the awareness contexts are moral—but rather a practical one: the activities and interactions of the professional flow from the awareness context in which he or she chooses to practice.

For example, closed, suspicion, and mutual pretense awareness contexts are inherently unstable and require close control by the clinician to manage the patient's assessment of clues and events about his or her dying. Clinicians, to maintain these types of contexts, must present a "situation as normal" picture and converse about the future, offering the patient a "fictional biography." Diagnostic dramas may take place; facial expressions and even the hospital location of a patient (e.g., ICU versus a terminal unit) have to be controlled to maintain the facade of "serious illness but not actually dying." Clinicians may also attempt to reduce clues about the patient's dying by restricting time and conversation with the patient. One paramount consequence of closed awareness, is that often clinicians, in order to preserve the context and avoid confrontation, feel they need to act as if they are still trying to save the patient's life when there is nothing more to do.[9]

Respect for the individual and basic honesty in human relations are best served by open awareness. An open awareness context—while it certainly does not eliminate complexity or difficulty—at least makes candid interchange possible. An experienced clinician has noted that it is simply less taxing, less demanding, and more rewarding to work with patients and families who are aware rather than deal with the stilted interactions necessitated by impaired awareness: "The thing I always say to anyone who asks, is that yes, I do tell the truth, and the reason I do is it is too hard to remember if I haven't told the truth, what I did say, or didn't say in the context of the patient discussion.[10]"

Open awareness means that the patient's dying is defined and this is critical because "dying must be defined in order to be reacted to as dying."[11] Through professional dominance the physician principally controls the awareness context and the defining of dying.[12] A burden is placed on others to accommodate a physician's will when he or she practices in contexts other than open awareness. For example, when a physician practices in closed awareness, nurses may feel pressure to lie to the patient and to lie for the physician—a burden of intolerable moral jeopardy.[13] In addition, nurses and families may become frustrated in their efforts to give appropriate dying care because the change from recovery care to comfort care is dependent upon the physician's announcement that there is "nothing more to do" and that dying is certain.

The problem is that when any health care clinician practices in any context other than open awareness, it leads to a situation in which decision making is unilaterally controlled by the clinician because *who knows what* principally determines *who will decide.* Such manipulation of information is incompatible with ethical practice because it conflicts with the values of respect for the person and basic honesty in human relations.

THE BIG LIE AND A REPLY

Choosing against open awareness is frequently seen by clinicians as protective of patients and thought to be in concert with benevolence and "doing no harm." Whatever the rationale, at least in these situations clinicians are intent against open awareness. A more insidious manipulation of open awareness arises when well-intentioned clinicians deceive themselves and their patients, when the truth is said to be told but in fact it is not. This serious problem has been labeled the "big lie" and can take five forms:

1. *The truthful lie.* The truthful lie avoids the guilt of lying. At the same time it avoids the discom-
fort of disclosure by telling the truth in such a complete and scientific way that in effect the patient is left in the dark, not comprehending.

2. *We'll never know for sure.* The fact that clinicians will never know precisely and without any doubt whatsoever is used as a reason for not telling a patient the truth. This rationalization is actually a red herring because it confuses the problem of accuracy of prognosis with the issue of honesty in human relations; "part of the truth which the doctor owes the patient is just that: that the doctor cannot be absolutely correct."[14] The most perverse form of self-deception has been labeled the "over-optimistic hope for the best." The over-optimistic strategy uses not only the truthful lie but adds a planned optimism that manipulates truth, leaving the patient hopeful and deceived.

3. *You can't tell a patient everything.* The claim that the facts about a patient's care are infinite, complicated, and impossible for a patient to understand is used to argue for professional control of information. The claim, however, in no way can justify withholding everything from the patient, especially that which is potentially meaningful or useful.

4. *Withholding information.* Omission is often felt to be more acceptable than an outright lie. Omission may, however, be even more morally reprehensible than lying, since telling the truth depends not merely on "telling it straight" but also on the patient's need and right to know.

5. *Indirect communication.* With this strategy, talking around the facts is substituted for plain, truthful talk. Such language is slippery because it provides no assurance against avoidance and self-deception.[15]

Against these "big lies," four fundamental reasons for the right of patients to know the medical facts about themselves are presented:

1. That as persons, human moral quality is taken away from the patient when he or she is denied whatever knowledge is available.

2. That the facts belong to the patient and that clinicians are entrusted by patients with what they learn.

3. That the fullest possibilities of medical treatment and cure in themselves depend on mutual respect.

4. That to deny a patient knowledge of the facts as to life and death is to assume responsibility

that cannot be carried out by anyone but the patient, with his or her own knowledge of the situation.[14]

Thus, the exigencies of the social situation and the values of respect for the individual and basic honesty in human relations come together to support a philosophy of open awareness in professional–patient relationships.

Openness about death does not automatically facilitate dying. Problems surrounding the timing and the manner of death still need to be resolved. However, existence of open awareness about terminality raises the question about the appropriate way of living while dying. This is the subject of the next section.

Patient Considerations

THE DYING TRAJECTORY

A patient's dying takes place over time during which the patient must go through a number of critical junctures that give shape to his or her dying. When considered together, the time and the critical junctures involved in dying are a patient's *dying trajectory*.[11]

The critical junctures in a patient's dying trajectory are (1) the patient is defined as dying, (2) preparations for death begin, (3) there is "nothing more to do" to prevent death, (4) the final descent takes place, (5) the last hours, (6) the death watch, and (7) death itself.[11]

Clinicians, with their access to prognosis, know that although the critical junctures of the dying trajectory will take place, they will occur differently for individual patients. Common variations of dying trajectories are:

1. *The lingering trajectory.* The patient is certain to die, but when is unknown, and the patient does not die for some while (e.g., death from cancer).
2. *The expected quick trajectory.* The patient is known to be dying and will almost certainly die in a few hours or at most a day or two (e.g., death from extensive burns).
3. *The unexpected quick trajectory.* A patient suddenly starts to die, completely surprising family, the professionals, and others (e.g., an operating room death).[11]

The shape of patient's dying trajectory is determined by key factors. The most critical factor is *who will decide* what shape the trajectory will take. Who decides is dependent on the awareness context operating (*who knows what* principally determines *who will decide*). A key related factor that determines the shape of the patient's dying trajectory is the decision to use or not use medical interventions.

In times of fewer available medical technologies, given the desire to "do something" about a dying situation, clinicians and patients could do less and so the natural course of the trajectory was likely to proceed undisturbed. Today, however, because of medical interventions, the issue becomes: " . . . who shall have what kinds and degrees of influence in shaping the end of the patient's trajectory? That issue involves not merely how the patient shall die, but also how he shall live while dying."[11]

One long-respected tradition in medical ethics distinguishes between ordinary and extraordinary means to sustain life. While all ill people are obligated to use ordinary means to maintain life, they are *not* obligated to use extraordinary means except in circumstances when the conditions of family responsibility and a high probability of success of the extraordinary treatment are present. Whether a medical intervention is classified as ordinary or extraordinary does *not* depend solely on the nature of the intervention under consideration, but also on the circumstances of the patient for which the intervention is intended. An ill person is under no obligation to undergo treatment which brings great suffering, excessive costs, disfigurement, or overtaxes the will and courage of the patient. Indeed, past moralists in making these distinctions were referring to patients whose lives could be meaningfully prolonged by radical or heroic interventions. That is why they called those measures extraordinary which the patient had good reason to refuse.[16]

The distinctions, ordinary and extraordinary, were not meant to apply to the patient who had already entered a dying trajectory and for whom such interventions could only be death-prolonging. For the dying patient, the duty to be treated ceases as therapy pales in the face of dying. Though clinicians should agree on the principle that dying extinguishes their duty to provide recovery-oriented medical interventions, they may not agree on when, in the care of the patient, this point occurs. This is when the clinician must turn to the patient to learn how the patient defines dying and which medical interventions are and are not of value while the patient, lives his or her dying trajectory.

Defining When Dying Comes

The modern response to the inevitability of death has been largely one of the trajectory prolongation through death-delaying technology. This response is now questioned by many and one approach has been to define a "natural death" in order to clarify what we owe as human beings to those who are going to die and to help develop rational limits to the use of medical technology:

My definition of "natural death" is this: the individual event of death at that point in a lifespan when, (1) one's life work has been accomplished; (2) one's moral obligations to those for whom one has had responsibility have been discharged; (3) the death will not seem to others an offense to sense or sensibility or tempt others to despair and rage at human existence; and finally, (4) the process of dying is not marked by unbearable and degrading pain.[17]

Although patients may not have anticipatory knowledge of or control over the diseases they may encounter and eventually die from, they may have very firm ideas related to when they wish to be defined as dying so that they may have control over their passage through the critical junctures of their dying trajectory. Different ways in which patients may define when dying comes are:

1. *The life is sacred at all costs definition.* For these patients, dying begins with the onset of biological death. These patients desire all possible technological interventions to be applied to prolong bodily existence. They view life as sacred under any circumstances and do not consider the qualitative differences of social as compared to biological death as relevant issues to their care.

2. *The quality of life is vital and dying begins after irreversible loss of capacity for social interaction definition.* For these patients, dying begins after severe irreversible impairment or the existence of a vegetative state occurs. These patients want to be treated as dying after such situations arise and would not wish any further recovery-oriented medical interventions undertaken. They would accept the basic comfort care of nursing measures.

3. *The quality of life is vital and dying begins with the likely potential for irreversible loss of capacity for social interaction definition.* These patients fall into two groups depending on the amount of risk they are willing to tolerate.

- The dying begins when there is *strong* likelihood of severe impairment or vegetative state resulting from medical interventions
- Dying begins when there is *any* likelihood of severe impairment or a vegetative state resulting from medical interventions.

Patients in these groups value a "natural" death more than a very small or practically non-existent chance for meaningful life and in such situations would not want recovery-oriented medical interventions initiated or continued.

In clinical practice, the challenge for the patient and the clinician is to identify the patient's perceptions of the ideal death and to integrate these values into the health care delivery system.

Elderly patients need to understand that they must make their values known, because without such information it is the nature of the present health care system to treat all patients as if they valued the first position—that of life at all costs.

THE EUTHANASIA ISSUE

A few authors would argue that the best way to approach the care of the dying is through euthanasia. Euthanasia is generally understood as the "action of bringing about a seriously suffering patient's death by at least one other person, where the motive for ending the life is merciful and the means chosen is as painless as possible."[18] Euthanasia can be described according to two variables: how the act is committed and whether or not it is voluntary. These variables come together in the clinical setting as illustrated by the following examples:

- Active–voluntary: a terminally ill patient chooses to ask the physician to directly end his or her life.
- Passive–voluntary: a terminally ill patient has directed that life-support measures be withdrawn.
- Active–involuntary: a comatose patient's life is directly ended without a present or past request (i.e., mercy killing).
- Passive–involuntary: a comatose patient's life-support measures are withdrawn without present or past request.

Passive–voluntary and passive–involuntary euthanasia are usually considered morally acceptable, particularly in cases of patients having severe, irreversible disease. Active euthanasia, whether voluntary or involuntary, is usually considered morally wrong and is illegal.

Euthanasia, however, by its very definition is a death-oriented solution to the problem of how to care for the dying; that is, the problem is resolved by focusing on death as an end. As such, euthanasia is a negative approach to the care of the dying and an admission of defeat in health care. The perceived need for euthanasia arises out of fear of dehumanized dying and death, which the primary care clinician must work to prevent. Focusing on euthanasia obscures the clinical and moral problem of how best to care for a patient who is living his or her dying trajectory. Relieving pain, desisting from useless medical interventions, comfort care, helping a patient cope with dying—these complex and positive health activities are the care due patients who are dying and primary care clinicians must not abdicate nor confuse such care with euthanasia.

In its "Declaration on Euthanasia," the Roman Catholic Church recently reaffirmed its condemnation of euthanasia while addressing the issues raised by modern medical technology: "Today it is very important to protect, at the moment of death, both the dignity, of the human person, and the Christian concept of life, against a technological attitude that threatens to become an abuse."[19] Because this document is expected to have impact beyond the Church itself, some of its key points are excerpted:

> It is . . . permissible to make due with the normal means that medicine can offer. Therefore one cannot impose on anyone the obligation to have recourse to a technique which is already in use but which carries a risk or is burdensome.[19]

When inevitable death is imminent in spite of the means used, it is permitted in conscience to make the decision to refuse forms of treatment that would only serve a precarious and burdensome prolongation of life, so long as the normal care due to the sick person in similar cases is not interrupted.[19]

In discussing the use of advanced and possibly experimental medical techniques, the Church stated that if there are no other sufficient remedies, it is permitted to use such means with the patient's consent. Furthermore, with the patient's consent, it is permitted to interrupt these means when the results fall short of expectations. In making such a decision, the reasonable wishes of the patient and the patient's family and the advice of physicians

would have to be taken into account. Physicians, in particular, may judge that the techniques applied impose strain and suffering on the patient out of proportion with the benefits the patient may gain.[19]

Refusal by the dying patient to use burdensome techniques is not the equivalent of suicide. On the contrary, such refusal "should be considered as an acceptance of the human condition."[19] In addition, as further stated by the Vatican, without in any way hastening the hour of death, patients and clinicians should be able to accept death with full responsibility and dignity.

DO NO HARM: LIVING WILLS AND
NATURAL DEATH ACTS

Living Wills are procedures whereby a person may provide in advance for the withholding or withdrawal of recovery-oriented medical care in the event the person should suffer a terminal illness or mortal injury. Living Wills are seen by many patients as a conscious effort to implement their personal choice in dying. These documents serve several functions. First, they represent an effort to retain individual choice and control over what happens when dying. Second, they attempt to enable patients to make choices about their dying while they are still competent. Third, they relieve the patient (or family) of the burden of choice at a time of crisis.[20] The legal status of these Wills has not been tested and proponents suggest discussion of the Will with the patient's physician to insure enforcement.

In some states, statutes, sometimes referred to as the Natural Death Act, which attempt to provide some legal basis for the implementation of the Living Wills, have been passed. The merits of these statutes, as well as the Living Wills, have been hotly debated. Whatever their pros and cons, these procedures are now a fait accompli and perhaps their chief value will have been to raise the issue of who controls the dying trajectory. For example, the California Natural Death Act creates a duty to desist from life-sustaining procedures when there is evidence of both valid refusal of care by the patient and when the physician has determined that death is imminent. Under this act, which appears to be patient-centered, control of the dying trajectory remains largely with the physician. Nevertheless, a major benefit may be that patients and clinicians will use the Act as an opportunity to discuss the issues surrounding the end of life.[21]

The developing public interest in Natural Death Acts, Living Wills, and the growth of organizations concerned with the patient rights in dying can be viewed as our society's attempt to operationalize guidelines for "natural death." Roles have become reversed. Patients are now saying to the clinicians, "Do no harm." The concept of "harm" as wrongful life—life continued against a patient's will and in a state incompatible with the patient's values—has emerged. The practical method of facilitating the injunction "do no harm" is the subject of the next section.

DECISION MAKING

Working Towards Resolutions

Once a philosophy of open awareness about dying has been adopted, the primary care clinician faces the challenge of making it *work*. Primary care clinicians have the unique opportunity to prevent the terrible ethical and psychological dilemmas that engulf specialists, the hospital, and the family. Our health care system is seriously burdened by patient situations that might have been avoided if a preventive approach was used when the patient still had the capacity to make decisions about the style of his or her own living while dying.

Working With Patients

In a primary care practice, the clinician has a unique opportunity to develop health care strategies for incorporating patient values about the use of medical interventions should a critical event or patient deterioration occur. Clinicians, however, have traditionally deferred such discussions about decision making on how to live while dying until the last days or hours of the patient's dying trajectory, that is, until a time when often a patient's competence is uncertain. Therein lies the crux of the problem, to which the only satisfactory solution is for the clinician to initiate a preventive approach. This responsibility for prevention belongs properly to the patient's primary care clinician and cannot be successfully abdicated to other health care providers. The skilled clinician will find it easier to deal with the issue of decision making at an early stage rather than to let things happen and to try to deal with events after they have occurred.

How the subject of decision making about the use of medical interventions is raised depends on the patient's health status. Additionally, as for any other

factor of health maintenance, although a full spectrum of information and discussion should be available, the clinician should anticipate patient participation in only those issues that the patient is able to take part in at the time. As a strategy it is often useful to link discussion of decision making related to this sensitive area with other subjects surrounding death, such as wishes regarding organ donations.

When using a preventive approach for healthy individuals, initiating the subject is facilitated by using printed materials easily accessible to patients in the office. The written material should contain these key elements: an introduction to the issue, a statement of the provider's philosophy, a statement of the patient's rights and responsibilities, specifics related to options at the end of life, discussion of the Natural Death Act and Living Wills, and an open invitation to discuss the subject.

The clinician can then, at the time of a health maintenance visit, ask patients if they have read the material. If not, encourage them to do so. If the patient has read the material, encourage discussion and after detailed inquiry, offer to incorporate his or her preferences into the medical record in a mutually acceptable format. It is essential that the patient's right to modify in any way or totally delete previous preferences be maintained. The subject should be raised annually and the patient encouraged to reaffirm his or her preferences in writing.

For patients already in a dying trajectory, a preventive approach must be implemented prior to the imminent ending of the trajectory. For example, for patients with severely compromised chronic obstructive pulmonary disease, at some uncertain point in time, the question of the use of a respiratory support system will arise. Part of the health care plan for these patients must be to introduce the prognostic and quality of life issues early so as to give patients the opportunity to discuss their values in the event that technological interventions could be considered for use. Failure to raise these issues until physiological processes deteriorate invites dilemmas related to patient competency and thus, subsequent dilemmas as to the fit of the dying process to patients' values.

Another challenge to the preventive approach is presented by those patients who have a disease but who are not yet in the dying trajectory. For example, patients suffering from transient ischemic attacks (TIAs) have several possible outcomes: total resolution of the TIA, continued TIA, or stroke. Outcomes from stroke range from mild impairment to severe impairment, a vegetative state, or rapidly impending death. The last three outcomes most often involve use of technological interventions, e.g., a respirator. In a preventive approach, patients with TIAs might be cared for in much the same way as those with terminal conditions—with incorporation of discussion of issues related to decision making about technology and dying in the patient's care plan.

At all times it is essential to allow sufficient time and circumstances for patient–clinician communication to develop. Most patients, given the opportunity, will indicate the amount and type of guidance they require. Skill in presenting this information to patients is crucial because the problems perceived as associated with open awareness about death and dying are more often related to lack of skill in communicating this sensitive material than to open awareness per se.

Working With Families

Patients have the right to decide *who* in their families should know *what* about their illness. The decision to tell or not to tell is based on at least two factors: does the patient want to share the open awareness with the family members and, if so, with whom; and, the timing of the disclosure. Timing of disclosure is a function of the patient's stage in the dying trajectory and of the perception the patient has of his or her own need and the family's needs. The primary care clinician may have important insights to offer the patient in this matter, but ultimately the decision is the patient's.

In an open-awareness context, the patient is in a unique position to determine with the clinician who in the family to include in the context. The patient needs to understand that choosing against open awareness will necessitate a burden of having to maintain a facade of "illness but not dying" and that this is extremely difficult to accomplish, especially if some family members know but others don't. Without open awareness, the patient may also lose significant support in his or her dying.

A useful strategy for the clinician is to obtain a clear picture of the patient's family and other significant support systems and then develop with the patient a plan for disclosure. The clinician must establish with the patient the preferred method for initially informing family members, and for dealing subsequently with family requests for information.

Often the patient will want to receive initial information with his or her spouse or other significant loved ones present. One approach to informing other family members is the conference in which the clinician informs the family as a group. It is preferable to speak to other family members with the patient present as this prevents misinterpretation and reassures the patient that he or she is in control. The clinician, because of knowledge of prognosis, can help the family to understand the rationale for choosing or not choosing certain types of medical interventions.

The clinician and the patient need to be aware that there will be well-meaning challenges by family members to the course the patient has chosen. This searching for hope through posing alternative medical interventions is a necessary step for the family to reassure itself that all is being done. The clinician must allow the family this type of questioning but must retain control for the patient by explaining what is and what is not in the patient's best interest. A good strategy is to disclose to the strongest family member, who then has the responsibility to relay information to the other family members according to his or her and the patient's best judgment.

Another issue in dealing with families is the timing of disclosure. For quick dying trajectories, there will be no choice about disclosure because the facts will speak for themselves. In these situations, the clinician must work quickly with the family to bring them into awareness and help them start the grieving process.

On the other hand, a lingering trajectory offers the patient and clinicians a degree of latitude in timing disclosure. Some patients will initially choose against awareness out of fear of unnecessarily burdening the family or of fear of becoming isolated and abandoned. Other patients will need to share the awareness early on because they need the physical, financial, and psychological support of their families. The factors guiding this decision are complex, and the patient will require the clinician's guidance in decision making.

The decision to postpone the sharing of awareness inevitably leads to the time when the patient's dying becomes visible and family members must be brought into awareness. This will be difficult because the family will then have to "catch up" with the patient in the grieving process. The patient will already have worked through his or her own grieving while the family will be in the earlier stages of denial and anger. The clinician must anticipate this and help the family to control its grieving. A useful strategy here is to correct any unfounded expectations family members have about the mode of dying and to assure them that events are taking place according to a plan worked out by their loved one. Clinicians can also help by retaining equanimity and assisting family members to provide comfort care for the patient.

Occasionally, a latecomer will arrive who, because of recently acquired grief, will upset the patient and family with demands that the professionals "do something." This family member may be shocked at the apparent "indifference" displayed by the family and raise once again the conflicts dealt with previously. Preparing the patient and family for this and reassuring them that they are "on schedule" with their grieving will help the family maintain unity. Faced with this situation, family members usually tend to come closer together and to discount the input of the latecomer.

Working in the Office

Practice strategies are those of good management and identical to those used to incorporate other ideas into the day-to-day office situation.

- Time: does the appointment system lend itself to discussions of such issues with the patient?
- Records: is the record system structured to remind the provider to raise the subject? Is there a method to keep the provider's knowledge about the patient's wishes up to date?
- Environment: is the office conducive to discussion? Acoustical privacy? Comfortable seating? Is there space to accommodate families?
- Materials: are printed materials readily accessible, current, and kept in stock?
- Associates: have the providers in the practice discussed their viewpoints on these issues? And have accommodations been made when philosophical differences exist?

Attention to practical details will make the difference between well-intentioned theoretical notions and actual implementation in practice. For example, Dr. Louis Baer, author of *Let the Patient Decide: A Doctor's Advice to Older Persons*, implements an open awareness by arranging the last hours of each office day for "just time to talk" and keeps copies of the Living Will in his waiting room.

Working With Specialists

Primary care clinicians frequently call on other specialists for assistance in patient care. The majority of these consultations are relatively straightforward requests for diagnostic or therapeutic aid. However, there will arise from time to time serious ethical dilemmas related to the consultation process for which the specialist is usually blamed. Primary care clinicians, while they may lament these dilemmas, must recognize that they share in their making.

Consider the restrictions within which specialists must operate: they do not know the patient intimately, they feel that they are being asked to utilize their technological expertise to "do something," and they are unsure of the interaction expected by the primary care provider. So, as well-intentioned as specialist might be, the context in which he or she practice does not have the advantage of the broad frame of reference available to the primary care clinician. It is the primary care clinician who, with an intimate history of the patient and responsibility for the patient's future, can ideally fit health care activities to the patient's values.

The primary care clinician, therefore, must carefully plan the consultation process. First, the reason for consultation must be clear. Obtaining an opinion is the first step: what is the diagnosis, the prognosis, or possible therapies? The consultant should be asked not only what is available but *what difference it will make*. What are the chances the proposed therapy would cure or greatly help the patient? What are the chances it could cause death? What are the major complications? What could happen with no treatment? For elderly patients, an additional question that is crucial must be asked: what are the chances that this therapy (whether routine or heroic) will neither kill nor cure the patient, but will leave the patient in limbo, existing biologically but with so much mental impairment or physical incapacity that the patient will be doomed to months or years in a nursing home with dying not life being prolonged?[22]

It is the proper role of the primary care clinician with the patient to maintain control of health care. Consultants should defer decision making about therapy with patients until they have discussed their opinions with the referring primary care clinician. The primary care provider must control requests for additional consultation. Primary care clinicians who deal in a straightforward manner with specialists will be able to develop a group of consultants who respect their approach. A working relationship can result in which the values of all professionals and of patients are considered, and the benefits of the specialty applied in a thoughtful manner.

Working With Hospitals

Primary care clinicians have the responsibility to be fully involved in the hospital care of their patients. A chief area of interface will be with the hospital emergency room. Emergency room physicians do not desire, nor should they bear, the burden of medical decision making for other physician's patients. To avoid dilemmas, the following guidelines should be followed:

- Instruct your patients verbally and in writing to notify the emergency room personnel that they are under the care of a primary care clinician:
- Instruct the emergency room personnel and constantly reinforce the fact that the primary care clinicians want to be notified when their patients reach the E.R.:
- The hospital should have as a policy that the patient's primary care physician has responsibility for the patient:
- The hospital should also have as a policy that decisions related to application of technological interventions or their discontinuation belong properly to the patients as exercised through their primary physician.

Primary care providers should participate in hospital procedure and policy making in so far as it affects the ethical dimensions of patient care. Currently, there is a growing movement among hospital-based professionals towards establishing committees and guidelines for the care of the critically terminally ill that go by such names as ethics committee, prognosis committee, optimum care committee, death committee, etc. Their functions are a matter of lively debate and it is unclear whether they will gain support and how they will evolve. However, any policies or committees that interfere with, minimize, or discount respect for the patient and basic honesty in human relations must be resisted. The point here concerns the locus of control for decision making: it is rightfully the patient's as worked out with due care over time with the guidance of a primary care clinician.

Working With Nurses

Ethical conflicts (while probably not consciously identified as such) are daily occurrences between hospital nurses and physicians engaged in the care of the critically terminally ill, particularly in speciality units. Nurses who deal intimately with the patient and family for prolonged hours each day often have a different perspective of the patient's needs than a physician who does not know the patient or family very well and only visits for a few minutes.

Indeed, in such situations, nurses and physicians may honestly differ in their estimation of the patient's stage in the dying trajectory. The difference is often dismissed as emotionalism of nurses versus scientific analysis by the physician, while in fact important information regarding trajectory estimation may be disregarded. In this respect, two aspects of prognosis are important: that of scientific prediction based on collective cases, and that of individualization based on the particular case. Nurses may have a superior ability to determine an individual trajectory secondary to their more intense exposure to the patient and his or her family: "I envy for medical students the advantages enjoyed by the nurses, who live in daily contact with the sick".[23]

The primary care clinician, who has an indepth knowledge of the patient's wishes for health care, has a unique opportunity to work with nurses and to integrate nursing observations about the patient's trajectory with patient values concerning the care the patient wants to receive. Such integration is facilitated by keeping the nursing staff appraised of and involved in the factors influencing decision making and developing mutual strategies for the care of the patient. Given the context of open awareness, which a primary care clinician can best implement, nurses in acute- or long-term care settings are better able to work towards fitting their skills to the patient's wishes, particularly the patient's need for the comfort care of good nursing.

Working With the Issue of Incompetency

Is the patient competent to decide? For the purposes of making an informed choice in medical treatment, competence is understood to "rest on the test of whether the patient understands the relevant risks and alternatives, and whether the resulting decisions reflect a deliberate choice by the patient."[24] A most delicate problem arises in those patient situations in which competency may be questioned because of pain, metabolic imbalance, or sedation from medication. These patients situations present a two-edged dilemma: while some clinicians would argue that patients are incompetent to decide because they are in the situation; others argue that the patient cannot decide competently until they are in the situation!

Issues of competency often spring from conflict between a professional's wishes and those of the patient. Patient incompetency is then used as camouflage by the physician to maintain control of the decision-making process. For example, a nephrologist who feels that dialysis should be undertaken may use impaired renal status and its effects on mentation to justify failure to honor the patient's request that therapy be discontinued or not be instituted in the first place. Such impingement on the patient's human dignity must be protected against by the primary care clinician and can best be accomplished by prevention.

When patients slip through the preventive defense, the primary care clinician must be prepared to work with the exponential problem of a patient no longer able to decide and who has not previously made any wishes known. Much attention has been given to this issue: Most of it, however, has involved those situations where the family and the physician have disagreed on the best course of action. One option for the primary care clinician is to present the facts squarely to the family members, with particular emphasis on eliciting their knowledge as to the wishes of the patient and to rely on their decision unless it conflicts with the values of the clinician. In cases of conflict, the wisest course may be to consider additional consultation (here is when a committee could be helpful) or to release the patient to a provider more sympathetic to the family's viewpoint.

An issue which frequently arises is the physician's and hospital's fear of legal reprisals. Recently, physicians have been seeking legal immunity in such situations. This strategy is subject to a serious challenge:

The medical community is arguing that, rather than take an almost nonexistent risk for terminating treatment on a terminally ill patient for whom there is no hope of a cure, they will actively and uselessly continue fruitless, painful, and extraordinary treatment unless they are granted legal immunity for terminating it. What an incredible self-indictment of the professional! . . . Physicians

have traditionally argued that they are special because they routinely deal with "life and death." The modern argument seems to be: "We are still special, but we won't make any medical decisions that involve life and death unless we are guaranteed immunity for the decision." Should we, as a society, give unreviewable life-and-death decision-making authority to a group of individuals who are afraid to take *responsibility* for their decisions?[25]

By their very nature, issues related to incompetency can never be completely resolved. As such, these issues represent a failure in health care and give compelling reason for primary health care clinicians to use a strategic preventive approach.

Working With Disappointment

Open awareness and a preventive approach are not a panacea protecting a clinician from dilemma. Indeed, because the approach is more demanding, disappointment attributed to its use is felt more acutely. Consider, for example, a patient who is told of his or her dying trajectory and who chooses to live his or her last weeks in an alcoholic oblivion, or a patient who denies that death is near, refusing to make preparations to the point of frustration for the dependent family. Certainly, these patients' dying styles challenge the unspoken professional ideal of the noble, serene death. Perhaps here the real issue at stake is not the patient's failure to conform to an ideal but the clinician's discomfort with the patient's nonconformity.

Compounding this reality conflict, other providers would add to a clinicians's discomfiture by stating that telling the truth in many cases is a poor and unrewarding practice. Is an individual patient style disheartening to a clinician a reason to discredit open awareness? No. Patients do not always act wisely, and imposed security through information control will not guarantee that they do so. It is far better to weather the disappointment than to abandon an ethical stance. In time, the positive results will justify what are perceived to be untoward effects.

CONCLUSION

For competency in clinical practice to be relevant to eldercare it must extend beyond the borders of scientific expertise and into the realm of ethical considerations in the delivery of health care. As has been said, the unexamined life is not worth living; so, too, the unexamined practice is not worthy of the stature awarded it. Developing an awareness of one's own ethical principles is a challenging endeav-

or. Awareness involves: raising the issues, articulating a position, and implementing the decision. The decision to practice in an open-awareness context is the foundation.

REFERENCES

1. Kieffer GH: Bioethics: A Textbook of issues. Reading, Addison-Wesley, 1979, pp 21–40
2. Hippocrates: Of the Epidemics, Book I, Section II, Second Constitution 5
3. Jonsen AR: Do no harm. Ann Intern Med 88:827–832, 1978
4. Amundsen DW: The physician's obligation to prolong life: A medical duty without classical roots. Hastings Center Report, August 1978, pp 23–30
5. Bacon SF: Advancement of Learning, Second Book IX 7
6. A definition of irreversible coma. Report of the ad hoc committee of the Harvard Medical School to examine the definition of brain death. JAMA 205:337–340, 1968
7. Imbus SH, Zawacki BE: Autonomy for burned patients when survival is unprecedented. N Engl J Med 297:308–311, 1977
8. Eliastam M, Duralde T, Martinez F, et al: Cardiac arrest in the emergency medical service system: Guidelines for resuscitation. JACEP 6:525–529, 1977
9. Glaser BG, Strauss AL: Awareness of Dying. Chicago, Aldine Publishing, 1965
10. Barnett R: Director family practice residency program, Sonoma County California. Personal communication, January 18, 1980
11. Glaser BG, Strauss AL: Time for Dying. Chicago, Aldine Publishing, 1968
12. Glaser BG, Strauss AL: Temporal aspects of dying as a non-scheduled status passage. Am J Soc 71:48–59, 1965
13. Yarling RR: Ethical analysis of a nursing problem: The scope of nursing in disclosing the truth to terminal patients. Supervisor Nurse 9:28–34, 1978
14. Fletcher J: Morals and Medicine. Princeton, Princeton University Press, 1954 pp 36–63
15. Veatch RM: Death, Dying, and the Biological Revolution, Our Last Quest for Responsibility. New Haven, Yale University Press, 1976, pp 204–248
16. Ramsey P: Ethics at the Edges of Life, Medical and Legal Intersections. New Haven, Yale University Press, 1978, pp 145–188
17. Callahan D: Natural death and public policy, in Veatch RM (ed): Life Span: Values and Life Extending Technologies. New York, Harper & Row, 1979, pp 162–175
18. Beauchamp TL, Perlin S: Ethical Issues in Death and Dying. New Jersey, Prentice-Hall, 1978, pp 216–220
19. Declaration on Euthanasia, issued by the Sacred Congregation for the Doctrine of Faith and approved by Pope John Paul II, in The New York Times, June 26, 1980
20. Bok S: Personal directions for care at the end of life. N Engl J Med 295:367–369, 1976
21. Jonsen AR: Dying right in California, the natural death act. Clin Res 26:55–60, 1978
22. Baer SL: Let the Patient Decide: A Doctor's Advice to Older Persons. Philadelphia, Westminister Press, 1978, pp 15–21
23. Osler: Aeqnanimitas: The Hospital as College
24. Rabkin MT, Gillerman G, Rice NR: Orders not to resuscitate. N Engl J Med 295:364–366, 1976
25. Annas GJ: After saikewicz: No-fault death. Hastings Center Report, June 1978, pp 16–18

RECOMMENDED RESOURCES

Baer SL: Let the Patient Decide: A Doctor's Advice to Older Persons. Philadelphia, Westminister Press, 1978 (in paperback)

Highly recommended. A thoughtful, concise book written by a family physician for clinicians and patients to acquaint them with the problems inherent in utilization of medical interventions in eldercare. Provocative section outlining the

possibilities open to the patient in controlling his or her dying trajectory. May be offered to patients as the best available discussion of the subject.

Concern for Dying. Educational Council, 250 West 57th Street, New York, New York 10019

Information about and copies of Living Wills are available from this group. The Council publishes a quarterly news-

letter reporting recent developments in the field of death and dying. Both patient and clinician oriented.

Jonsen AR, Cassel C, Lo B, Perkins HS: The ethics of medicine: An annotated bibliography of recent literature. Ann Intern Med 92:136–141, 1980

Annotated bibliography dealing with ethical problems likely to be encountered by clinicians, stressing practical, current, and available resources. Divided according to content areas, e.g., death and dying, informed consent,

ethics of medication, etc. Very helpful guide to a rapidly expanding field of literature.

Lo B, Jonsen AR: Ethical decisions in the care of a patient terminally ill with metastatic cancer. Ann Intern Med 92:107–111, 1980

First in a series of presentations authored by members of the Bioethics Program of the University of California at San Francisco. Presentations adapted from actual patient situations.

3

Physical Changes in the Aged

Roger Jacobs, Ph.D.

Physiologic aging is a process (or processes) that occurs in such an insidious manner as to provide no evidence of change on a daily basis. Nevertheless, it is quite certain that over the years profound changes will occur in individuals and ultimately will result in their demise. Regardless of the nature of the aging process, the manifestations of aging are manifold and various.

STRUCTURAL CHANGES

Stature and Posture

Throughout life our stature and posture change. With aging the stature decreases in most individuals about 1.2 cm for each 20 years.[1] The major change becomes obvious at about the fiftieth year. This decrease is dependent upon several factors acting in concert with aging, such as sex, race, environment, etc. The extremities, however, remain relatively unchanged, as the long bones do not shorten significantly. The appearance is one of disproportionately long arms and legs in the elderly individual. The main cause of the decrease in stature appears to be a thinning of the vertebral disks in addition to a lessening of vertical size of the vertebrae.

Postural changes with increasing age may also apparently further decrease height. The elder person assumes a stooping, bent forward characteristic. The knees and hips are flexed somewhat and the arms may be bent at the elbows to raise the hands. In order to maintain the gaze level, the head may be tilted backward, producing a jutting forward appearance of the head. Shoulder width decreases,

while chest depth and pelvic width increase.[2] A decrease in the depth of the abdomen also occurs.[2]

The nature of changes in stature and posture involve developmental, as well as aging, processes, and the cause of these changes lies primarily in the skeletal and muscular systems, and the subcutaneous tissues, such as fat, and other dermal structures, which are mainly those that do not replace themselves in the course of normal events.

Bone is a dynamic tissue constantly undergoing resorption and renewal. In aging bone, a changing equilibrium results from a greater resorption and lesser deposition of calcium. The structural and postural changes occur primarily because calcium is lost from the bones (resulting in osteoporosis), and cartilage and muscle tissue undergo atrophic processes. The osteoporosis probably gives rise to compression of the bones, while degeneration of the cartilage appears to underlie the decrease in intervertebral distance. Osteoporosis may become particularly significant in women in the postmenopausal period (resulting in an increased probability of fracture). See Fig. 3-1. Muscle shrinkage and loss of tone contribute to the forward-leaning posture and a flaccid appearance of the limbs, sometimes accompanied by a decrease in limb circumference. Osteoarthritic changes lead to decreased mobility and/or mobility with pain and may add to postural decline.

Weight Changes and Subcutaneous Fat

In the male, the average weight remains more or less constant from about the mid-twenties through the mid-forties.[2] Thereafter, an age-related decline

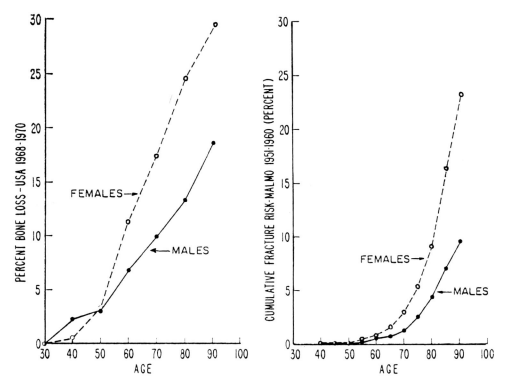

Fig. 3-1. Bone loss (left) and fracture risk (right) in humans as a function of age. [From Garn SM: Adult bone loss, fracture epidemiology and nutritional implications. Nutrition 27:107–115, 1973. (Fracture risk data after Alffram, 1964.) With permission.]

of about eight pounds per decade occurs through the mid-seventies and beyond. In contrast, females do not appear to lose weight with age. Overweight individuals of both sexes, on the other hand, tend to lose weight with increasing age. Often persons in the "middle age" group gain weight only to lose it later as they age.

Subcutaneous fat distribution changes markedly throughout life. For example, fat deposition in the abdomen and hips may increase, while that of the face may decrease with age.[3] Forearm subcutaneous fat loss with age is usually dramatic even in somewhat overweight persons.

Women's breasts undergo atrophy of the fatty tissues as well as of the glandular components. The result is a sagging, flattening, and loss of turgor. The nipples may also invert because of shrinkage and fibrotic changes.[3]

Skinfold thickness (the skin is folded manually and may be measured with a caliper), which is one measure of subcutaneous fat content, is greatly reduced in the forearm with age, whereas that of the pubis, umbilicus, and waist does not undergo much change.[4] The skinfold of the back of the hand

of the female lessens rapidly after 45 years of age even where total weight is increasing. The onset is delayed in males.[5]

Skin, Hair, and Nails

Aging of skin is of psychological as well as physiological importance because the skin, particularly of the face and hands, is readily observable by others. Skin creasing and sagging becomes more prevalent with age. The general direction of change in the thickness of the epidermis is controversial,[6,7] but variability of thickness does occur. The mitotic index is decreased in aging epidermis[7,8]; healing response time to injury and rate of healing are also reduced.[7] Tanning response to light lessens with age.[7]

The dermis becomes thinner primarily as a result of the decrease in subcutaneous fat. The content of collagen, an important constituent of dermal tissue, has been reported by some investigators to decrease with age[9] and by others to increase.[10] At this time, therefore, the contribution of collagen to dermal thinning is unresolved. Elastin concentration increases,[7] but both elastin and probably the collagen fibers become more cross-linked[11,12] with age, leading to a decrease in elasticity of the skin. The decrease in elasticity may also be related to the degree of exposure of the skin to environmental factors, such as sunlight, wind, and drying conditions. In aviators and others who spend many hours at high altitudes, ozone may also be a contributing factor in development of wrinkling and loss of elasticity. Skin wrinkling most likely results from thinning and shrinking of the dermis as well as loss of tone in underlying musculature. Creases usually form in the skin at 90-degree angles to the axis central to the muscle fibers (direction of contraction), in some cases near the insertion of the muscle tendon. Flat pigmented spots (freckles, nevi) appear, become more numerous, and enlarge especially with increased exposure to intense natural or artificial sunlight.

With advancing years, the sweat glands decrease in density and size.[13] The rate of sweat production also declines as well as the time of response to activity or thermal stress. The thermal threshold for sweat production increases. The sebaceous glands, which are often associated with hair follicles, decrease in number and function, but their structural integrity is probably retained.[7]

The vascular bed of the dermis declines after 20 years of age. Vascular hyperplasia, however, increases. Veins may become more pronounced as varicosities and benign cherry hemangiomas and venous lakes (particularly on the head) frequently appear.

The hair undergoes graying and is lost to some extent from the body in later years. The color change is apparent in 50 percent of the population by age 50 regardless of the sex or the hair colorization of the young adult.[14] Hair becomes gray because of decreased melanin production in the follicle. Hair loss is observed most prominently in some males and is manifested as the inherited characteristic pattern baldness. Recession of hair in men may begin as early as 20 years of age. Women also show these changes but generally to a much smaller extent. The density of hair follicles decreases from 615/cm² at age 30 to 500/cm² at 50 years of age and thereafter remains relatively constant.[15] The cross sectional diameter of the individual scalp hairs decreases with advancing age. By 40 years of age, the hair of the body, as well as that of the axillary and pubic regions, has reached its pattern limit and then recedes with increasing age.[6] The

axillary and pubic hair of postmenopausal women is decreased.[7] According to some investigators,[16] a progressive loss of axillary and pubic hair occurred with age with a higher proportion of females showing this loss. Coarse hair in areas of skin such as the ears (in the external canals and on the pinnae) in both sexes, on the chin, and around the lips of women may proliferate and thicken with advancing age—in some cases beginning as early as the third decade.

The nails of the fingers at about age 30 grow at an average rate of 0.8 mm/week. This rate decreases by nearly 40 percent at 90 years of age.[17,18] The nails of the toes, which grow at a rate of about 15 percent of that of the finger nails, also probably undergo a decline in growth rate with age. Longitudinal striations of the nails increase in depth and prominence as aging occurs.[7]

Facial Changes

The face is nearly always exposed to observers. Changes that occur as a result of aging processes are thus readily apparent, at least superficially. The most profound of these changes are the wrinkles, creases, and folds that the skin presents with age. These creases generally form in a direction 90 degrees to the axis of muscle contraction. Once a fold line is established, it tends to remain and increase in depth with age. The depth is determined by a number of factors, including the amount of subcutaneous fat, the elasticity, dermal thickness, and amount of lateral surface compression (from underlying muscular contraction) of the skin. Characteristic wrinkles that form with age are those of the forehead parallel to the mouth, the "crow's feet" at the external canthi of the eyes, creases around and at either side of the mouth, and wrinkles at right angles to the axis of the neck. Skin creasing can begin as early as the second decade, and the fold depth slowly increases throughout life.

The loss of bone mass, particularly from the mandible, produces a decrease in the size of the lower part of the face which accentuates the size of the upper mouth, nose, and forehead. Tooth loss causes an indented "loss-of-lip" look to the mouth[17] when uncorrected by prosthesis. Redistribution of fat leads to a baggy appearance of the lids—in part from increasing fat deposits—and a sunken appearance of the eyes, as orbital fat declines.[3]

The loss of dermal tone—from loss of elasticity, subcutaneous fat, thickness, and underlying muscle

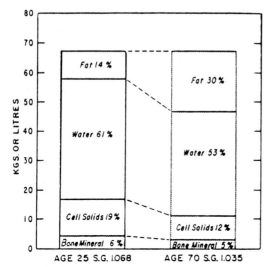

Fig. 3-2. Variations of human selected body components with age. S.G. is specific gravity. [From Fryer JH: Studies of body composition in men aged 60 and over, in Shock N (ed): Biological Aspects of Aging. New York, Columbia University Press, 1962, p 59. With permission.]

tissue—leads to a drooping character of the skin. This accentuates the jowls, elongates the ears,[19] causes stasis of the upper eyelids, contributes to bagginess of the lower eyelids,[3] and may also take part in formation of a "double chin" in some individuals.

Skin color in many cases decreases in intensity because of a loss of pigmentation and vascularity. Darkly pigmented spots such as freckles and flat nevi, however, may appear and enlarge with time; exposure to ultraviolet light, a component of sunlight, may lead to their increased numbers.

Body Composition

Shifts in body composition occur with age, and the most outstanding of these changes are variations in fat and water content. Fat concentration increases by about 16 percent from 25–75 years of age, while in the same period water content decreases by 8 percent (see Fig. 3-2); but the extracellular component of body water does not vary appreciably with age, remaining at about 20 percent of the total body water.[20,21] Other constituents such as cell solids and bone decline with advancing age (see Fig. 3-2).

The specific gravity of the body decreases with age (Fig. 3-2), and this corresponds to the increasing fat content; fat is the only body component less massive than water.[22]

Isotope studies involving measurement of exog-

enous and endogenous concentrations of potassium[23,24–26] and sodium have indicated that, in general, a decrease in the lean body mass occurs.[22] This reduction was found to be about 25 percent in males and 15 percent in females.[25]

Other changes in composition occur at the intercellular matrix and intracellular levels, in particular in normally nondividing cells such as those of the nervous system. In the intercellular space containing the ground substance where collagen and elastin are present, increasingly cross-linked, more rigid types replace the original resilient materials. Among intracellular changes occuring with age are variations in the concentration of certain structural proteins, enzymes, chromosomal components including deoxyribonucleic (DNA) and ribonuclic acids (RNA) and other constituents. Another most impressive cellular compositional change is the accumation of lipofuscin pigments in nervous and other nonrenewing (cardiac muscle, for example) tissues. Lipofuscin is a brown fluorescent substance that has been referred to as "age pigment." It is distributed within the cell as discrete separate particles or aggregates. Many investigators have claimed that the age-related accumulation of lipofuscin may be the most constant morphological age change at the cellular level. The effect of the increasing presence of this pigment in cellular and whole body physiology is not understood. It has been suggested that it may be intrinsic to or a byproduct of the aging process.

FUNCTIONAL CHANGES

General

In general, the functions of the body decline with increasing age. Figure 3-3 shows the changes that occur in a few selected parameters.

Important considerations are the decline in homeostatic capacity: the rapidity and degree of reaction to stress, including wound healing, immune response, toxin clearance, blood pH variation and glucose tolerance metabolism and thermoregulation, muscular strength, and reaction time. The maximum duration of response to a challenge also decreases with age.

Cardiovascular

The heart and blood vessels have been intensively studied in regard to effects of aging, because cardiovascular failure is the primary physiological cause of death in humans. Changes in the heart and blood vessels are probably highly interdependent. The heart undergoes a number of changes with age that result in decreased performance. These manifestations have been summarized previously[27]: cardiac output decreases by 1 percent/year as compared to an average 5-liter/minute baseline for individuals. This decrease in output results from a lower heart rate and smaller stroke volume. The work performed by the left ventricle in an aging person at rest is estimated to be lessened, although the heart rate is essentially unchanged under this condition. Increased delay in the recovery of irritability and contractility develops with age. Response time to sudden stressful conditions in lengthened and cardiac reserve capacity is decreased. The influence of the vagus is increased. Atropine has a lowered effectiveness on cardiac tissue but sensitivity to stimuli from the carotid sinus rises. Metabolic capacity (utilization of oxygen) is lessened and it appears that cold pressor response is increased with age. The electrocardiogram shows little change in aging[28]; however, a small lengthening in the P-R, QRS and Q-T intervals, as well as a decrease in the QRS complex amplitude and a left shift of the QRS axis, may occur in some individuals.[7]

The size of the heart may vary with age, but the left ventricular capacity is decreased. The aorta becomes less elastic and enlarges. Stenosis of the cardiac valves is common in aging. The histologic changes that occur are similar to those observed in the vascular tissues.

Vascular changes with age have been stated[27] to include: a decrease in coronary arterial circulation of about 35 percent in 60-year-old individuals as compared to young adults; an increase in resistance to peripheral blood flow amounting to about 1 percent/yr; and an increase in pulse wave velocity with age. These changes can be generally attributed to decreased elasticity in the arteries and arterioles.

Hypertension, an abnormal increase in blood pressure, affects up to 50 percent of the population at age 80 and, therefore, bears mention as a phenomenon associated with aging. Hypertension is defined as systolic pressure of 160 mm Hg and/or diastolic pressure of 95 mm Hg or greater.[29] Hypertension probably results from a combination of hereditary and environmental factors involving the entire cardiovascular system and also such organs as the kidneys and liver, the pituitary gland, and the nervous system, as well as lipid, cholesterol, carbohydrate, and possible salt ingestion.

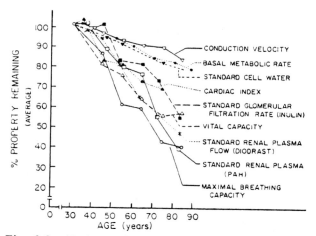

Fig. 3-3. Various selected parameters measured as a function of age in humans. [Adapted with permission from Shock NW: Discussion on mortality and measurement, in Strehler BL, Ebert JD, Glass HB, et al (eds): The Biology of Aging: A Symposium. Washington, DC, American Institute of Biological Sciences, 1960.]

Whether hypertension is caused by arteriosclerosis or atherosclerosis or the reverse is not clear. An increase in both appears to be concomitant. It is understood, however, that an increased mortality rate is associated with both hypertension and arterio- or atherosclerotic processes.

Causative factors probably forming the basis for decreased functionality of the cardiovascular system with age consist mainly of: lessened elasticity because of collagen and elastin deposition and crosslinking and binding of calcium, cholesterol plaque formation in arteriosclerosis, fatty deposits in and degeneration of vascular tissue in atherosclerosis, deposition of amyloid (hyaline material resembling starch with eosinophyllic and iodine staining properties), vascular and myocardial fibrosis secondary to infarction. On the cellular level, many changes in enzyme concentration are noted and lipofuscin pigments accumulate, though the functional significance of the latter is unclear.

Kidneys

The kidneys are the organs primarily responsible for the homeostatic regulation of fluid volume and soluble solids in the body. Extensive studies have shown that in aging, kidney function declines.[30-33]

The aging kidney progressively loses the ability to replace damaged or lost nephrons, resulting in a gradual decrease in renal function capacity. Figure 3-4 shows the relationship of a composite of glo-

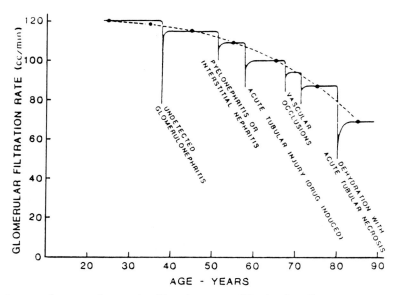

Fig. 3-4. Average human glomerular filtration rates. The broken line represents a proposed steady decline in renal function, whereas the solid line alternatively represents stable renal function until a pathologic condition causes some degree of irreparable damage to the glomeruli. [From Lindeman RD: Age changes in renal function, in Goldman R, Rockstein M (eds): The Physiology and Pathology of Human Aging. New York, Academic Press, 1975, p 29. With permission.]

merular filtration rate data to age along with indications of causitive factors associated with reduced kidney function. Generally, the capacity of the kidney to provide homeostatis of the body fluids remains adequate. In old age, a challenge to the kidneys may exceed their reduced capacity, whereas

a youthful individual may retain adequate renal function to meet such a challenge.

The other components involved in excretion—the ureters, bladder, and urethra—undergo changes with age. These changes consist mainly of prostatism (in males) and increased frequency of infections (which may cause scarring and stricture of the ureters or urethra), leading to reduced urinary elimination and nocturia. Severe restriction of urinary flow results in decompensation of the bladder and, ultimately, complete renal failure, if it is not corrected.

Respiratory

Decrease of pulmonary function in the aging individual has been well documented.[34–36] Figure 3-5 shows some of the changes in respiratory parameters measured as a function of age. Although the total lung capacity (TLC) remains constant, the vital capacity decreases and the residual volume (RV) thus increases.[34]

Morphological variations in the pulmonary system that underlie the changes in ventilation with age consist primarily of decreases in elasticity of the pleural tissues, weakening of the intercostal muscles and perhaps the diaphragm, and, in some individ-

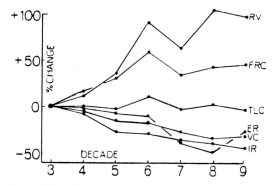

Fig. 3-5. Variations in selected lung capacities in normal individuals by decades relative to the third decade. RV is the residual volume, FRC is the functional residual capacity, TLC is the total lung capacity, ER is the expiratory reserve, VC is the vital capacity and IR is the inspiratory reserve. [From Mithoefer JC, Karetzky MS: The cardiopulmonary system in the aged, in Powers JH (ed): Surgery of the Aged and Debilitated Patient. Philadelphia, WB Saunders, 1968, p 144. With permission.]

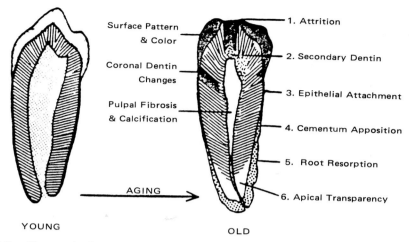

Fig. 3-6. Change in human tooth structure with age. [From Nalbandian J, Sognnaes RF: Structural age changes in human teeth, in Shock NW (ed): Aging, Some Social and Biological Aspects. Washington, DC, American Association for the Advancement of Science, publication no. 65, 1960. Copyright 1960 by the American Association for the Advancement of Science.]

uals, obesity and/or rib cage changes. A loss of alveoli occurs with age,[37] even though the lung regenerates well, usually with little scarring. The frequency of upper respiratory viral infections decreases, but the lungs become increasingly vulnerable to disease processes, such as emphysema, with age.[7]

Oral Cavity and Gastrointestinal System

The oral cavity and the gastrointestinal system, consisting of the esophagus, stomach, small intestine, and colon, their components and the accessory components—the liver, biliary tract, and pancreas—display various changes in aging, some of which are profound. The consequences of serious oral or gastrointestinal impairment range from severe discomfort to severe malnutrition and potentially life-threatening conditions.

In the oral cavity, taste sensation diminishes (threshold and response intensity), salivation decreases and the gums, mandible, and maxilla suffer degenerative changes (periodontal disease and osteoporosis, respectively), while the teeth become worn, develop caries and are lost. Structural decline in teeth occurs chiefly as a result of abrasion of the enamel and dentin, particularly at the mastication surfaces. Some other changes involve compensatory increase of internal dentin and the supporting cementum. Age differences in the teeth are illustrated in Fig. 3-6. An interesting finding concerns the racemization of amino acids in the teeth and its close relationship to the chronological age of the individual.[38]

The chief age change in the stomach, small intestine, and colon is decreased motility; however, decreased gastrointestinal blood supply, secretion in the stomach, and absorption of digested nutrients in the small intestine are also significant.[39,40]

The liver becomes smaller after 40 years of age. Regeneration after hepatic injury is probably slower to begin and is probably completed more slowly as well. Most serum indicators of liver status and function such as bilirubin,[41] the enzymes serum glutamic oxalacetic transaminase (SGOT), serum glutamic pyruvic transaminase (SGPT), and alkaline phosphatase remain unchanged in the normal individual from youth.[42] Total protein also remains essentially unchanged, but some variation in the protein moiety occurs.[7] Liver function capacity decreases with age as evaluated with the bromsulfonphthalein (BSP) clearance test.[7]

Biliary changes most likely result from hepatic alterations of bile composition often with saturation of cholesterol or less frequently precipitation of calcium in the bile, and these changes can lead to formation of calculi. About 10 percent of men and 20 percent of women at age 60 have cholelithiasis (gallstones). This incidence rises to nearly 40 percent of the population by age 80.[43,44] Treatment is usually surgical involving cholecystectomy (removal of the gall bladder) or cholecystostomy (removal of the stones in poor risk cases), although stone solvents which appear safe, chenodeoxycholic acid (CDCA),[45] ursodeoxycholic acid (UDCA)[46] and various combinations of terpenes[47] are under current investigation for toxicity.

The pancreas shows changes with age at the microscopic level, but weight differences are controversial. The most important change in the pancreas is decreased β-cell insulin elaboration response to increased blood glucose.[48] Glucagon response by the α-cells is probably also decreased. Pancreatic digestive enzymes are also decreased in output volume and concentration in aging, but with the non-diseased pancreas, this secretion appears adequate for normal digestion.[7]

Many other diverse gastrointestinal abnormal and disease processes may occur with aging.[49] Some of these include reflux esophagitis, hiatus hernia, atrophic gastritis, peptic ulcer, obstruction, bleeding, diverticulosis, colitis, and benign and malignant tumors.

Endocrine

Endocrine changes with age are, in some instances, conspicuous (some reproductive hormones) and in other cases nonexistent or unclear. This may be due in part to the complex feedback mechanisms and hormonal interrelationships in the endocrine systems. These systems are currently being intensively investigated. Some aspects, however, have been elucidated.

Diabetes mellitus becomes more prevalent with age.[50] This has prompted a good deal of study of the effects of aging on insulin production. As indicated in the previous section (Oral Cavity and Gastrointestinal System), the response of the pancreas to elaborate more insulin to higher glucose levels is decreased.[48,50] A suitable method for determining this characteristic change has been the glucose tolerance test,[48] which has been said to be abnormal in all elderly individuals. Insulin in the older person contains a relatively higher concentration of serum proinsulin (the insulin precursor), which is less active in glucose metabolism than insulin, although the total resting concentration of insulin and proinsulin remains little changed throughout life.[51] The relationship of aging and glucagon response and effectiveness is not yet clarified.

The thyroid, important in metabolic regulation, shows microscopic alterations with age. The functional capacity for elaboration of thyroid hormone,

however, appears to remain unchanged, even in very old individuals.[52,53] The basal metabolic rate (BMR) does decrease, but this seems to be related to the decrease in biomass with age[54] or possibly a decreased target tissue response.

The adrenal hormones consist of steroids elaborated by the cortex and amines produced by the medulla. Regulation of secretion of cortisol, an important glucocorticoid, does not appear to be affected by aging.[55] Daily production of cortisol, however, declines 25 percent in old age.[56] The response of the adrenal cortex to adrenocorticotropic hormone (ACTH) decreases. Urinary excretion of androgenic 17-ketosteroids (17-KS) is diminished to less than 50 percent of the youthful level,[56] but when considered in terms of creatine excretion, it is curious that a nearly linear relationship is observed (see Fig. 3-7).[57] The function of the adrenal androgens has not been elucidated and so the importance of the age-related change in 17-KS is not known.[53] The adrenal medulla produces slightly less epinephrine and norepinephrine with age, but dopamine is increased.[58] The significance of these changes is not clear.

The kidney also has endocrine function in the regulation of blood pressure via the renin–angiotensin II-aldosterone system.[29] The kidney may be involved in the development of hypertension in aging.[29]

Parathyroid hormone and calcitonin secretion has been said by some investigators to increase and by others to decrease in aging. The effects of these hormones in aging has not been investigated. Estrogen may inhibit parathyroid hormone mediated bone loss of calcium, and these low estrogen levels may be a causative factor in postmenopausal osteoporosis.[59]

The thymus is now definitely recognized as an endocrine organ. It appears that several hormones are elaborated by the thymus, and these hormones exercise some control over the development and function of the immune system.[60] Growth hormone and thyroid stimulating hormone of the pituitary influence thymic function.[60] In aging, the thymus becomes atrophic and involuted, and an associated decrease in thymic hormones occurs. This is probably involved in the observed age-related decrease in immune response.

The reproductive hormones of the female undergo significant change at the menopause. Ovarian estrogen production ceases, but some plasma estrogen precursor (androstenedione) is still elaborated by the adrenals, and this is converted into estrone, which is then the chief remaining estrogen.[61] The loss of ovarian estrogen production occurs as the ovary becomes fibrotic and involuted, with atretic corpora lutea and corpora albicantia.[62] The oocyte population drops to a few thousand.[62] Although these oocytes are still intact, they have been said to be much less responsive to pituitary gonadotropic hormone stimulation.[62] Periodic menstruation ceases and subjective "hot flashes" may occur.

After the menopause, androgen is produced by the ovary, but the androgen level is comparable to that of premenopausal women. The plasma concentrations of both the estrogens and androgens in older females are maintained in part by the reduced clearance rates of these hormones.

Progesterone secretion also decreases significantly after the menopause. The remaining 40 percent is probably maintained by the adrenals.[7]

After cessation of the reproductive cycle, the changes accompanying the cycle end. The component organs of the reproductive system are altered in a manner consistent with this nonreproductive phase of life.

Testosterone concentration in plasma probably does not change appreciably, but reports conflict. The secretion and clearance rates decrease, however.[7] In some instances ideopathic Leydig cell failure in the testes may give rise to a slow onset of impotency.[63]

The pituitary is a composite secretory organ with a surprising number of diverse functions. It plays a central role in complex hormonal feedback control mechanisms. In aging, the pituitary may lose up to 20 percent of its mass,[64,65] but the importance of this change is not understood because the plasma concentrations of its hormones do not change appreciably. There are some variations in the rhythmicity of release of anterior pituitary hormones such as growth hormone (GH). Others—adrenocorticotropic hormone (ACTH), thyroid stimulating hormone (TSH), their releasing factors (RFs), prolactin, the posterior pituitary secretion vasopression and antidiuretic hormone (ADH)—do not show a significant change in concentration with age. The status in aging of oxytocin or the melanocyte stimulating hormone of the pars intermedia of the pituitary is unclear. Follicle stimulating hormone (FSH) and lutenizing hormone (LH) also remain relatively constant in the male, but a significant increase in FSH and a moderate increase in LH

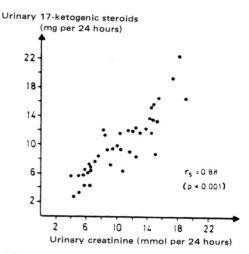

Fig. 3-7. Urinary 17-ketosteroid (17-KS) excretion plotted relative to urinary creatinine clearance. [From Bleichert-Toft M: The adrenal glands in old age, in Greenblatt R (ed): Aging. New York, Raven Press, 1978, vol 5, p 86. With permission.]

plasma levels occur in postmenopausal females. This probably results from a loss of negative feedback control over secretion of these hormones when the ovarian estrogen production ceases. The relationship of the pineal hormone melatonin to the aging individual has not been clarified.

Changes in neuroendocrine control involving the pituitary and target tissues occur in aging.[66-69] The best understood alteration resides in the neuroendocrine-pituitary-ovarian axis.[67] Evidence derived from ovarian transplantation studies may indicate that brain centers elaborating gonadotropin RF's may control the time of menopause.[67]

Target tissue responsiveness to hormonal stimulation may be lessened. Hormonal receptors may be involved, although this does not necessarily follow.[70,71] At the molecular biology level, it may be possible that inhibition of genomic expression, normally responsive to hormonal signals, occurs in aging.

Nervous System and Neurotransmission

The nervous system consists of complex interrelated components employing electrical, ionic, and endocrine processes to carry out the function of information transmission in the body. Various aging changes may be observed in nervous tissue characteristics, and the sum of these changes is a general decline in function.

The brain and central nervous system (CNS)

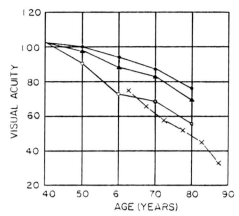

Fig. 3-8. Visual acuity as a function of age. [From Friedenwald JS: The eye, in Cowdry EV (ed): Problems of Aging. Baltimore, Williams & Wilkins, 1942, p 535. Reprinted with permission, © 1942, The Williams & Wilkins Company, Baltimore.]

sometimes, and only in certain areas, lose cells with age,[72] and total brain mass may decrease up to 25 percent in old age. The cells in the CNS are post-mitotic, that is, they are not replaced if lost, and so, at present, neuronal loss is permanent. In some cases, where alternate neuronal systems exist, they may take up the function of destroyed original pathways. Numerous morphologic cellular changes occur in aging neurons. An important manifestation is the progressive dendritic dearborization of neurons with aging.[73] Perhaps the best known morphologic change is the accumulation of lipofuscin pigment. The functional significance of accumulation of lipofuscin pigment in neurons is, however, unknown. Nerve depolarization conduction velocity has been demonstrated to decrease about 15 percent in persons 90 years old as compared to young adults.[7]

Neuroendocrine synaptic transmission via multi-synaptic pathways seems to be significantly slowed with age.[74] Reflex responses and voluntary reaction times are thus decreased. Monamine metabolism in the brain is altered in aging, and changes in mon-amine oxidase (MAO), as well as serotonin concentration in the brain, may be involved in the development of parkinsonism in older persons.[75]

Psychological disturbances, such as senile dementia, that occur in aging individuals may be either a functional expression of aging or an age-related disease process. In any event, the CNS changes observed in the elderly suggest a relationship to this type of psychological abnormality.

The Eye, the Ear, and Other Sensory Receptors

In general, sensitivity to stimuli is diminished with age. The response threshold to stimuli is decreased; that is, the intensity and duration of a stimulus must be increased to evoke a sensory receptor response. A variety of causal factors are responsible for this lowered sensitivity.

The eye displays several age changes and age-associated disease processes, some of which are closely related to the passage of time. These aging variations lead to decreased visual acuity (see Fig. 3-8). Among these changes are: glaucoma, an increase in intraocular pressure that occurs with increasing frequency from 50 to about 65 years of age[76]; macular degeneration and retinopathies secondary to diabetes mellitus, glaucoma and vascular occlusions; vitreous debris; occular muscle problems; optic nerve and CNS disturbances. Dark and light adaptation is reduced, and visual acuity is decreased. The most prevalent and consistent ocular age changes, however, occur in the crystalline lens. With age, the lens becomes increasingly rigid and less able to be focused (see Fig. 3-9), usually resulting in presbyopia. Lenticular polypeptides form aggregates called high molecular weight protein, associated with increasing pigmentation, light absorption,[77] scatter and increasing concentrations of fluorescent materials.[78-80] The increasing pigmentation may lead to opacification in the form of brunescent cataract of the lens nucleus. Another less age-related type of cataract is the white cortical cataract. If the cataract becomes extensive, complete loss of useful vision can result. The only practical treatment at present is surgical removal of the lens followed by prescription of appropriate corrective lenses. The formation of arcus senilis, a corneal ring, often develops with aging, but it does not interfere with vision.

Auditory function declines with age. The sound threshold increases[7,81] and the audio frequency range decreases (see Fig. 3-10).[82] This is probably the result of ossification, causing decreased articulation of the ossicles, and of decreased auditory nerve function. The ability to discern frequencies at the high end of the audio spectrum steadily declines and sound above 4000 Hz is typically unappreciable by age 60.[7] Tinnitus sometimes develops in old age.

Olfaction and taste also undergo similar changes

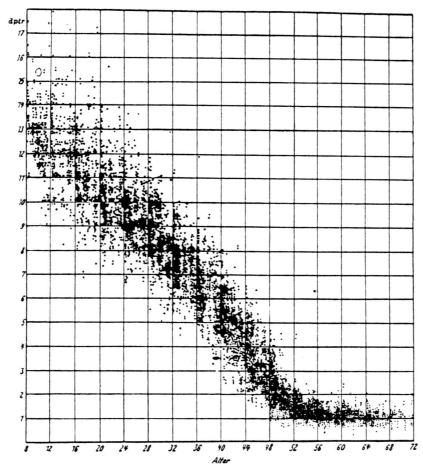

Fig. 3-9. Accommodation ability of the human eye as a function of age. [From Friedenwald JS: The eye, in Cowdry EV (ed): Problems of Aging. Baltimore, Williams & Wilkins, 1942, p 513 (after Duane). Reprinted with permission, © 1942, The Williams & Wilkins Company, Baltimore.]

with age[83]; that is, increased thresholds of sensitivity and decreased response to various stimuli. In the elderly, 80 percent of the taste buds may be lost.[7] In addition, CNS changes may be involved in these reduced sensitivities.

Tactile stimulation is less effective in providing sensory responses (increased thresholds),[84] and the same is apparent for pressure and pain reception.[7] Thermal, proprio-, and kinesthetic sensation probably are also reduced with age. These reductions might result from significant numerical decreases and changes in the receptor cells. CNS disturbances may also play a role in decreased sensory receptor effectiveness.

Biochemical and Genetic

Molecular structure and function form the basis for the characteristics of the organism. Thus, aging is ultimately an expression of alteration occurring at the molecular level. Investigations designed to elucidate biochemical changes that underlie aging phenomena have often been directed towards substances associated with the control of such phenomena. Since the chromatin containing genetic material and the apparatus involved with the transfer of genetic information are central in the elaboration of proteins and enzymes, these entities have been a focus of interest.

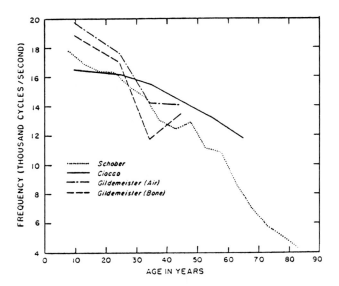

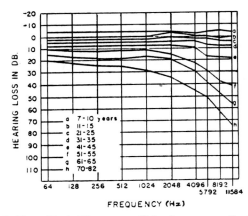

Fig. 3-10. (Top) Upper audible frequency limit as a function of age as measured by several investigators. [From Weiss AD: Sensory functions, in Birren JE (ed): Handbook of Aging and the Individual. Chicago, University of Chicago Press, 1959, p 520 (adapted from Gildemeister, 1908; Ciocco, 1932; and Schober, 1952).] (Bottom) Hearing loss of different age groups as a function of acoustic frequency. [From Weiss AD: Sensory functions, in Birren JE. (ed): Handbook of Aging and the Individual. Chicago, University of Chicago Press, 1959, p 521 (after Rosée, 1953).]

Certain changes in chromatin occur with age.[83–89] These changes may reflect changes in the operation of DNA repair mechanisms. Whether the apparent changes in DNA and associated information translating apparatus represent a primary cause of aging

or are the result of an aging mechanism remains unresolved.

The importance of genetic factors in aging should not be minimized, however. One need merely observe the differences in the life span of different species or different strains (mice, for example) to understand that a relationship between genetic determination and aging most probably exists. This relationship is not as clear in human intraspecific aging. The uncertainty exists because of the relatively long life span of humans, which makes obtaining information on aging characteristics from one generation to the next difficult. Nevertheless, the pedigree method, population sampling, and samples of twins and twin-families have been employed in an effort to shed some light on the subject.[90] Long-lived families, for example, seem to have ancestral longevity, and women appear to outlive men.

The study of twins, monozygotic (identical) compared with dizygotic, has probably provided the best information on genetic determination of human longevity. Of these twins, it is found that on the average they die within nearly five years of one another.

Some disorders associated with aging can be inherited or genetically predisposed. These may include: cardiovascular diseases such as hypertension and coronary artery disease; neoplasias; psychological disturbances such as Creutzfeldt-Jakob syndrome, Pick's disease, Huntington's chorea, Alzheimer's disease, senile progressive idiopathic dementia, vascular dementia, and late paraphrenia; and "normal" decline in mental function and capacity.

These examples of aging and age-associated disorders are often the result of polygenic inheritance.[91] The rare diseases, Progeria (Hutchinson-Gilford syndrome) and adult progeria (Werner's syndrome), have many characteristics in common with aging but occur at a greatly accelerated rate. The Hutchinson-Guilford syndrome has a usual onset between birth and 2 years of age with death occurring at between 7 and 27 years. Werner's syndrome begins later, at about 20, and death is 20 or 30 years earlier than the normal life expectancy. These disorders appear to be inherited as a single gene with autosomal recessive characteristics.[92] The conclusion is that longevity is determined in part by the endowment of genetic information inherited by the individual.

THEORIES

Observation and description of aging phenomena are important in that they aid us to understand the limitations aging imposes upon us and indicate what types and degrees of therapy are appropriate in age-associated disorders. This is not enough, however, to provide an understanding of the mechanism or mechanisms that are the basis of the aging process. Such an understanding must depend not only on observation and description, but also upon cognitive processes combined with experimental examination of hypotheses.

Numerous theories of aging have been proposed, possibly dating back to the time of the first awareness of the aging process. Diversity in theories about aging and its inevitable consequence—death—has come about mainly as a result of the tendency of theorists to favor their primary field of involvement. Most of these theories have become untenable in light of modern knowledge of biology. Some, however, are interesting or appear promising, at least as precursors of a lucid understanding of aging and may therefore merit consideration.

The wear and tear theory has been one of the longest held and most popular ideas. This is largely due to the ease of making human aging analogous to the functional and cosmetic decline with time of common entities such as machinery or clothing, etc. The wear and tear theory as a basis for aging appears unlikely because the living cells and tissues have many types of repair mechanisms, the most basic of which is probably the mechanism for the maintenance of the integrity of the genetic informational macromolecule, DNA. Additionally, in many instances, severe stress and decreased food intake, which would be expected to accelerate aging, do not. On the contrary, they may prolong life (exercise and caloric restriction). Theories involving protein deterioration, immunity, accumulation of debris (clinkers), free radicals, biomolecule crosslinking and changes in and repair of damage to DNA, have been investigated.[93–102]

Cells grown in tissue culture (in vitro) were once thought to be immortal.[103] Normal cells, however, have been shown to die out after several generations.[104] The reason for this limitation is unknown, but a relationship to aging in multicellular organisms has been suggested by some and argued against by others. Abnormal transformed cells are freed of this growth limitation.

Perhaps the most promising of the theories of aging is the concept of an evolved genetic program. Evolution works toward the selective advantage of the species rather than the individual. If the individual benefits from inherited characteristics, it is fortuitous. The theory diverges at this point. It has been suggested that in aging the organism simply runs out of program.[105] Some proponents argue that a program has evolved to give the individual (and, hence, the species) the best chance of survival against the multitudes of hostile environmental factors.[106] The other concept considers that the primary cause of aging is a program that selectively controls the expression of characteristics which limit the longevity of the individual. One possible but by no means the only selective advantage of such a program would be to limit the population size to prevent outgrowing the food supply.

Caloric restriction experiments,[107] essential amino acid (tryptophan) deficient diets,[108] L-dopa,[109] and possibly procaine[110] increase the life span of animals (rodents) and may have similar effects in man. These manipulations appear to limit the production of serotonin or some other neuroendocrine intermediate that is hypothetically important in the timing of the "reading" of an aging program. This operation may produce a slowdown in this reading, the result being a decrease in aging rate and thus a lengthening of the lifetime.

Since the animals in these experiments did not survive indefinitely, this particular type of attack on the question cannot provide the entire answer. Tissue competence to respond to endocrine signals might also be regulated by a program for aging. Deeper probing of genomic aging mechanisms may involve the nuclear receptor–acceptor complexes or regulation of the effectiveness of such complexes to act on genomic expression.

An extension of the aging program idea is the "gene latch" concept, that is, as the reading of the genetic program in a cell proceeds, the cell is latched into a more advanced stage of differentiation. The cell then becomes incompetent to react to signals (hormones, etc.), meaningful at previous stages. Examples of cell types displaying these characteristics are the postmitotic neurons and cardiac cells. Exceptions exist in the mitotic cells, for example, epithelial and endothelial cells, and whether or not these cell types age in the manner of multicellular organisms is controversial. The aging process then would be primarily concerned with tissues comprised of postmitotic cells with secondary effects occurring in other tissues. A great deal of investigation remains to be carried out before a clear understanding of the mechanisms of aging can be achieved.

REFERENCES

1. Trotter M, Gleser GC: Trends in stature of American whites and negroes born between 1840 and 1924. Am J Phys Anthropol 9:427–440, 1951

2. Damon A, Seltzer CC, Stoudt HW, et al: Age and physique in healthy white veterans at Boston. Aging and Human Devel 3:202–208, 1972

3. Rossman I: The anatomy of aging, in Rossman I (ed): Clinical Geriatrics, ed 2. Philadelphia, JB Lippincott Company, 1979, p 3

4. Wessel JA, Ufer A, VanHuss WD, et al: Age trends of various components of body composition and functional characteristics in women aged 20–69 years. Ann NY Acad Sci 110:608–622, 1963

5. Ryckewaert A, Parot S, Tamisier S, et al: Variations, selon l'âge et le sexe, de l'epaisseur du pli cutané mesuré au dos de la main. Rev Franc Études Clin Biol 12:803–806, 1967

6. Hanna MJD, MacMillan: Aging and the skin, in Brockelhurst JC (ed): Textbook of Geriatric Medicine and Gerontology, ed 2. Edinburgh, Churchill Livingstone, 1978, p 626

7. Goldman R: Decline in organ function with aging, in Rossman I (ed): Clinical Geriatrics, ed 2. Philadelphia, JP Lippincott Company, 1979, p 23

8. Forbes GB, Reina JC: Adult lean body mass declines with age: Some longitudinal observations. Metabol 19:653–663, 1970

9. Shuster S, Black MM, McVitie E: Influence of age and sex on skin thickness, skin collagen and density. Bri J Derm 93:639–643, 1975

10. Cannon DJ, Davison PF: Cross-linking and aging in rat tendon collagen. Exp Gerontol 8:51–62, 1973

11. Bakerman S: Quantitative extraction of acid-soluble human skin collagen with age. Nature (London) 196:375–376, 1962

12. Bjorksten J: Theories, in Bakerman S (ed): Aging Life Processes. Springfield, Charles C Thomas, 1969, p 147

13. Silver AF, Montagna W, Karacan I: The effect of age on human eccrine sweating, in Montagna W (ed): Advances in Biology of Skin. Oxford, Pergamon Press, 1965, vol 6, p 129

14. Keogh EV, Walsh RJ: Rate of greying of human hair. Nature 207:877–878, 1965

15. Giacometti L: The anatomy of the human scalp, in Montagna W (ed): Advances in Biology of Skin. Oxford, Pergamon Press, 1965, vol 6, p 97

16. Melick R, Taft HP: Observations on body hair in old people. J Clin Endocrinol 19:1597–1607, 1959

17. Bean WB: Nail growth: 30 years of observation. Arch Int Med 134:497–502, 1974

18. Orentreich N, Sharp NJ: Keratin replacement as an aging parameter. J Soc Cosmet Chem 18:537–547, 1967

19. Fleischer K: Das Alternde Ohr. Aesthet Med 16:95–98, 1967

20. Edelman IS, Haley HB, Schloerb PR: Further observations on total body water, I. Normal values throughout the life span. Surg Gynecol Obstet 95:1–12, 1952

21. Rathbun EN, Pace N: Studies on body composition, I. Determination of body fat by means of the body specific gravity. J Biol Chem 158:667–676, 1945

22. Rossman I: Anatomic and body composition changes with aging, in Finch CE, Hayflick L (eds): Handbook of the Biology of Aging. New York, Van Nostrand Reinhold Company, 1977, p 189

23. Moore F, Olesen KH, McMurrey JD, et al: The Body Cell Mass and Its Supporting Environment. Philadelphia, WB Saunders, 1963, p 535

24. Meneely GR, Heyssel RM, Ball COT, et al: Analysis of factors affecting body composition determined from potassium content in 915 normal subjects. Ann NY Acad Sci 110:271–281, 1963

25. Burmeister W, Bingert A: Die quantitativen Veränderungen der menschlichen Zellmasse zwischen dem 8 und 90 Lebensjahr. Klin Wshr 45:409–416, 1967

26. Misner JE, Boileau A, Massey BH, et al: Alterations in the body composition of adult men during selected physical training programs. J Am Geriat Soc 22:33–38, 1974

27. Harris R: Cardiac changes with age, in Goldman R., Rockstein M (eds): The Physiology and Pathology of Human Aging. New York, Academic Press, 1975

28. Simonson E: The effect of age on the electrocardiogram. Am J Cardiol 29:64–73, 1972

29. Crane M: Hypertension in the aged, in Greenblatt R (ed): Aging. New York, Raven Press, 1978, vol 5, p 115

30. Davies DF, Shock NW: Age changes in glomerular filtration rate, effective renal plasma flow, and tubular excretory capacity in adult males. J Clin Invest 29:496–507, 1950

31. Wesson LG: Physiology of the Human Kidney. New York, Grune & Stratton, 1969

32. Miller JH, McDonald RK, Shock NW: The renal extraction of p-aminohippurate in the aged individual. J Gerontol 6:213–216, 1951

33. Van Zonneveld RJ: Some data on the genito-urinary system as found in old age surveys in the Netherlands. Gerontol Clin 1:167–173, 1959

34. Klocke RA: Influence of aging on the lung, in Finch CE, Hayflick L (eds): Handbook of the Biology of Aging. New York, Van Nostrand Reinhold Company, 1977, p 432

35. Brody AW, Johnson JR, Townley RG, et al: The residual volume. Predicted values as a function of age. Am Rev Respirat Dis 109:98–105, 1974

36. Muiesan G, Sorbini CA, Grassi V: Respiratory function in the aged. Bull Physio-Pathol Respir 7:973–1007, 1971

37. Thurlbeck WM: Internal surface area and other measurements in emphysema. Thorax 22:483–496, 1967

38. Maugh II TH: Any horse trader could have told you. Science 205:574, 1979

39. Geokas MC, Haverback BJ: The aging gastrointestinal tract. Am J Surg 117:881–892, 1969

40. Soergel KH, Zboralske FF, Ambert JR: Presbyesophagus: esophageal motility in nonagenarians. J Clin Invest 43:1472–1479, 1964

41. Calloway NO, Merrill RS: The aging adult liver, I. Bromsulphalein and bilirubin clearances. J Am Geriat Soc 13:594–598, 1965

42. Papanayiotou P, Papinicolaou NT, Dontas AS: Étude coamparée de l'epuration de la BSP chez l'adult jeune et le sujet âgé. Sem Hop Paris 45:235–239, 1969

43. Friedman DK, Kannel WB, Dawber TR: The epidemiology of gall bladder disease: Observations in the Framingham study. J Chronic Dis 19:273–292, 1966

44. Newman HF, Northrup JD: The autopsy incidence of gallstones. Int Surg 109:1, 1959

45. Pearlman BJ, Marks JW, Bonorris GG, et al: Gallstone dissolution—A progress report. Clin Gastroenterol 8:123–140, 1979

46. Fedorowski F, Salen G, Colallilo A, et al: Metabolism of ursodeoxycholic acid in man. Gastroenterol 73:1131–1137, 1977

47. Bell GD: Medical treatment of gallstones. J Roy Coll Physicians of Lond 13:47–52, 1979

48. Andres R: Aging and diabetes. Med Clin N Am 55:835–846, 1971

49. Straus B: Disorders of the digestive system, in Rossman I (ed): Clinical Geriatrics, ed 2. Philadelphia, JB Lippincott Company, 1979, p 266

50. Williams TF: Diabetes mellitus in the aged, in Greenblatt R (ed): Aging. New York, Raven Press, 1978, vol 5, p 103

51. Duckworth WC, Kitabchi AE: Direct measurement of plasma proinsulin in normal and diabetic subjects. Am J Med 53:418–427, 1972

52. Gregerman RI: The age-related alteration of thyroid hormone metabolism in man, in Gitman L (ed): Endocrines and Aging. Springfield, Charles C Thomas, 1967, p 161

53. Gregerman RI, Bierman EL: Aging and hormones, in Williams RH (ed): Textbook of Endocrinology, (ed 5). Philadelphia, WB Saunders, 1974, p 1059

54. Denckla WD: Role of the pituitary and thyroid glands in the decline of minimal O_2 Consumption with age. J Clin Invest 53:572–581, 1974

55. Blichert-Toft M: Secretion of corticotrophin and somatotrophin by the senescent adenohypophysis in man. Acta Endocrinol 78:15–154, 1975

56. Gherondache CN, Romanoff LP, Pincus G: Steroid hormones in aging men, in Gitman L (ed): Endocrines and Aging. Springfield, Charles C Thomas, 1967, p 76

57. Romanoff LP, Morris CW, Welch P, et al: The metabolism of cortisol-4-C^{14} in young and elderly men, I. Secretion rate of cortisol and daily excretion of tetrahydrocortisol, allotetrahydrocortisol, tetrahydrocortisone and cortolone (20α and 20β). J Clin Endocrinol 21:1413–1425, 1961

58. Horky K, Marek J, Kopecka J, et al: Influence of age on orthostatic changes in plasma renin activity and urinary catecholamines in man. Physiol Bothemoslov 24:481, 1975

59. Heaney, RP: Age-related changes in calcium metabolism in perimenopausal women and their relationship to the development of osteoporosis. Endocrine Aspects of Aging sponsored by NIA, the Endocrine Society, and the Veterans Administration, Bethesda, 1979

60. Makinodan T: The thymus in aging, in Greenblatt R (ed): Aging. New York, Raven Press, 1978, vol 5, p 217

61. Siiteri P: Interaction of androgens, estrogens and the sex hormone binding globulin. Endocrine Aspects of Aging sponsored by NIA, the Endocrine Society, and the Veterans Administration, Bethesda, 1979

62. Asch RH, Greenblatt R: The aging ovary: Morphologic and endocrine correlations, in Greenblatt R (ed): Aging. New York, Raven Press, 1978, vol 5, p 141

63. Albeaux-Fernet M, Clorinda SSB, Karpas AE: Tes-

ticular Function in the aging male, in Greenblatt R (ed): Aging. New York, Raven Press, 1978, vol 5, p 201

64. Bourne GH: Aging changes in the endocrines, in Gitman L (ed): Endocrines and Aging. Springfield, Charles C Thomas, 1967, p 66

65. Verzar F: Anterior pituitary function in age, in Donovan BT, Harris GW (eds): The Pituitary Gland. Berkeley, University of California Press, 1966, p 444

66. Timiras P: Neuroendocrine strategies to modify aging. Endocrine Aspects of Aging sponsored by NIA, the Endocrine Society, and the Veterans Administration, Bethesda, 1979

67. Finch CE: Neuroendocrine and autonomic aspects of aging, in Finch CE, Hayflick L (eds): Handbook of the Biology of Aging. New York, Van Nostrand Reinhold Company, 1977, p 262

68. Clemens JA, Amenomori Y, Jenkins T, et al: Effects of hypothalmic stimulation, hormones, and drugs on ovarian function in old female rats. Proc Soc Exp Biol Med 132:561–563, 1969

69. Finch CE: Endocrine and neural factors of reproductive aging—a speculation, in Terry RD, Gershon S (eds): Aging. New York, Raven Press, 1976, vol 3, p 335

70. Roth GS: Hormone receptor changes during adulthood and senescence: Significance for aging research. Fed Proc 38:1910–1914, 1979

71. Roth G: Hormone action and receptors during aging. Endocrine aspects of aging sponsored by NIA, the Endocrine Society, and the Veterans Administration, Bethesda, 1979

72. Brody H: Aging of the vertebrate brain, in Rockstein M, Sussman M (eds): Development and Aging in the Nervous System. New York, Academic Press, 1973, p 121

73. Scheibel ME, Scheibel AB: Differential changes with old and new cortices, in Nandy K, Sherwin I (eds): The Aging Brain and Senile Dementia. New York, Plenum Publishing, 1977

74. Wayner MJ, Emmers R: Spinal synaptic delay in young and aged rats. Am J Physiol 194:403–405, 1958

75. Robinson DS, Niles A, Davis JN, et al: Aging, monoamines and monoamine-oxidase levels. Lancet 1:290–291, 1972

76. Kornzweig AL: The eye in old age, in Rossman I (ed): Clinical Geriatrics, ed 2. Philadelphia, JB Lippincott Company, 1979, p 369

77. Said FS, Weale RA: The variation with age of the spectral transmissivity of the human crystalline lens. Gerontologia 3:213–231, 1959

78. Satoh K, Bando M, Nakajima A: Fluorescence in the human lens. Exp Eye Res 16:173–182, 1973

79. Spector A, Roy D, Stauffer J: Isolation and characterization of an age-dependent polypeptide from human lens with nontryptophan fluorescence. Exp Eye Res 21:9–24, 1975

80. Jacobs R, Krohn DL: Variations in fluorescence characteristics of intact human crystalline lens segments as a function of age. J Gerontol 31:641–647, 1976

81. Coros JF: Auditory perception and communication, in Birren JE, Schaie KW (eds): Handbook of the Psychology of Aging. New York, Van Nostrand Reinhold Company, 1977

82. Rockstein M: The biology of aging in humans—an overview, in Goldman R, Rockstein M (eds): The Physiology and Pathology of Human Aging, Proceedings of a Symposium on the Physiology and Pathology of Human Aging. New York, Academic Press, 1975

83. Strehler BL: Introduction: Aging and the human brain, in Terry RD, Gershon S (eds): Aging. New York, Raven Press, 1976, vol 3, p 1

84. Konshalo DR: Age changes in touch, vibration, temperature, kinesthesis, pain sensitivity, in Birren JE, Schaie KW (eds): Handbook of the Psychology of Aging. New York, Van Nostrand Reinhold Company, 1977

85. Hydén H: The neuron, in Brachet J, Mirsky AE (eds): The Cell, vol 4. New York, Academic Press, 1960, p 215

86. Chaconas E, Finch CE: The effect of aging on RNA/DNA ratios in brain regions of the C57BL/6J male mouse. J Neurochem 21:1469–1473, 1973

87. Kurtz DI, Sinex FM: Age related differences in the association of brain DNA and nuclear protein. Biochem Biophys Acta 145:840–842, 1967

88. Carter DB, Chae C: Composition of liver histones in aging rat and mouse. J Gerontol 30:28–32, 1975

89. Sinex FM: The molecular genetics of aging, in Finch CE, Hayflick L (eds): Handbook of the Biology of Aging. New York, Van Nostrand Reinhold Company, 1977, p 37

90. Jarvik LF: Genetic aspects of aging, in Rossman I (ed): Clinical Geriatrics, ed 2. Philadelphia, JB Lippincott Company, 1979, p 86

91. Upton AC: Pathobiology, in Finch CE, Hayflick L (eds): Handbook of the Biology of Aging. New York, Van Nostrand Reinhold Company, 1977, p 513

92. Epstein CJ, Martin GM, Schultz AL: Werner's syndrome: A review of its symptomatology, natural history, pathologic features, genetics and relationship to the natural aging process. Medicine (Baltimore) 45:177–221, 1966

93. Orgel LE: The maintenance of the accuracy of

protein synthesis and its relevance to aging. Proc Nat Acad Sci 49:517–521, 1963

94. Walford RL: The Immunologic Theory of Aging. A/S Copenhagen, Munksgaard, J Jørgensen, 1969

95. Bjorksten J: Recent developments in protein chemistry. Chem Industr 48:746, 1941

96. Bjorksten J: Aging, primary mechanism. Gerontologia 8:179–192, 1963

97. Harman D: Free radical theory of aging: Effect of free radical reaction inhibitors on the mortality rate of male LAF mice. J Gerontol 23:476–482, 1968

98. Sinex MF: Aging and the lability of irreplaceable molecules. J Gerontol 12:190, 1957

99. Watson JD: The Double Helix. New York, Atheneum, 1968

100. Cutler R: Redundancy of information content in the genome of mammalian species as a protective mechanism determining aging rate. Mech Age Dev 2:381–408, 1973

101. Curtis HJ: Biological mechanisms underlying the aging process. Science 141:686–694, 1963

102. Hart RW, Setlow RB: Correlation between deoxyribonucleic acid excision-repair and life-span in a number of mammalian species. Proc Nat Acad Sci 71:2169–2173, 1974

103. Carrel A: On the permanent life of tissues outside of the organism. J Exp Med 15:516–528, 1912

104. Hayflick L, Moorhead PS: The serial cultivation of human diploid cell strains. Exp Cell Res 25:585–621, 1961

105. Comfort A: Ageing: The Biology of Senescence. New York, Holt, Rinehart & Winston Inc, 1964, p 53

106. Sacher GA: Longevity, aging, and death: An evolutionary perspective (1976 Robert W Kleemeier Award Lecture). Gerontologist 18:112–119, 1978

107. McCay CM, Crowell MF, Maynard LA: The effect of retarded growth upon the length of life span and upon the ultimate body size. J Nutr 10:63–79, 1935

108. Segall PE, Ooka H, Rose K, et al: Neural and endocrine development after chronic tryptophan deficiency in rats, I. Brain monoamine and pituitary responses. Mech Age Dev 7:1–17, 1978

109. Cotzias GC, Miller ST, Nicholson AR Jr, et al: Prolongation of the life-span in mice adapted to large amounts of L-dopa. Proc Nat Acad Sci 71:2466–2469, 1974

110. Aslan A: Novocain als eutrophischer Faktor und die Möglichkeit einer Verlängerung der Lebensdauer. Ther Umschau Bern 9:165–173, 1956

4

Psychological Aspects of Aging

William M. Whelihan, Ph.D.

Psychological changes do occur with aging in the way older people process information, respond emotionally, and behave in the context of a particular social and physical environment. There is a fairly common sentiment that with aging an overall, inevitable decline in these psychological functions takes place with negative results. Butler[1] provides us with a fairly elaborate stereotypic sketch of old age:

An older person thinks and moves slowly. He does not think as he used to or as creatively. He is bound to himself and to his past and can no longer change or grow. He can learn neither well nor swiftly, and, even if he could, he would not wish to. Tied to his personal traditions and growing conservatism, he dislikes innovations and is not disposed to new ideas. Not only can he not move forward, he often moves backward. He enters a second childhood, caught up in increasing egocentricity and demanding more from his environment than he is willing to give it. Sometimes he becomes an intensification of himself, a caricature of a life-long personality. He becomes irritable and cantankerous, yet shallow and feeble. He lives in his past. He is behind the times. He is aimless and wandering of mind, reminiscing and gregarious. Indeed he is a study in decline, the picture of mental and physical failure. He has lost and cannot replace friends, spouse, job, status, power, influence, income. He is often stricken by diseases which in turn restrict his movement, his enjoyment of food, the pleasures of well-being. He has lost his desire and capacity for sex. His body shrinks, and so too does the flow of blood to his brain. His mind does not utilize oxygen and sugar at the same rate as formerly. Feeble, uninteresting, he awaits his death, a burden to society, to his family, and to himself.*

*Reprinted with permission from Butler RN: Why Survive? Being Old in America. New York, Harper & Row, 1975, pp 6–7.

This stereotype, though clearly a myth, must affect how older people perceive themselves and, to that degree, how they subsequently think, feel, and behave.

Changes in attitudes toward elders may be more important in influencing psychological functioning than new knowledge. In contrast to the prevailing myth, most of the "normal" aged (70–75 percent of those over 65 years of age) are intellectually and socially able, productive (given the opportunity), mentally vigorous, interested in their surroundings, and eager to participate in the social life of family, kin, and community. Where there are decrements and apparent declines, the cause is not necessarily the biological process of aging, but other, often controllable, impositions only partially related to age. Among these are:

1. Physical health status
2. Ability to perform activities of daily living
3. Degree of participation in meaningful activity
4. Amount and quality of social contacts and supports
5. Quality of the physical environment—residence and neighborhood
6. Degree to which basic needs are met (e.g., nutrition)
7. Economic status

The inability of some aged persons to cope intellectually and socially is usually due to stresses associated with aging rather than caused by it. This view, that at least some declines are not inexorably bound to the normal pattern of human development, forces the conclusion that it is possible to prevent or treat many of the intellectual, social, and emotional problems of a significant proportion of the aged population. Moreover, it emphasizes the ability of many of the aged to lead independent, self sustaining, and satisfying lives.[2]

The importance of looking at the older person holistically cannot be overemphasized. Though we are beginning to understand how dysfunction in one area can influence many others, there still remains much to be learned about these interactions before a clear picture of the concomitants of the aging process per se can be had. Many of the psychological changes that have been attributed to aging may be due to disease states or various other trauma associated with longevity. There is in fact a good deal more to learn about psychological functioning in the elderly despite centuries of observation and comment on the aging process.

RESEARCH IN THE PSYCHOLOGY OF AGING

Research studies have produced very different findings on psychological functioning thus far. Most research designs have been cross-sectional and have overemphasized decrements with age. These designs compare groups of older and younger people at one point in time and hence do not take into account the different life and educational experiences of older people as compared to young people. Other designs have been longitudinal; that is, they study a group of people over a rather long period of time and measure functions periodically. This latter type of design perhaps presents too rosy a picture of the aging process due to a selective drop-out and survivor bias; that is, only the higher motivated, the healthier, and those who remain alive are available for subsequent testing. These designs also have the problems of using a standard set of measures which may become outdated in the course of a long study. In addition, historical change over the course of time may influence the results at subsequent testing and therefore distort the interpretation of age-change. Results of many of these longitudinal studies show little or no decline with age in psychological functions.

The remainder of the chapter will provide a perspective on some of the controversial assertions and research findings that appear across studies which address the issue of psychological changes with aging. The focus will be on age-related changes in sensory, psychomotor, cognitive, emotional, personality, and sexual processes. These psychological changes affect the behavior of the older person perhaps more intensely than does the aging of their bodies. Here also lurk most of the myths, stereotypes, and cruelties that characterize younger peoples' vision of age: supposed mental rigidity, declining intelligence, inability to learn, and inevitable senility.[3]

ENVIRONMENTAL IMPACT ON BEHAVIOR

Over the past decade, a general reintroduction of "the environment" into the thinking of social science has occurred, representing a considerable break with the tradition in psychology whereby explanations for behavior have typically been sought within the individual, to the exclusion of what goes on around the individual.[3] So while the main focus of this chapter will be on changes that occur with aging within the older person, consideration will also be given to the impact of environmental variables on the older person's behavior and the ways in which these variables may be manipulated to facilitate adaptive functioning.

A principle in this area of person–environment transactions that has particular relevance for the elderly has been labeled by Lawton the "environmental docility hypothesis."[4] It states that as competence or status of any kind decreases, the probability becomes greater that behavior will be influenced by environmental constraints or facilitators. The corollary of this is that a small environmental improvement may produce a disproportionate amount of more adaptive behavior in a low-competent individual.

With aging, the potential for decreased competence or status becomes greater due to age-related changes in biological health, cognition, sensory-motor behavior, social interaction, and so on. To that degree, many older people are more vulnerable to their environmental context than younger adults. Recent research[5,6] involving the collaborative efforts of geropsychologists and architects has suggested many practical interventions focused on design or redesign of the older person's environment to optimize orientation, functional activity, and safety. The environment can be modified to optimize functioning by enhancing and amplifying stimulus qualities and by providing feedback mechanisms for the sensory- or cognitively impaired older person.[4] A number of these are included as examples in the sections that follow.

SENSORY PROCESSES

The decline of sensory processes is one of the most familiar, general, and troublesome aspects of psychological aging. The older person receives less sensory information and the information which is received tends to be ambiguous.[3] Visual and hearing deficits in particular can lead to sensory isolation if left uncorrected. As a result, the older person can become frustrated, phobic, paranoid, or just "out of touch" with his or her physical and social environment. It is even possible that confusional states or disorientation can be present much like the responses seen in sensory-deprivation experiments with younger people. All too often these behaviors can be attributed to senility (or in professional circles, to organic brain syndrome, a label which has been flagrantly overused).

In the visual area, the following changes have been noted with aging:

1. The lens becomes less transparent affecting the transmission and refraction of light.
2. The size of the pupil decreases with age. This along with reduced transparency of the lens affects the quantity of light reaching the retina.
3. Visual acuity (ability to see clearly at a distance) decreases appreciably from age 60 onwards.
4. Dark adaptation threshold changes: decreased ability to see clearly when illumination is low.
5. Color discrimination: with age, an increased difficulty discriminating hues of short wavelengths (blues, blue-green, violet).

Once recognized, these sensory deficits can be compensated for, at least to some degree, by environmental modifications. For example, visual deficits can be ameliorated by the provision of sufficiently bright, glare-free light especially for reading. Since the older person can generally see warmer colors more readily (red, yellow, orange), these might be incorporated aesthetically into the residential environment to mark hazards (for example, the top step of a landing) or to facilitate orientation in general. Accidents during the night might be dramatically reduced by providing a nightlight in the bedroom to ease the problem of adjustment to rapid changes in illumination such as when the older person wakes up to use the bathroom.

Hearing loss, particularly of the higher frequencies, is a common problem. Consonant sounds are affected more so than vowel sounds. Therefore, speech can be heard but not always understood. Hearing aids are only effective if the older person is willing to wear one; resistance to their use is fairly widespread. Also, some hearing loss cannot be corrected with hearing aids. Shouting is not only ineffective, but also frustrating (and tiring) to carry on in any long-term conversation. At least as important as auditory sensitivity in conversation is the pace at which verbal communication is directed at the elderly. Too rapid speech is unintelligible partly because of the stimulus-persistence effect that seems to characterize the aged nervous system; a longer time is required before the stimulation from one sound leaves the sensory mechanism free to be stimulated by the next sound. The lower flicker-fusion threshold of the elderly is a visual example of stimulus persistence;[7] in the auditory area, words run together and comprehension difficulty is exacerbated by the shorter attention span shown by many older people. Perhaps, then, the best way to compensate for these hearing deficits is to enunciate clearly and to speak more slowly when conversing with the older person.

PSYCHOMOTOR FUNCTIONING

Once a sensory receptor has been adequately activated, there is, in addition, evidence that suggests the older person is slow to interpret, process, and act upon the stimulus with an appropriate response. This psychomotor response slowing is probably the most prominent characteristic which has been documented in gerontological research. Response time increases with age across all sensory modalities and is evident even in subjects selected for excellent health status.[8] The cause is most probably due to changes in the efficiency of central nervous system functioning.

The dominant alpha rhythm, as measured by the EEG, decreases with age even in the healthiest of aging individuals.[9,10] In fact, since scientists first began thinking about the EEG, the e alpha rhythm has been associated with speed and timing in the nervous system.[11,12]

Woodruff[13] has attempted to test the degree to which alterations in alpha rhythm by means of biofeedback approaches can lead to changes in reaction time in younger and older subjects. Her research demonstrated that modifications in both alpha rhythm and reaction time could be effected in both subject groups in predicted directions. Although the findings were not conclusive, they challenge our perception of these phenomena as being fixed and inevitable consequences of aging. This research also demonstrates the potential for behavioral interventions in assuaging performance deficits in the older client.

Other psychophysiological researchers have focused on the impact of arousal state on performance in the older subject. Obviously, too high or too low a level of arousal will adversely affect performance. The ideal level is somewhere in between the extremes. We have seen some evidence for a low arousal level in the alpha slowing and concomitant reaction time slowing in the elderly. The sensory-persistence effect and studies of evoked potentials add additional support for this lower arousal level. Eisdorfer[14] presents evidence that older people may be hyperaroused when demands are placed upon them to perform, and they may remain at this hyperaroused state for longer periods than younger people after completion of a demanding task. In fact, in older people, both overarousal and underarousal may be present simultaneously. The latter is associated with central nervous system measures; the former with autonomic nervous system measures. Thompson and Marsh[15] have suggested a desynchronization hypothesis: with age, the integration between the central and autonomic nervous systems may deteriorate. Research studies[16,17] using varied central and autonomic measures have lent initial support to this hypothesis.

From an intervention perspective, it appears that overarousal diminishes over time as the older person becomes more familiar with the experimental procedures and setting.[18] Therefore, giving the older person an opportunity to become accustomed to novel environments, to understand the nature of a task, to interact with others, to relax and to be comfortable should enhance performance in educational, clinical, research, and other settings.[19,20,21] Underarousal of central nervous system functions may be reversed to some degree by increasing the meaningfulness or relevance of tasks (thereby increasing motivation to perform), by increasing levels of sensory input, and by encouraging risk-taking behavior to counter the overly-cautious response style that we often see in the current generation of older people.

Birren[22] has emphasized that slowness of behavior is the independent variable that sets limits for the older person in such processes as memory, perception, and problem solving. To some extent this slowing can be ameliorated, but the differences in this area between young and old subjects will tend to persist.

COGNITIVE PROCESSES

Cognition is concerned with how individuals retain their experiences and integrate this knowledge with information from their present circumstances to generate ways of behaving which are appropriate to those circumstances, as well as to move beyond both existing knowledge and present circumstances to inferences and to the production of truly creative acts.

Intellectual Functions

In commenting on research in the cognitive area, David Wechsler,[23] the author of the most widely used intelligence test today (Wechsler Adult Intelligence Scale) has stated that nearly all studies have shown that most human abilities decline progressively after ages 18 to 25. Baltes and Schaie,[24] current lifespan development researchers, are at the other end of the pendulum in their belief that there is little or no cognitive decline with age. The truth probably lies closer to a middle point. Much of the research which produced results consistent with a decline model was based on cross-sectional research designs which have limitations.

Botwinick,[25] in a review of both the old and new literature, found that a decline in intellectual ability is clearly part of the aging picture; however, declines may start later in life than heretofore thought and they may be smaller in magnitude. They may also include fewer functions.

Traditionally, intelligence has been measured by a battery of verbal and perceptual-motor tests. Older people today show more of a decline on the perceptual-motor speeded tests and, in general, little or no decline on the verbal measures relative to a younger reference group. This classic aging pattern constitutes one of the best replicated results for normal aging populations.[26] Much of the decline noted is a result of a slowing down of performance speed, which seems to be a relatively pure age-related change as noted earlier. Additional difficulties are probably due to task demands requiring the solving of new and unfamiliar problems for which accumulated experience is of little help. Kimmel[27] suggests that the typical elderly person is likely to be somewhat "slow" at intellectual tasks, somewhat impaired at mastering new problems in his or her daily life (such as Medicare forms), but relatively unimpaired in many aspects of ordinary intellectual functioning.

It should be noted that individual differences among older people are large. The correlation between age and intelligence test scores is in the neighborhood of .4–.5; only about 20 percent of intelligence test scores can be predicted by age. There are a large number of test-performance modifiers which may be more important than age. Among these are health, education, socioeconomic status, and cultural-generational factors.[28,29]

In the Human Aging Study,[8] a multidisciplinary investigation of a small group of older men at the National Institute of Health, noninstitutionalized subjects were chosen for excellent health status. Subsequently, it was found that a portion of the group had subclinical health problems, difficulties that were only apparent after intensive medical workups. It is significant that of 23 psychological tests given to all subjects, scores were poorer for those subjects with asymptomatic health problems than for the "healthier group" in all but two tests. But even for these exceptionally healthy older subjects, the classic pattern of higher verbal and lower perceptual-motor scores was apparent.

Granick and Friedman[30] demonstrated that education is a cogent factor in intellectual functioning during later life. Education serves to stimulate intellectual interest and helps to set up habit patterns that perpetuate such interests throughout the lifespan. Studies have suggested that the educational level of a person is more important than age in regard to mental ability. The failure to control or remove the effects of education by statistical or experimental means exaggerates the detrimental effects of aging since the elderly tend to have fewer years of schooling than the young.

Memory Functioning and Learning

In the area of memory functioning, many older people retain and recall earlier events in their lives more efficiently than more recent ones. This may be due to the fact that this early information has been with them for longer periods of time, has been reviewed periodically, and has greater emotional significance than more recent input. In addition, current information may not be retained as effec-

tively due to its amount and the speed with which it is disseminated in our present technologically accelerated and advanced environment. Deficits have been documented in short-term memory and in the search-and-retrieval aspects of retention, particularly under the stress of time. But once learning has occurred, according to the same criterion as for younger people, the deficit is reduced.[31] Many older people experience considerable anxiety about specific instances of memory failure, seeing these lapses as possible harbingers of malignant decline.[20] Reassurance that such instances are not symptomatic of feared senility and provision of accurate data on the prevalence of organic brain syndrome in community elderly (5–12 percent) are usually sufficient to alleviate concern. From a clinical standpoint, the older person who presents with memory complaints is, upon testing, often found to show symptoms of depression or lack of environmental stimulation and subsequent withdrawal, rather than poor performance on the memory tests in the psychological battery.

There have been a number of demonstrations of particular difficulties experienced by elderly subjects in the area of problem solving. Jerome,[32] for example, used a concept-learning task. Successful solution required the subjects to inquire systematically for further information. Older subjects took longer to formulate the goal, repeated their requests for the same information more often, had difficulty in applying the information to the solution, and could not utilize notes taken on the information as well as younger subjects. On the other hand, problem solving and other kinds of learning have been shown to be facilitated in older people by the use of more concrete and more familiar stimuli.[33,34]

From an intervention standpoint, note taking and list making are worth suggesting to offset the inevitable benign form of forgetting. Learning, in turn, may be enhanced by slowing the pace of presentation, reducing psychophysiological arousal, increasing task meaningfulness, and by teaching the older person to organize material effectively to meet task demands.

PERSONALITY

Research approaches to the study of personality and aging have not been very helpful in shedding light on this complex domain. Most studies again have been cross-sectional and therefore do not take

Table 4-1
Adaptive and Maladaptive Qualities in Elders

Adaptive Qualities
    A.   Candor, ease of relationships, dependence, affirmation, positive
         self-concept, sense of usefulness.
    B.   Defense mechanisms: Insight, denial, use of activity. Some of these
         defense mechanisms are more useful than others. Naturally,
         insight is a valuable aid in alleviating anxiety and guilt by
         realistically appraising the changed circumstances of life and
         body. Denial can be beneficial if it does not interfere with
         needed medical or emotional care and if it facilitates
         relationships and activity. Older people "keeping busy" in order
         to counteract fear or depression also have a defense that is an
         asset. Less adaptive are the counter-phobic defenses, wherein
         some older people undertake excessive activities, dangerous to
         life and limb, in order to prove their continued prowess,
         youthfulness, and fearlessness.

Maladaptive Qualities
    A.   Paranoid isolation: Paranoid personality features have a particular
         maladaptiveness in old age, since so much happens to reinforce
         the notion that the problems are all "out there." In addition,
         hearing and other sensory losses increase the inability to deal
         with threatening forces and compound the isolation of the
         person with paranoid tendencies. A defensive use of perceptual
         loss, such as "hearing what one wants to hear," may be present.
         Tendencies to use age, disease, or impairment as a defense (by
         action more helpless than is warranted) are common problems.
         Personality characteristics of rigidity, despair, depression, and
         the whole range of psychopathological reactions can further
         hamper adaption to old age.

Maladaptive in Early Life—Adaptive in Late Life
    A.   Obsessive-compulsive features
    B.   Schizoid mechanisms
    C.   Dependent personality

into account different life and educational experiences of the older person as compared to the younger person and the obvious impact of these experiences on personality functioning. As a result, many contradictory findings have been reported in the literature.

Refined research designs will ultimately provide a better understanding. For now, the consensus is that aging affects personality and personality affects aging.

The classic studies of healthy, community elderly living in the Kansas City area[35] in the 1950s and subsequent cross-sectional analyses have provided the best available evidence for age-related changes in intrapsychic dimensions of personality. These are:

1. A shift in sex-role perceptions. Older men seemed more receptive than younger men to their affiliative, nuturant, and sensual promptings; older women to their aggressive and egocentric impulses.

2. A shift towards increased interiority—a withdrawal, a turning inwards, and a decreased interest in external events.

3. A shift from active to passive mastery in relating to the environment. Subjects tended to see the environment as complex and dangerous, no longer to be reformed with one's own wishes, and to see the self as conforming and accommodating to outer-world demands.

These same studies indicate that, in the 50–80 age range, and in relatively healthy individuals, age does not emerge as a major variable in the goal-directed, purposive qualities of personality. In other words, while consistent age differences occur in covert, intrapsychic processes (those not readily available to awareness or to conscious control and which have no direct expression in overt social behavior), they do not appear on those variables which reflect attempted control of the self and of the life situation. Age-related changes, then, appear earlier and more consistently in the internal than in the external aspects of personality.[36]

How does personality affect aging? Neugarten and Maddox[37] note that personality traits have been shown to be powerful predictors of adaptation. Also, coping styles appear to remain highly consistent as an individual moves from middle-age through old age. In studying survivorship as an index of adaptation, a few investigators have suggested that grouchiness or combativeness, while not ordinarily viewed as a measure of psychological health at other periods of life, is a survival asset among the very old. Other studies based on broader typologies have indicated that some personality types adjust well (those with high degrees of self-acceptance or those who employ strong psychological defenses), and others poorly (those who are chronically angry, dissatisfied, or depressed) to the biological and social changes that accompany aging. Butler and Lewis,[38] using data from the NIH Human Aging Study, have elaborated adaptive and maladaptive qualities. See Table 4-1.

EMOTIONAL FUNCTIONING

Older people are subject to the same range of psychopathology as young and middle-aged adults and there does not seem to be much difference in the incidence of neuroses and psychoses with age.[39] Yet, with aging, the impact of physical illness and social trauma often make rather severe demands on the coping abilities of the older person. Butler and Lewis[38] feel that loss is the predominant theme characterizing the emotional experiences of older people. The older person is confronted with multiple losses that may occur simultaneously: death of marital partner, older friends, colleagues, relatives; decline of physical health and coming to personal terms with death; loss of status, prestige, and participation in society; and, for large numbers, additional burdens of marginal living standards. These inevitable losses of aging and death are compounded by potentially ameliorable cultural devaluation and neglect. It is amazing how well most older people function in light of the losses they sustain and the attitudes of the society in which they live.

Depression

The most common response to these losses is depression, although other reactions are also prevalent: grief, guilt, rage, and a sense of impotence and helplessness.[38] Even in the presence of good physical health, 20 percent of the subjects in the Human Aging Study[40] had a mild reactive depression by psychiatrists' ratings, and this diagnosis represented the largest single pathology. When one considers that suicide death rates increase dramatically with age for white males, it becomes clear that an understanding of the causes and treatment of depression in the elderly is a major task for gerontologists to address.

Busse[41] states that depression in older people differs from depression in younger people in that it results from a loss of self-esteem directly related to the loss of roles in our youth-oriented society. Ageistic attitudes stereotype the elderly as useless, mindless, sexless, etc. These attitudes are contagious to the extent that older people succumb to the self-fulfilling prophecy and acknowledge these characteristics in themselves.

Intervention

Treatment for the emotional problems of older people is still almost nonexistent. Again, the attitude of many in the society is that the elderly cannot benefit from counseling and are not capable of insight or behavioral change. Lawton[42] has provided interesting data on mental health treatment for this age group. These data allow one to conclude first that institutions are the treatment environments of choice for the elderly; second, that there has been an overall trend away from treatment of the elderly within the mental health system; and, finally, that no trend toward increased use of outpatient mental health facilities is discernable at this point. In addition, only 3 percent of the patients seen by psychiatrists for ambulatory office care in 1975–1976 were 65 and over.[43]

On the bright side, there are indications that psychodynamically and behaviorally oriented therapeutic techniques can be productively employed to deal with the emotional problems of the older person.[44,45] With appropriate modifications of therapeutic approaches,[20] both therapists and older clients have been gratified with the outcome.

Butler[46] has suggested one therapeutic approach that focuses on a "life review." This review is stimulated by recognition in the older person that one's life will inevitably end. In this process, the person recapitulates the past in its positive and negative aspects as a mechanism to maintain the self in the face of the threat of death. According to Butler, this life review is usually stressful but, if successful, it strengthens the self to endure the deprivations of old age and the finality of death.

There are several coping strategies or personality styles that may modify emotional response in the older person. Although many defense mechanisms may be employed, the most common response is denial.[47] Lawton[20] has suggested that denial of unpleasant facts by the elderly serves as a positive adaptive mechanism in maintaining morale. It may well be that this defensive style characterizes this particular generation of older people rather than the aging process per se. Nonetheless, denial seems to be the style of today's elderly, and it should be respected.

Similarly, assertiveness or the appropriate expression of dissatisfaction or anger should not be discouraged. Several studies[48,49] have demonstrated a positive relationship between these traits and survival in the elderly.

The presence of a confidante is particularly important for maintaining morale in the older person. The opportunity to engage in a meaningful manner with another person is something we need throughout life. For the older person who experiences multiple losses, this need is particularly critical.

Certain psychopathology can become increasingly adaptive as people age. Obsessional maneuvers fill the emptiness of retirement, schizoid detachment apparently insulates against loss, and dependency can result in a welcoming of greater care and help from others.

SEXUALITY

Most younger people assume that older people have no interest in sex and most certainly do not engage in any sexual activity. Like the other prejudices against the elderly, this attitude is contrary to the facts. A review of sexuality in elders is found in Chapter 7.

CONCLUSIONS

The psychology of aging is clearly too new a field to present definitive findings in all of the many areas traditionally of interest to the psychologist. The early research has been fraught with methodological difficulties. While knowledge has been advanced, interpretations of these findings must be cautious.

Along with upgrading our research approaches, it is important to work towards changing the attitudes of society and in particular the attitudes of care providers towards the elderly person.

Ollie Randall, an octogenerian herself, provides a final optimistic note[50]:

Beyond our numbers we have the new dimensions of length in that many more of us are living much longer than we ever expected to do; and we also have depth, a new awareness of ourselves as people who count as members of our society. And, given the opportunity which was denied to most of us for far too long, we know we can, by our own efforts, create a place in society for ourselves. We have diversity in the membership of what society calls "older Americans." We have all races, creeds, colors, and cultures to call upon. We also have a separateness which society itself brought into being, and this gives us the right and the power to think and act independently in our own behalf. We now accomplish this through many avenues of activity formerly denied to us because of our years. But most of all we have the dimension of experience in living through the radical changes of this century and discovering that we have the ability and flexibility to cope with change—with success. An eminent psychiatrist at a meeting once asked recently whether older people can learn. The reply was "of course we can, or how otherwise would we have survived at all."*

*From Randall OA: Aging in America today: New aspects in aging. Gerontol 17(1):6–11, 1977. Reprinted by permission of The Gerontologist.

REFERENCES

1. Butler RN: Why Survive? Being Old in America. New York, Harper & Row, 1975, pp. 6–7
2. National Insitute of Aging: Our Future Selves: A Research Plan Toward Understanding Aging. Washington, DC, US Government Printing Office, DHEW Publ No. 77:1086, 1977
3. Manney JD: Aging in American Society. Ann Arbor, Michigan, University of Michigan-Wayne State University 1975, pp 35–36
4. Lawton MP: Sensory Deprivation and the Effect of the Environment on Management of the Senile Dementia Patient. Paper presented at NIMH Con-

ference on Clinical Aspects of Alzheimer's Disease, December 1978

5. Lawton MP, Newcomer RJ, Byerts TO: Community Planning for an Aging Society. Stroudsberg, Pennsylvania, Dowden, Hutchinson & Ross, 1976

6. Schooler KK: Environmental change and the elderly, in Altman I, Wohlwill JF (eds): Human Behavior and Environment. New York, Plenum Press, 1976, vol 1, pp 265–298

7. Botwinick J: Aging and Behavior, ed 2. New York, Springer, 1978

8. Birren JE, Butler RN, Greenhouse SW, et al: Human Aging: A Biological and Behavioral Study. Washington, DC, US Government Printing Office 1963, pp 283–316

9. Obrist WD: Cerebral physiology of the aged: Relation of psychological function, in Burch NR, Altshuler H (eds): Behavior and Brain Electrical Activity. New York, Plenum Press, 1975, pp 421–430

10. Obrist WD: The Electroencephalogram of healthy aged males, in Birren JE, Butler RN, Greenhouse SW, et al (eds): Human Aging: A Biological and Behavioral Study. Washington, DC, US Government Printing Office, 1963, pp 88–89

11. Woodruff DS: A physiological perspective of the psychology of aging, in Woodruff DS, Birren JE (eds): Aging: Scientific Perspectives and Social Issues. New York, Van Nostrand, 1975, p 186

12. Surwillo WW: Timing of behavior in senescence and the role of the central nervous system, in Talland GA (ed): Human Aging and Behavior. New York, Academic Press, 1968, pp 1–35

13. Woodruff DS: Biofeedback control of the EEG alpha rhythm and its effect on reaction time in the young and old. Doctoral dissertation, University of Southern California, 1972

14. Eisdorfer C: Psychophysiologic and cognitive studies in the aged, in Usdin G, Hofling C (eds): Aging: The Process and the People. New York, Brunner & Mazel, 1978, pp 105–106

15. Thompson LW, Marsh GR: Psychophysiological studies of aging, in Eisdorfer C, Lawton MP: The Psychology of Adult Development and Aging. Washington, DC, American Psychological Association Press, 1973, pp 112–148

16. Thompson LW, Nowlin JB: Relation of increased attention to central and autonomic nervous system states, in Jarvik LR, Eisdorfer C, Blum JE (eds): Intellectual Functioning in Adults. New York, Springer, 1973, pp 107–123

17. Lacey JI, Lacey B: Some autonomic-central nervous system interrelationships, in Black P (ed): Physiological Correlates of Emotion. New York, Academic Press, 1970, pp 205–207

18. Froehling S: Effects of propranolol on behavioral and physiological measures of elderly males. Unpublished doctoral dissertation, Duke University, 1974

19. Eisdorfer C, Nowlin J, Wilkie F: Improvement in learning in the aged by modification of autonomic nervous system activity. Science 170:1327–1329, 1970

20. Lawton MP: Geropsychological knowledge as background for psychotherapy with older people. J Geriatr Psychiatr 10:221–233, 1977

21. Botwinick JA: Cautiousness in advanced age. J Gerontol 21:347–353, 1966

22. Birren JE: The Psychology of Aging. New Jersey, Prentice-Hall, 1964, p 129

23. Wechsler D: The Measurement and Appraisal of Adult Intelligence, ed 4. Baltimore, Williams & Wilkins, 1958, p 135

24. Baltes P, Schaie KW: Aging and IQ: The myth of the twilight years. Psych Today 7:35–40, 1974

25. Botwinick J: Intellectual abilities, in Birren J, Schaie KW: Handbook of the Psychology of Aging. New York, Van Nostrand, 1977, pp 580–605

26. Eisdorfer C, Busse EW, Cohen LD: The WAIS performance of an aged sample: The relationship between verbal and performance IQs. J Geront 14:197–201, 1959

27. Kimmel DC: Adulthood and Aging: An Interdisciplinary View. New York, Wiley, 1974, p 378

28. Eisdorfer C, Wilkie FW: Stress, disease, aging and behavior, in Birren JE, Schaie KW: Handbook of the Psychology of Aging. New York, Van Nostrand, 1977, pp 251–275

29. Jarvik LF, Kallman FJ, Falek A: Intellectual changes in aged twins. J Geront 17:289–294, 1962

30. Granick S, Friedman AS: Educational experience and maintenance of intellectual functioning by the aged: An overview, in Jarvik LF, Eisdorfer C, Blum JE (eds): Intellectual Functioning in Adults. New York, Springer, 1973, pp 59–64

31. Hulicka IM, Weiss RL: Age differences in retention as a function of learning. J Consult Psychol 29:125–129, 1965

32. Jerome EA: Decay of heuristic processes in the aged, in Tibbits C, Donahue W (eds): Social and Psychological Aspects of Aging. New York, Columbia University Press, 1962, pp 808–823

33. Arenberg D: Concept problem solving in young and old adults. J Geront 23:279–282, 1968

34. Rowe EJ, Schnore MM: Item concreteness and reported strategies in paired-associate learning as a function of age. J Geront 26:470–475, 1971

35. Neugarten BL: Adult personality: Toward a psychology of the life cycle, in Neugarten BL (ed): Middle Age and Aging. Chicago, University of Chicago Press, 1968

36. Neugarten BL: Personality and aging, in Birren JE, Schaie KW (eds): Handbook of the Psychology of Aging. New York, Van Nostrand, 1977, pp 626–649

37. Neugarten BL, Maddox GL: Our Future Selves: Report of the Panel on Behavioral and Social Sci-

ences Research. Washington, DC, National Institute of Health, DHEW Publ No. (NIH) 78-144, pp 9–10

38. Butler RN, Lewis MI: Aging and Mental Health. St. Louis, CV Mosby, 1977, pp 203–204

39. Kimmel DC: Adulthood and Aging: An Interdisciplinary View. New York, Wiley, 1974, p 324

40. Perlin S, Butler RN: Psychiatric aspects of adaptation to the aging experience, in Birren JE, Butler RN, Breenhouse SW, et al (eds): Human Aging: A Biological and Behavioral Study. Washington, DC, US Gov't Printing Office, 1963, vol 1, pp 162–163

41. Busse EW, Pfeiffer E: Behavior and Adaptation in Late Life, ed 2. Boston, Little Brown & Co, 1977, p 172

42. Lawton MP: Clinical geropsychology: Problems and prospects. Master lecture, American Psychological Association, Toronto, Canada, August, 1978

43. Provisional Data on Federally Funded Community Mental Health Centers, 1976–1977. Rockville, MD, National Institute of Mental Health, 1978

44. Whelihan WM: Traditional modalities can work for older people too. Generations 3:18–19, 1979

45. Hoyer WJ, Mishara BL, Riedel RG: Problem behaviors as operants. Geront 15:452–465, 1975

46. Butler RN: The life review: An interpretation of reminiscence in the aged. Psychiatr 119:721–728, 1963

47. Revere V: The remembered past: Its reconstruction at different life stages. Doctoral dissertation, University of Chicago, 1971

48. Lieberman MA: Some issues in studying psychological predictors of survival, in Palmore E, Jeffers FC (eds): Prediction of Life Span. Lexington, Massachusetts, Heath, 1971, pp 167–180

49. Gutmann D: Navajo dependency and illness, in Palmore E, Jeffers FC (eds): Prediction of Life Span. Lexington, Massachusetts, Heath, 1971, pp 181–198

50. Randall OA: Aging in America today: New aspects in aging. Gerontol 17:6–11, 1977

5

Caring for Elders

Len Hughes Andrus, M.D.
Mary O'Hara-Devereaux, Ph.D.

Effectively caring for elders demands comprehensive health care services. Clinicians must have a prospective that is more broad than only the medical approach with its focus on the diagnosis and treatment of disease. Eldercare involves more than titrating antihypertensive drugs, digitalizing cases of congestive heart disease, or regulating insulin dosage in diabetics. Improving health status in elders usually depends on changes in the physical, social, and total living environment.

PHYSICAL ENVIRONMENT

Medical Setting

A comprehensive approach includes attention to the physical aspects of the office and other clinical settings. The clinical setting is often arranged in a manner that makes it difficult for elders to manage. What is created in this clinical environment should reflect thoughtfulness, concern, and sensitivity towards the needs of elders. Ideally, a clinic or office should be located near a public transit stop; there should be adequate parking in proximity to the facility, as well as safe access walks and ramps for wheelchairs and for people with ambulatory problems. Wide, non-slip walkways with minimal longitudinal slope (less than 5 percent), with level landings on each side of wide, manageable doors are needed; hand-activated doors in the path of travel should be operable with a single effort by lever-type hardware, panic bars, push-pull activating bars, or other means not requiring the ability to grasp. Such hardware should be of proper height and the doors should have bottom kickplates or be made of material that withstands the abuse of canes, crutches, and wheelchair wheels or foot platforms.

Lighting should be adequate for safety, easily read directional signs should be properly placed, and wide hallways with safe stairways and elevators, which are easily operated and will accommodate a stretcher and wheelchairs, are necessary. Elevator call buttons, car controls, emergency telephones and public telephones should be the proper height and should have braille and marked arabic numerals. In new buildings, the state and federal building codes regulate public use facilities serving the handicapped and ensure proper construction for usage by elders. State regulations may, however, vary and the American National Standards Institute at 1430 Broadway, New York, New York 10008 can provide excellent guidelines.

The office setting should be attractive and the decor warm and relaxing. There should be room for movement of wheelchairs, as well as for people with crutches and walking devices. Furniture should be comfortable but with special attention given to height and armrests, which facilitate sitting and rising of elders with limited mobility. The waiting room should neither be overcrowded nor a dangerous place for the frail elderly. It is advisable to have seating areas for older people separate from pediatric patients in a family practice office. When waiting room space is a problem and when it is impossible to provide for quiet, isolated waiting areas, special scheduling of elders can be arranged to avoid waiting in a confused, noisy, and contaminated waiting room.

Acoustics is important and noise contamination should be at a minimum; there should be no loud background music, and all attempts should be made to reduce multisources of noises. The waiting room should have reading materials appropriate for older people, some with large print and with subjects that elders enjoy reading.

Ideally, there should be separate toilet facilities for each sex with adequate space, proper lavatories, toilets, and urinals for people in wheelchairs. Grab bars, mirrors, towels, and soap dispensers should meet the needs of the handicapped. The toilet facilities should be designed so that urine and stool specimens can be obtained without great difficulty. This should apply to other office procedures such as drawing blood and taking cardiograms.

The back office space should be designed to include multiple examining rooms (preferably three per provider) and arranged to facilitate patient flow since older patients take more time disrobing and dressing and, as such, should be allowed enough time without feeling hurried.

Sociologists, architects, behavioral scientists, and others interested in elders and their physical environment are doing much to improve the quality of life through new facility design. Taking into consideration the decreased sensory perceptions and motor functions associated with aging, particular attention is being paid to glare, color, and acoustics. In addition, the elder's decreased emotional adaptation is being accommodated by decreasing confusing designs such as long hallways, indistinct colors and shade changes between walls, doors, rooms, and floors. Where possible, the cultural and ethnic background of older patient groups are reflected in the design.

CLINICAL APPROACH

The nature of the social interaction that takes place in the clinical setting is especially critical to the quality of care for the elderly. *People* are the most significant part of that therapeutic environment; that is, people who show concern not only for the older patient but also for the family and friends who may accompany them; people who demonstrate a helpful, pleasant approach, who speak clearly and directly to patients, who are willing to repeat directions, who repeatedly check to see how things are going for patients and those accompanying them; and above all, people who *listen* to what elders, their families, and friends have to say are of utmost importance to the kind of

therapy an elder receives and should include the *entire* staff.

For many elderly patients, the visit to the doctor's office is an important event, sometimes their only social contact outside the home. In anticipation, they get all "dolled-up" for the occasion—best dress, hair freshly coiffured, and jewelry are the order of the day. It is important for the staff to acknowledge this with comments on how they look and compliments on their attire. This warm and friendly response usually enhances the efficient management as well as the quality of care elders receive. By filling in for something that is missing in the patient's life, however, this interaction can occasionally be burdensome due to unrealistic demands upon personnel time. The resourceful staff can identify community resources that meet these social needs. Arrangements can be made for the mobile patients at such services as daycare centers, senior citizen activities, church groups, etc. For the patient confined to home, such activities as telephone reassurance services, Meals-On-Wheels, skilled nursing, home health care aides and/or choreworkers, occupational and physical therapists, friendly visitors (from agencies or church), senior companions, etc., can fill this social void. The social worker, when available, is especially qualified to arrange and coordinate these services in such a way as to monitor the patient's well-being and at the same time guard against sponsoring unnecessary dependency.

The office receptionist, a key contact person, can also reflect the practice's sensitivity and concern for older patients by how he or she schedules appointments. For example, in the family practice setting, special time can be used to schedule older people similar to that scheduled for obstetrical and well-baby visits that minimizes contact with younger patients with acute illnesses. This is particularly important in practices with heavy pediatric cases. Time, in relation to transportation such as bus or streetcar schedules and the availability of friends for transportation, is an important consideration. The time of day is relevant to some elders in that they function better and have greater lucidity during certain time periods.

The duration of an office visit should not be overtaxing or wearing to fragile, older persons with chronic ailments. There is no direct relationship between time spent with a patient and the quality of care. Prolonged waiting in a waiting room, followed by prolonged interviews and examination may be more detrimental to an older patient's well-being than can be countered by the therapeutic interventions. A limited amount of time spent in a supportive environment with a sensitive and skilled clinician constitutes a higher quality of care than a more prolonged visit. If delays and long waits are unavoidable, patients should be given periodic updating as to what is happening. Often serial visits to care for multiple chronic problems is better than one long visit.

The Providers

The interest and attitude of health care providers is critical and unfortunately may constitute the greatest barrier to quality health care services for elders. It is appropriate for all clinicians dealing with elders to examine their own attitudes and feelings concerning the care of geriatric patients: "Do I enjoy working with elders and can I deal with their complex, multisystem, often progressive medical problems with equanimity?" The ease, or "disease" with which health care providers contact patients is contagious. Providers should learn to contact elders from a position of "ease." The need for the clinician to have a positive holistic approach to the patient is critical in that the strict "scientific approach," with emphasis on diagnosis and treatment, may be much less important to the patient's quality of life and total health status than the supportive attitudes of those with whom he or she relates. Many times our efforts in medicine are best channeled in trying optimistically to help patients cope, accept, and live with disabilities and variations from normal, rather than in attempting the impossible task of trying to *restore* function to normal.

Since confusion is frequently a part of the older patient's life, it is important that all encounters begin with clarity and understanding. A clinician should always properly identify him- or herself and make sure that the older patient knows whom he or she is. The stage must be set so that the patient understands what is being done and what, in the encounter, are the goals.

We often demonstrate "ageism" by talking down to the patient rather than to show respect for and recognition of the older person's uniqueness and individuality. The elder should have a sense that the clinician is listening to what he or she has to say. Then the patient is a participant in what is happening and in the decision to be made that will affect his or her life. Therapeutic decisions should not be made on the basis of what the provider considers

best for the patient, but on what is determined best *with* the patient. Whenever possible, have family and friends involved to the extent of their concern and actual responsibilities for the patient. The family, friends, and intimate social groups, who make up a network, are the most overlooked and underutilized resource available.

The Team

Clinical care of elders is best carried out by a team. Trying to keep a patient comfortable and fairly well adjusted with a disease that is progressing on a course doomed to eventual deterioration and death can be very frustrating and wearing to a solo provider. Much of the frustration and dissatisfaction experienced by physicians in caring for older, chronically ill patients comes from the stress of the doctor–patient interaction. This one-to-one relationship often results in a protracted and overwhelming self-imposed burden on the physician. An intimate clinical team sharing responsibility makes the life of the physician much less burdensome and more stimulating and at the same time helps maintain a personalized and humanistic approach. The quality and scope of the health care of elders is enhanced by the team approach.

The team composition will vary with the size of the providership, the location, and the economics of the setting. The medical leader of such a team legally and traditionally is the physician. The rest of the primary health team may only consist of one or two other providers. These may be an office nurse, nurse practitioner, or physician's assistant, or several others, such as a social worker, clinical pharmacist, health educator, family and/or community aides, psychologist, occupational therapist, physiotherapist, etc. Much depends on what the setting will support, the philosophy and experience of the physician, and those in control. Although it makes for a close relationship, all members of the team do not necessarily need to be employees of the physician or clinic. Formal working relationships with social workers, psychologists, physical therapists, etc., can be developed even for the solo practitioner office.

There are some models of comprehensive approaches to eldercare in which the medical aspects are not the major focus and the central coordinating team member is a nonphysician, such as a social worker. In these situations, two major factors are operating: one is a reaction to the traditional medical profession's focus on "diagnosis and treatment," and the second factor is that purely medical problems are only a *part* of the elder's needs for health and quality of life. Too often the physician is focused on the medical problem facing the patient and his or her treatment recommendations when, because of social or living circumstances, it may be impossible to carry out the therapy prescribed. Frequently, appropriate resolution of these circumstances also solves the medical problem because of the interaction of both on the general well-being of the elderly patient.

The health care team's involvement and utilization of the total resources available to elders is discussed in Section 3.

Home, Nursing Home, and Institutional Visits

Through home visits, the clinician can obtain a clearer picture of the patient's physical environment and gain insight into the patient's personality and the daily interpersonal relationships affecting his or her life. In assessing the physical environment, one can note the availability of good nutrition, the adequacy of shelter and maintenance of an acceptable temperature range, the state of sanitation, the spacial relationships, and the room for mobility. The clinician may also note the presence of safety hazards and appraise the feasibility of remodeling alterations that would improve safety and adapt the environment to the patient's physical limitations. A more accurate inventory of both prescription and nonprescription medications, that are available and used by the patient can be done by direct observation rather than by history gathering or asking the patient to bring all drugs to the office for inspection. A sense of the patient's well-being and personal identity is afforded by this first-hand experience in the home. The patient is seen in his or her territory while the clinician is the guest or visitor. The interplay between the patient and his or her physical environment and the interpersonal dynamics operating among all those in the home setting can be observed. A home visit also communicates to the family and patient that what happens in the home is terribly important to the care of the patient. Through these observations, a broader assessment of the patient's health status and the problems that involve therapeutic compliance can be obtained.

More effective utilization of the primary health care team, the family, and other community resources would allow most patients to be adequately cared for at home. Most effective therapeutic modalities can be carried out at home as can the measurements needed to monitor patient care properly. Most of these can be done without the presence of the physician, who can then supervise the medical management through proper teamwork, communications, and a good record system. The necessary physical changes in the home can usually be accomplished through minimal remodeling that would make use of special hardware, such as hand rails; minimize hazards; facilitate patient movement; change scenery, and ensure comfort. The social worker coordinating community resources is often the best team member to accomplish these physical alterations.

Tragic errors can be made in response to home visits if the clinician, especially the physician, inappropriately interjects his or her value system into the decisions affecting an elder's life. An elder may be emotionally and medically better off in what to us is a filthy house with inadequate heating, poor sanitation, poor ventilation, disorganized and cluttered with trash, abundant with dog and cat hair, than in the clean, sterile confines of the hospital, nursing home, or other institution. A practical working knowledge of how to improve the home situation and the appropriate utilization of family and community resources may be much more beneficial than dislocating medical intervention.

The clinician must always ask, "What is in the best interest of the patient?," not, "What is the easiest way for *me* to manage this case?" Unfortunately, lesser time demands and greater remuneration may point to institutionalization. In addition to being sensitive about their own attitudes and financial incentives, clinicians should recognize those incentives of the institutions in which they commit their geriatric patients. Those incentives often determine what kind of care setting the patient is in and whether the patient should be transferred to another institution. Institutions protect their own interests and service industries may grow without interservice controls. Often there are few incentives for increasing the independence of elders or for transferring them to less costly institutions or service programs. The primary health care team must accept the responsibility for managing and coordinating the total care in the best interest of the patient.

Institutionalization, especially hospitalization, is costly and in itself may be dangerous and life-threatening. Older people may decompensate and become disoriented, compounding their exposure to drugs, injuries, hospital infections, and all the serious medical complications of inactivity. Whenever institutionalization or any change of residence is contemplated, elders should be properly advised and emotionally prepared and supported; this will both enhance their adaptation and lower morbidity and mortality. The clinician's active involvement in patient-care affairs and good relationships with the staff will also enhance the quality of care delivered by the institution.

In caring for elders in a setting such as a nursing home or hospital, the physician may have to see many patients in a very limited time. Even so, the encounter should be one of quality. Two physicians spending exactly the same amount of time with a patient may be perceived differently: one as if on roller skates, rolling from one patient to another, hurried and uncaring; and the other being present, listening, involved, interested, and caring.

Monitoring chronic illness at home or in an institution is often best carried out by nurse practitioners or physician's assistants, visiting nurses, social workers, home and community aides, and others working under the medical supervision of a physician. Not only is the quality of care increased, but it is much more cost-effective for nonphysicians to render this service whenever possible.

The conscientious clinician must be particularly assertive in preventing patients with adverse changes in their physical status from being "dumped" from their homes into nursing homes or from nursing homes into hospitals in order to avoid the responsibility of more intensive care regimens. Inappropriate dumping may occur when death is impending and those at home feel inadequate or when those in the nursing home wish to minimize the perceived stigma of death in their institution. For those patients to whom the rest home has become "home" and for those who care for them, "family," it is perfectly logical for the elder to desire to spend the last days and to die in that setting. We should allow them their dignity by supporting them in this wish and persuading the institution to help death occur peacefully. Many communities, urban and rural, have home hospice programs that make dying at home easier for the patient and family to manage.

The Record System

The common communication tool for all members of the health care team is the medical record. Information should be organized, accurate, and concise. The problem-oriented record system advocated by Weed is the most appropriate and is particularly important in the long-term management of older patients.[1] There are many record forms and formats derived from the problem-oriented approach, and several of these are available commercially. One system that is helpful and well organized is the Andrus/Clinic-Rec.*

Older people are more likely to suffer from chronic conditions and to have multisystem involvement and are proportionately less likely to have acute medical conditions. Good records are of central importance in the monitoring of chronic illness. Progress notes are organized in the "SOAP" format, listing subjective data, objective data, appraisal, and the plan on one sheet. The flowsheet is a special form of progress notes and constitutes a concise, easily read, and easily understood common communication system for following chronic ailments. The parameters to be followed, symptomatic and objective data, therapeutic measurements, and the patient education plans should be worked out with all members of the health care team. The protocols for specific conditions, such as hypertension, are available but should be "tailored" to each case. Parameters can be developed for the multiple diseases, as well as the psychological and socioeconomic problems facing elders and can be organized on a flowsheet that is adaptable to most any situation. For economic reasons, the information is usually handwritten, particularly on progress notes and flowsheets; acceptable marks and abbreviations are important in saving time and space.

A separate, updated medication sheet for careful monitoring of the number and kinds of drugs, prescription and over-the-counter, is a critical part of the record. Older people take twice the drugs and have more than three times the adverse reactions than the rest of the population. These problems are discussed in Chapter 6.

All members of the health care team directly participating in patient care should record in the same progress notes. It is essential that they be trained to be organized and concise in their recordings. This is especially true for social workers and others who may be in the habit of writing voluminous notes. The problem list should be complete and contain the input of the entire primary health care team, consultants, and other health care personnel, and should be continuously updated through team conferences. Thus, the patient's re-

---

*Andrus/Clinic-Rec may be purchased through Bibbero Systems, Inc., 36 Second Street, San Francisco, CA 94105.

6

Pharmacology: Drug-Related Problems of the Elderly

James W. Cooper, Jr., Ph.D., F.C.P.

A careful and thoughtful approach to drug use with elders is essential if appropriate therapy is to be prescribed. Drugs are especially hazardous to elders because of age-related or altered physiology and pharmacokinetics, the high incidence of drug interactions, inappropriate prescribing practice, inadequate monitoring of long-term medication, and inaccurate patient compliance. Choosing a safe and effective course of action, balancing drug use between the benefits and risks, calls for special knowledge and management strategy for the primary care clinician.

The purpose of this chapter is to provide perspective and knowledge that promote appropriate drug use. Most common drug-related problems are presented along with the relevent physiologic, pharmaceutic, and pharmacologic factors.

RATIONALITY OF GERIPHARMACOTHERAPY

There is a basis for the belief that drugs are not wisely used in the elderly. Part of the problem is a poor attitude towards elder care by physicians.[1] A look at drug use patterns, problems, and diagnostic accuracy lends credence to this belief.

In 1972, Americans 65 and over received 22 percent of all R_x drugs even though they comprised only 9 percent of the population.[2] The most frequently prescribed drug classes are cathartics, analgesics, antipyretics, and tranquilizers.[3] See Table 6-1. It has been estimated that 84–87 percent[4,5] of elderly ambulatory and 95 percent[10] of institutionalized elderly patients are taking prescription drugs.

Seventy to eighty percent of drug reactions are considered preventable.[7] Still, in patients over 60–70 years of age, the risk of drug reaction is almost double that in adults 30–40 years of age.[7] Several studies have found that elderly patients had a higher frequency of drug-related admissions to hospitals than younger patients.[8,9] Up to a third of the elderly patients admitted to two small community hospitals had drug-related problems (DRPs) that contributed to their admission.[9] Fully two-thirds of these DRPs were misuse and the other third were adverse reactions and interactions. Compound drug problems may be overlooked or missed because problems caused by drug reactions are not readily apparent, or symptoms are vague such as forgetfulness, weakness, confusion, or anxiety.

The number of drugs prescribed for an individual influences the rate of adverse reactions and noncompliance.[7] Despite the high risks, overprescribing both in large numbers and dosages is common for elders. In one nursing home, the patients received an average of 5–7 drugs.[6,10] Almost a fourth of the drugs prescribed were found to be unnecessary and/or ineffective.[6] In a second study, up to a fourth of the patients were placed at risk of potential drug interaction by multiple drug usage.[10] When multiple drug therapy is unavoidable, such as with multiple-problem patients, extreme care must be exercised in monitoring for drug interaction and side effects.

Drugs are frequently prescribed for symptoms rather than for diagnoses in the elderly (i.e., for

Table 6-1

Number and Percent of Patients Receiving Drugs by Drug Category in
Rank Order in a 250,000-Patient Skilled Nursing Facility Population

Drug Category	Patients		
	Number	Percent	Rank
Cathartics	1,839	53.3	1
Analgesics and antipyretics	1,645	47.7	2
Tranquilizers	1,549	44.8	3
Other	1,258	36.4	4
Diuretics	1,169	33.8	5
Vitamins	1,149	33.3	6
Sedatives and hypnotics	1,147	33.2	7
Cardiac drugs	1,000	28.9	8
Skin and mucous membranes	613	17.7	9
Anti-infectives	539	16.9	10
Antacids and absorbents	489	14.2	11
Antihistamines	479	13.8	12
Hypotensives	428	12.4	13
Eye, ear, nose, and throat	408	11.8	14
Spasmolytics	394	11.4	15
Insulin and antidiabetic agents	384	11.1	16
Controlled substances (Schedule II)	372	10.7	17
Electrolyte replacements	345	9.9	18
Vasodilating agents	298	8.5	19
Antidepressants	289	8.4	20
Anticonvulsants	257	7.4	21
Estrogens/androgens	121	3.5	22
Thyroid replacements and antithyroid agents	87	2.5	23
Adrenals	77	2.2	24
Anticoagulants	37	1.0	25

Category reference: American Society of Hospital Pharmacists Formulary Service, Washington, DC. Reprinted from Long-Term Care Facility Improvement Study: Introductory Report. USDEHEWPHS, Office of Nursing Home Affairs, July 1975, p 52.

temperature, pain, restlessness, rigidity, sleeplessness, and/or agitation).[11] One study found 64 percent of patients had incorrect admission diagnoses—primarily concerning psychiatric problems. The inadequate performance in identifying clinical and therapeutic problems of the chronically ill aged were remarkably consistent, regardless of whether patient referral was from a general or psychiatric hospital, the patient's home, or another nursing home.[12] If the preadmission diagnosis is incorrect in so many patients admitted to long-term care facilities, how can the preadmission drug therapy be rational? Another problem is the use of tranquilizers to control the behavior of patients in an elder care facility.

Often the least mentally impaired and most physically active nursing home patients were the most heavily "drugged" with neuroactive substances.[11]

BIOPHARMACEUTIC AND PHARMACOKINETIC FACTORS

The altered physiology of the elder affects action and excretion of drugs. Most drugs are carried and distributed by the water-containing areas of the body. Both total body water and intracellular water decrease with age. Furthermore, the albumin—the principal serum protein which binds highly bound drugs such as phenytoin, warfarin, and salicylate—has been shown to decrease with age and to impaired liver function. At the same time, much muscle tissue is being replaced by fat. Drugs distributed in muscle (most drugs) would therefore have less mass for distribution (e.g., digoxin) and those with high lipid solubility would be stored for longer periods (e.g., phenothiazines and glutethimide).

Thus, as a person ages, there is less water and muscle tissue in which to distribute the drug and less albumin to bind those drugs significantly bound by plasma protein, the net result is higher total tissue and free drug levels. The liver is the primary site of drug metabolism. With aging there is a decrease of hepatic cells at aged 50–60. These functional declines may not be evident from the usual liver function tests. Marked differences in elderly patients' metabolic capability have been shown for phenylbutazone and benzodiazepines (e.g., Valium and Dalmane).[13] Most likely the duration of action of most of the commonly administered drugs is longer in elders. For those with impaired liver function, who take drugs that are extensively metabolized by the liver (e.g., digitoxin, tetracyclines, chloramphenicol, macrolides, and most CNS depressants), the risk of toxic accumulation is great.

Functional reduction in renal excretory rates in the aged may be balanced to a degree by slower absorption, altered transport, and cell utilization. Significant toxicity can result with drugs such as digoxin. This results in increased concentration. It is important to realize that the linear decline in functional nephrons that occurs with aging may be paralleled by decreased lean muscle mass and protein intake, so that the serum creatinine and blood urea nitrogen (BUN) may appear to be normal even though there is significant decrease in renal function. The Jeliffe formula[14] gives an approximation of creatinine clearance (CrCl) from stable serum creatinine:

$$CrCl \ (male) = \frac{98 - 0.8 \ (aged \ 20)}{serum \ creatinine \ (mg\%)}$$

$$CrCl \ (female) = 0.9x$$

Where x = CrCl (male). Mild renal impairment is 50–80 ml/min, moderate 10–50 cc/min, or severe renal impairment less than 10 cc/min. These calculations should not be used if the kidney has been subjected to direct insult (e.g., nephrotoxic drugs, stones, or crush injury) or indirect injury (e.g., shock). A tabulation of recommended dosage intervals[15] along with the use of nomographic methods for dosing digoxin and gentamicin may help to reduce renal-related adverse reactions. Table 6-2 lists those drugs that require dosage and/or dosing interval modifications in function or organic renal and/or hepatic impairment.

In terms of drug dosing, from 25–30 percent of body cells and functional capacities are lost from aged 30 to old age at a persistent and irreversible rate of about 1 percent per year.[16] This suggests that whenever medications are definitely needed in the elderly, their dosage should be tapered by 20–50 percent or more. When this factor is not taken into account, higher tissue levels and increased incidence of adverse effects are seen especially with digoxin, anticoagulants, phenylbutazone, and the aminoglycosides. Dosing of all drugs should be by lean body weight (5' = 100 in females; or 110 in males, pounds plus 5 pounds per inch).

There is some evidence that supports that elders have an increased sensitivity of certain receptor sites. The decline in autonomic function increases postural hypotension with the use of hypotensive drugs[17] as well as the risk of hypothermia, particularly with the phenothiazines.[18] (See Chapter 12.)

IMPAIRED HOMEOSTASIS AND DRUG RESPONSE

The key principle in understanding drug effects in the elderly patient is that their homeostatic response to any stress (pharmacologic in this case) is either delayed and/or reduced. Drugs that change CNS status, blood pressure and/or cardiovascular system may cause profound changes in the individual. Drugs calling for special precautions are found in Table 6-3.

IMPLICATIONS FOR PATIENT CARE

The potential for drug-related problems in the elderly is high. Methods for reduction of these problems include complete drug history, patient education, and dosing by lean body weight and renal–hepatic function with attention to special consideration for particular drugs.

Table 6-2
Some Drugs to be Used With Caution (e.g., Dosage and/or Dosing Interval Changes) in the Elderly

Amikacin†: Amikin
Allopurinol†·¶: Zyloprim
Amphetamines
Antidepressants
Aspirin*·§
Atropine, Scopolamine
Antihypertensives
Barbiturates§
Bishydroxycoumarin*·¶: Dicumarol
Bromides
Chloramphenicol§: Chlormycetin
Chlordiazepoxide§: Librium
Clofibrate*·**: Atromide-S
Chlorpropamide§: Diabinese
Codeine
Colistin†: Colmycin
Cortisone-related agents*
Diazepam§: Valium
Dextrothyroxine**: Choloxin
Digotoxin†·§·#
Digoxin†·#: Lanoxin
Epinephrine
Flurazepam#: Dalmane
Gentamycin†·#: Garamycin
Guanethidine†: Ismelin
Haloperidol: Haldol
Heparin‖
Hydralazine: Apresoline
Indomethacin: Indocin
Isocarboxazid§: Marplan
Kanamycin†·#: Kantrex
Lidocaine§
Lithium salts†
Liothyronine: Cytomel

Methyldopa†·§: Aldomet
Mineral oil (prolonged regular use)
Morphine†
Nalidixic acid†: Negram
Nitrates (long acting): Peritrate, Isordil
Neomycin†
Oxyphenylbutazone*·†: Tandearil
Pargyline: Eutonyl
Phenothiazines§: Thorazine Compazine, Mellaril, Separine, etc.
Phenytoin§·¶: Dilantin
Phenylbutazone*·†·¶: Butazolidin, Azolid
Pipradol: Meratran
Polymyxins†
Procainamide†: Pronestyl
Propranolol: Inderal
Quinidine†
Rauwolfia alkaloids: Reserpine, etc.
Spironolactone†: Aldactone
Sulfonamides†: Triplesulfas, Gantrisin, Gantanol
Testosterone
Tetracyclines†·§
Tobramycin†: Nebcin
Tolbutamide*: Orinase
Thiazides: Diuril
Thyroid
Trimaeternee†: Dyrenium
Tranylcypromine: Parnate
Trihexylphenidyl: Artane
Warfarin*·¶: Coumadin

*Especially with oral anticoagulants.
†If renal function is diminished.
§If hepatic function is diminished.
‖Women over 60 years in particular.
¶Genetic variation in metabolism exists.
#Prolonged half-life in "healthy" elderly.
**Increased cardiovascular morbidity and mortality shown in some studies.
Adapted from Holloway DA: Drug problems in the geriatric patient. Drug Intell Cl Pharm 11:597–603, 1977; Wallace DE, Watanabe AS: Drug effects in geriatric patients. Drug Intell Cl Pharm 8:632–640, 1974; O'Malley K, Judge TG, Crooks J: Geriatric clinical pharmacology and therapeutics, in Avery GS: Drug Treatment. Sydney, ADIS Press, 1976, pp 124–142; Stanaszek W: The hospital pharmacist and the geriatric patient. Hosp Form Mgt 9:18–24, 1974; Solomon F et al: Sleeping pills insomnia and medical practice. N Engl J Med, 300:803–808, 1979; American Hospital Formulary Service: American Society of Hospital Pharmacists, 4630 Montgomery Avenue NW, Washington, DC.

Table 6-3
Special Drug Considerations for the Elderly Patient

Analgesics	Special Consideration
Acetaminophen: APAP (Tylenol, Datril)	Preferred analgesic in elderly with noninflammatory pain. As effective as propoxyphene and codeine. Chronic daily ingestion of more than 4–5 g can lead to liver damage.
ASA: aspirin	Least expensive, preferred over APAP in inflammatory pain. Also as effective as propoxyphene and codeine. GI blood loss in 3/4 who take it of concern in PUD HX and borderline anemia; concomitant liquid antacid minimizes. Antiplatelet effect may be of benefit in prevention of recurrent MI and TIA.
Phenacetin	Never use chronically, as well known to lead to analgesic nephropathy, especially in combination analgesics, both prescription (Darvon-Compound-65^R) and OTC
Propoxyphene and Propoxyphene combinations (Darvocet-N-100 and Darvon compounds)	Single ingredient propoxyphene not as effective as ASA or APAP alone. Combination as effective as ASA or APAP. Confusional reactions increased in elderly. Avoid long-term full-dose use.
Codeine and Codeine combination (Tylenol No.^{QZZ})	Codeine has equal potency with ASA and APAP. Combination has greater potency. Nausea, vomiting, and constipation more common in elderly.
Pentazocine (Talwin)	Less effective than ASA. Also prone to cause confusional reactions.
Injectable analgesics Meperidine (Demerol) Morphine, anileridine (Leritine) Hydromorphone (Dilaudid)	Use 1/3 to 1/2 usual adult dose, as much more potent in elderly patient. No side effect differences in equilanalgetic doses, but incidence increases with age.
Antiinflammatories–analgesics Phenbutazone (Azolid, Butazolidin) and Oxyphenylbutazone (Tandearil)	Longer half-life. Higher incidence GI upset and severe toxic reactions in older patient. Must be given with meals and/or liquid antacid to minimize GI effect. Not recommended in those over 60 by some authorities. Also causes fluid retention and blood dyscrasias as well as increased oral anticoagulant effect. Avoid full daily dose for more than 7–14 days.
Indomethacin (Indocin)	GI effects similar to phenlbutazone but more insidious. CNS effects of lightheadedness and headache also more common. Avoid full dose use greater than 7–14 days.
Tolectin, Nalfon, Clinoril, Motrin, Naprosyn	All nonsteroidal anti-inflammatory analgesics less effective than ASA in inflammatory disease but lower incidence of GI side effects. Much more expensive than ASA.
Injectable oral corticosteroids Hormones (Prednisone, Decadron) (Medrol)	Use should be reserved for crippling inflammatory diseases (rheumatoid arthritis) or disabling allergic disease, (asthma) and always taper dose. Greatly increased risk of GI bleeding and loss of diabetes

(continued on next page)

Table 6-3 *(continued)*

Analgesics	Special Consideration
	control, infection, osteoporosis and myopathy with tissue mobilization to central compartment, catarracts, psychic disturbances, and fluid retention with long-term use.
Other hormones	
Thyroid replacement	Cautiously use lower doses and increase gradually; otherwise increased risk of cardio- and cerebrovascular morbidity.
Antidiabetic Agents	Weight reduction and dietary measures control up to 70% of maturity-onset diabetics. Oral agents may increase cardiovascular morbidity. Hypoglycemic signs of tremor, sweating, and tachycardia not as readily discernible in elderly. Chlorpropamide (Diabenese) and acetohexamide (Dymelor) active metabolite have prolonged half-lives in elderly.
Cardiovascular drugs	
Digitalis preparations	Digoxin (Lanoxin) preferred glycoside. Avoid digitoxin and digitalis leaf (long hepatic and renal half-lives). Although of benefit in low output failure and atrial fibrillation, successfully withdrawn in up to 3/4 of patients. Subacute toxicity of anorexia with weight loss more common initial signs than other GI or cardiovascular effects. Baseline and follow-up ECG essential. Dose on lean body weight and creatinine clearance with attention to electrolyte and thyroid status. One-third to one-half patients noncompliant.
Quinidine	Higher serum levels both drugs with concurrent digoxin use. Half-life prolonged in elderly. "Cinchonism," (GI effects, lightheadedness, tinnitus) occurrence more commonly in elderly with low body weight. Decrease loading dose by 1/3 in significant heart failure.
Procainamide (Pronestyl)	Similar reduction in loading dose. Usually has to be dosed q4h to attain therapeutic levels.
Propranolol (Inderal)	Toxic effects more common in elderly along with reduced beta-blocking responsiveness in older patient. Aggravates bronchospastic tendency in COPD and can precipitate heart failure. Also affects diabetic control at higher doses. Increased tendency to "cold limb" effect in lower extremities in those with peripheral vascular or vasospastic diseases.
Lidocaine (Xylocaine)	Reduce bolus and continuous infusion doses in older patients especially those with organic liver disease.
Nitroglycerin tabs (Nitrostat)	Nitrostat most stable form. Caution to sit down before sublingual dose placement. Beware of orthostatic effect of all vasodilators.
Nitroglycerin ointment (Nitrol)	Never rub into skin. Headache may be relieved with ASA or APAP.
Long-acting nitrates (Isordil, Sorbitrate, Peritrate)	Variable effectiveness in older patients. Caution about blood pressure lowering effect.

Analgesics	Special Consideration
Central cerebrovascular and peripheral vasodilators (Vasodilan, Nylidrin) (Cyslospasmol, Hydergine) and niacin	May be worthy of one to three month trial in senile dementia or peripheral vascular disease. Beware concurrent alcohol enhancement of vasodilatation.
Antihypertensives Diuretics (all increase incontinence)	(Evaluate dose reduction if pressure less than 120/70)
Thiazides (many, no significant difference use hydrochlorthiazide generic)	Start with lowest possible dose. Patients must drink sufficient liquids. Watch volume, serum electrolyte urate and glucose effect. Ineffective with CrCl < 30–40 cc/min.
Furosemide (Lasix)	Most potent diuretic, effective with CrCl < 30 cc/min. Should be held until thiazides no longer effective. Does promote calcium excretion. Thiazides and furosemide profoundly deplete sodium, potassium, and chloride. Cautious use of potassium supplements and salt substitutes necessary as with decreased muscle mass elderly tend to have lower total body potassium.
Spironolactone (Aldactone)	Potassium-sparing diuretic often used in combination with thiazide (Aldactazide). Special caution if concurrent potassium supplement or salt substitute in use. Fatal hyperkalemia reported.
Triamterene (Dynenium)	Potassium-sparing diuretic most often used in combination with thiazide (Dyazide) with similar precaution as spironolactone.
Sympatholytic antihypertensives	(Beware continued pressure below 120/70, orthostatic effects, impaired male sexual function, and drowsiness or sedation.)
Methyldopa (Aldomet)	Reduced dosage in combination with thiazide (Aldoril); sodium retention seen when diuretic not used. Once-a-day bedtime dosing may take advantage of sedative effect, with therapeutic effect equivalent to multiple daily doses.
Propranolol (Inderal)	Only sympatholytic not requiring diuretic to prevent sodium retention. See cardiovascular section. Pulse less than 50–60 poorly tolerated.
Guanethidine (Ismelin)	Profound sympotholytic with long second-phase half-life. Use in small doses. Tricyclic antidepressants can interfere with antihypertensive effect.
Clonidine (Catapres)	Avoid in poorly compliant and patient with renal hypertension.
Reserpine	Avoid in those with depression, sinusitis, peptic ulcer disease, and history of breast cancer.
Vasodilator antihypertensives Hydralazine (Apresoline)	Reflex tachycardia aggravates angina; effect may be blocked by Inderal.
Prazosin (Minipres)	No reflex tachycardia but profound first dose effect—

(continued on next page)

Table 6-3 *(continued)*

Analgesics	Special Consideration
	have patient lie down. Both vasodilator and alpha-blocker.
Combination antihypertensives	
Ser-Ap-Es	Generally effective combinations with reduced diuretic
Aldoril	sympatholytic and/or vasodilator doses to minimize
Esimil	full dose side effects, but always start with step 1
Salutensin	diuretics and titrate to combination if necessary.
Hydropres	
Potassium chloride supplements	Beware functional/organic renal disease potassium
Liquid KCl	conservation with all sufficient water to prevent
	osomotic diarrhea must be used with liquid KCl.
Salt substitutes	Patients must be trained to carefully measure as each
(Neocurtasal, CoSalt)	teaspoonful has about 65 mEqKCl.
Effervescent	Expensive but tastes better than diluted liquid KCl.
(K-lyte)	
Solid (Slow K, Kaon-Cl)	Expensive but well tolerated except in esophageal or
	pyloric obstruction, or delayed GI transit time.
Anticoagulants	
Heparin	Increased risk of bleeding with age especially in
	females over 60.
Warfarin (Coumadin)	Increased risk of bleeding with age, due to altered
	sensitivity with genetic, nutritional and liver factors.
	Carefully evaluate use and do serial protimes.
	Beware risk of hemorrhage, especially with possible
	hemorrhagic stroke, peptic ulcer disease, hiatal
	hernia, and diverticulosis or any bleeding diathesis.
	No concurrent ASA usage except possibly with heart
	valve prostheses.
Anticonvulsants	
Phenytoin (Dilantin)	Increased neurologic and hematologic effects with
	lower serum albumin or renal impairment.
Sedative–Hypnotics and minor tranquilizers	
Barbiturates (Phenobarbital,	With the exception of phenobarbital as an
Butisol, Nembutal, Seconal)	anticonvulsant, continual use of other barbiturates is
Amytal	irrational due to prolonged half-lives, paradoxical
	exitation in some, tolerance and sleep pattern
	abberations in all.
Antihistamines	
(Benadryl, Atarax, Vistaril)	May be useful for intercurrent prn use for sedation
Dimetane	and hypnotic effect. Beware anticholinergic and
(Chlor-Trimeton)	tolerance effect with long-term use.
Meprobamate	No better than placebo with narrow therapeutic index.
(Equanil, Miltown)	Continual use not recommended.
Benzodiazepines (BZs)	Prolonged half-lives and cumulation of all BZ's
(Librium, Valium,	reported with all except Ativan and Serax.
Tranxene, Vestran, Ativan,	Prolonged daily sedative (1–3 months) or hypnotic
Serax and Dalmane)	(7–14 days) use not recommended due to
	depression of normal sleep pattern and resultant
	confusion, delirium and psychologic changes. Serax

Analgesics	Special Consideration
	best choice due to short half-life. No hypnotic should be used nightly longer than 14 days. Skip a night to every third night.
Chloral hydrate (Somnos, Noctec)	Excellent hypnotic in absence of liver disease.
Nonbarbiturate hypnotics (Valmid, Qualude, Noludar, Doriden, Placidyl)	None recommended due to same types of problems as in barbiturates.
Major Tranquilizers—antipsychotic agents	(Use lowest dose possible and titrate approximately)
Phenothiazines (Mellaril, Slelazine, Vesprin, Prolixin)	Increased incidence of extrapyramidal symptoms (EPS) in elderly. Postural (orthostatic) hypotension a problem. Temperature control and tardive dyskinesia more common with higher doses.
Butyrophenone (Haldol)	Highest incidence of EPS.
Thioxanthenes (Navane)	Potent antipsychotic with low order of side effects.
Antiparkinsonian agent (Artane, Kemadrin, Cogentin) Benadryl	Prophylactic use with antipsychotic agents generally not recommended. When EPS appear, 1–3 month use may be beneficial. Watch for constipation, tremors, delirium on prolonged use, especially with Cogentin.
Carbidopa-levodopa (Sinimet)	Generally better tolerated than levodopa alone with less side effects. (Hypotension, syncope, anorexia, nausea, emesis.)
Antidepressants	(Useful only in endogenous depression in up to 1/2 usual dosages.)
Elavil, Aventyl, Tofranil, Pertofrane, Vivactyl, Sinequan	Can exacerbate tremors, psychosis, constipation, postural hypotension, BPH, delayed micturation, and arrhythmias). Prolonged half-life, caution in full-dose bedtime use especially with Elavil and Tofranil.
Monoamine oxidase inhibitors	Not recommended in elderly.
Antibiotics Penicillins, erythromycins and cephalosporins	Generally same type of problems as younger patients.
Aminoglycosides Kantrex, Garamycin Nebcin, Amikin	Must be dosed on lean body weight and creatinine clearance to prevent oto- and nephrotoxicity.
Tetracyclines Vibramycin, Minocin Aureomycin, Terramycin Rondomycin, Tetracycline	Caution in doses with renal and/or hepatic impairment. Oral dosage form must be given with full glass of fluids to prevent esophageal or stomach irritation.
Clinamycin (Cleocin)	Incidence of diarrhea and pseudomembranous coloitis increase with age.
Chloramphenicol (Chlormycetin)	Hematologic toxicity more likely in elderly with impaired hepatic function.

(continued on next page)

Table 6-3 (*continued*)

Analgesics	Special Consideration
Nitrofuration (Furadantin, Macrodantin)	Useful only in chronic lower UTIs. Caution in CrCl less than 40 cc/min, (as increased hematologic and pulmonary reactions possible). Must be given with meals or antacid.
Methenamine complexes (Mandelamine, Hiprex)	Not rational in catheterized patients as only active in bladder urine.
Sulfonamides (Gantrisin)	Prolonged half-life reported. Adequate hydration essential.
Isoniazid (INH)	Liver toxicity more common in those over 50.
Laxative usage	Avoid mineral oil due to lipid aspiration and pneumonitis possibility. Regular use of irritant (Dulcolax, Ex-Lax, Modane) or saline (MOM, Epsom Salts) should be discouraged due to laxative habit. Stool softeners (Colace, Surfak) and bulk laxatives (Psyllium as Metamucil, Silac, Effersyl or Konsyl) produce most "physiologic" stool. Bulk type may be of benefit in chronic diarrhea. Take careful drug history in history of chronic constipation.
Vitamin–hematinic usage	Vitamin supplements may be of benefit, especially where diets may be marginal. Anemia should always be carefully evaluated prior to hematopoietic therapy initiation.

Adapted from Holloway DA: Drug problems in the geriatric patient. Drug Intell Cl Pharm 11:597–603, 1977; Wallace DE, Watanabe AS: Drug effects in geriatric patients. Drug Intell Cl Pharm 8:632–640, 1974; O'Malley K, Judge TG, Crooks J: Geriatric clinical pharmacology and therapeutics, in Avery GS: Drug Treatment. Sydney, ADIS Press, 1976, pp 124–142; Stanaszek W: The hospital pharmacist and the geriatric patient. Hosp Form Mgt 9:18–24, 1974; Solomon F et al: Sleeping pills insomnia and medical practice. N Engl J Med, 300:803–808, 1979; American Hospital Formulary Service: American Society of Hospital Pharmacists, 4630 Montgomery Avenue NW, Washington, DC.

Each elder should be approached as a unique individual and a correct diagnosis made for each problem. The drug prescribed or recommended should have a readily definable endpoint of effect (beneficial–toxic) that should be reached within a specified period of time. Review of the *total* patient-problem list every time a new drug is added can reduce unnecessary therapy. An example would be to keep in mind the fact that diphenhydramine (Benadryl) is not only an antihistamine but also has antiemetic, anticholinergic, antitussive, and sedative properties that make it useful on an intermittent basis for a number of symptomatic complaints of the elderly. Always look at the patient-problem and drug list and ask, "Would removing a drug benefit the patient more than adding a drug," or, "Could this problem/complaint be caused by a drug(s) the patient is taking." Some eminent geriatricians feel that the elder is best managed with five or fewer chronic-use drugs, so we will always encourage trying to taper the patient to this "magic number." Several reasons are given for this: cost, rationality, and the fact that, as the number of medications per patient exceeds this number, the likelihood of poor compliance and adverse reaction increases in *geometric* (not arithmetic) fashion.

DRUG HISTORY

Guidelines for taking and maintaining good drug histories includes an updated drug list, good history technique, and frequent reevaluation.

On first and subsequent visits the drug history

must be gained and updated, especially if the patient is seeing multiple prescribers. The medication survey instrument in Fig. 6-1 can aid in this process. It is essential to determine compliance between visits. Calling the pharmacist to confirm refill dates is an excellent method for determining both refill patterns and other drugs the patient may have obtained from other prescribers. Dosage form counts and prodding (e.g., "We all miss doses from time to time, how many times per week or month do you miss?"), as well as open-ended questions (e.g., "How have you been doing" or "taking your medication?"), may be necessary to gain an accurate history. This is especially important in chronic disease states where compliance is known to be a problem—hypertension, congestive heart failure, chronic lung disease, and peptic ulcer disease.

Never overlook what "remedies" (folk medicine or over-the-counter drugs) the patient is taking. Most elders regard these as beneficial. A sensitive and sincere approach to their perceptions may gain a wealth of knowledge helpful to total patient management. Many patients have "tried-and-true" remedies passed down through their families and friends that may or may not be regarded as "drugs or medicines." A careful history emphasizing "all remedies, potions, medications, cures, tonics, and relievers" may help to reveal some of these agents. There are potential drug interactions between these medications. The greatest danger in folk-medicine practice, however, is probably the delay in obtaining scientifically sound treatment of the valid problems of the patient.

The clinician should keep alert to symptoms of adverse reactions. Most inpatient adverse reactions consist of functional GI disturbances (nausea, vomiting, and diarrhea), which, together with sensitivity reactions (rash, itching, and fever), account for up to 70 percent of symptoms in adverse reactions. More serious reactions do occur with drugs known to be toxic to bone marrow, kidney, or liver. On the other hand, one study of healthy persons on medi-

Fig. 6-1.
Drug survey instrument

Health Care
Facility _____

Patient's Name _____
Physician(s) _____

TO: The Patient or Your Family

MEDICATION SURVEY

1.   The purpose of this survey is to gather as much data as we possibly can concerning the medications you have taken over the past several months. This information will be tabulated and communicated to your physician so that a complete picture of your medication history will be available to him or her.

All data furnished is solely hospital or nursing home property and will be treated with strict confidentiality. Please provide as much information as you can.

2.   Please list the names and addresses of pharmacies or drug stores where you have had prescriptions filled in the last six months:

NAME   ADDRESS

_____   _____
_____   _____
_____   _____
_____   _____

3.   Please list the names of all doctors, dentists, podiatrists, or other persons whom you have seen for health needs in the past six months.

_____   _____
_____   _____
_____   _____

4.   Please list the medications, both prescription·and nonprescription, that you have been taking over the last (year, month). If you do not know the name of the medications, please list the prescription number and pharmacy where obtained, and give the best physical description of the drug (color, size, shape, etc.). If possible, please bring in all your current medications for identification. They will be returned to you after they have been identified.

The following list may help you to remember some of the medications, drugs or patent medicine, or "cures" you have taken. Please give as much information as possible. Thank you.

Have you, in the last 6 months, taken or been advised to take any of the following for:

(continued on next page)

Fig. 6-1.
Drug survey instrument (*continued*)

	Symptoms		Drugs	How long (days, weeks, months)

4.1   "Irregularity"   ——— Milk of Magnesia
      "Constipation"   ——— Ex-Lax, Dulcolax
                          ——— Mineral Oil, Haley's MO
                          Other _____

4.2   "Diarrhea"   ——— Kaopectate, Pepto-Bismol
      "Runny Stools"   ——— Donnagel, Lactinex, Lomotil
                          Paregoric

4.3   "Upset Stomach"   ——— Alka-Seltzer, Bromo-Seltzer
      "Ulcer Medication" ——— Baking Soda
                          ——— Tums, Rolaids
                          ——— Gelusil, Maalox, Mylanta
                          Other _____

4.4   Aches and pains   ——— Aspirin, Anacin, Empirin
      "Headaches"   ——— Bufferin, BC Powders
      "Arthritic and   ——— Codeine, Darvon, Demerol
        rheumatic pain"   Decadron, Cortisone,
                          Prednisone
                          ——— Other _____

4.5   Eye preparations   ——— Phospholine-Iodide, Timoptic
      "Glaucoma"   ——— Humersol, Isopto-Carpine
      "Red, irritated   ——— Visine, Pilocarpine
        eyes"   Other _____

4.6   Ear preparations   ——— Auralgan, Debrox
                          ——— Other _____

4.7   Colds   ——— Antihistamines
      Hayfever   ——— Aspirin, Tylenol
      Stuffy nose   ——— Neo-Synephrine, Afrin
                          ——— Cold Tablets, Contac
                          ——— Cough Syrup, Nyquil
                          Other _____

4.8   Birth Control   ——— Oral contraceptives
      Hormones   ——— Estrogens, Premarin
      GYN "the pill"   ——— Other _____

4.9   "Heart medications" ——— Digitalis
                          ——— Nitroglycerin, Nitrol
                          ——— Quinidine, Pronestyl
                          ——— Other _____

4.10 "High blood   ——— Diuril (Water Pill)
        pressure"   ——— Reserpine, Ser-Ap-Es
      "Water pills"   ——— Aldomet, Minipres
      "Potassium"   ——— Esimil, Lopressor
                          ——— Catapres, Inderal
                          ——— Kaochlor
                          Klorvess
                          Slow-K, Kaon-Cl

4.11 Asthma, bronchitis ——— Tedral, Amesec, Bronkotabs
      Emphysema   ——— Prednisone
                          ——— Isuprel Aerosol, Metaprel
                          ——— Epinephrine Aerosol
                          ——— Decadron, Cortisone
                          Other _____

4.12 "Nerve pills"   ——— Librium, Thorazine, Serax
                          ——— Valium, Mellaril, Ativan
                          Meprobamate (Miltown,
                             (Equanil)
                          ——— Other _____

4.13 Insomnia   ——— Sominex, Nytol, Dalmane
                          ——— Seconal, Doriden, Quaalude
                          ——— Nembutal, Noludar, Noctec
                          ——— Chloral Hydrate
                          Other _____

4.14 Antibiotics   ——— Penicillin
      "Infections"   ——— Tetracycline
                          ——— Erythromycin
                          ——— Sulfa, Septra
                          Other _____

4.15	Blood clotting "Blood thinners" "Anticoagulants"	___ Coumadir. ___ Heparin ___ Other _____	
4.16	"Blood builders" Anemia drugs	___ Iron tablets, Geritol ___ Fem-Iron ___ Folic Acid ___ B_{12} Shots ___ Vitamins ___ Other _____	
4.17	Diabetes	___ Insulin ___ Orinase ___ Diabinese, Thyroid ___ Other _____	
4.18	Hemorrhoids	___ Anusol ___ Preparation H ___ Medicine, Tucks ___ Other _____	
4.19	Skin Conditions—dry eczema, psoriasis athletes foot, corns dandruff, infections	___ Neosporin ___ Tegrin, Mazon ___ Keri, VioForm ___ Other _____	
4.20	Other Conditions		

5. Do you or have you ever had:

5.1 Any problems with drugs? ____Yes ____No (Please list)

_____

_____

5.2 Any allergies to foods, drugs, pets, environment? ____Yes ____No

5.3 A family history of allergy? ____Yes ____No

5.4 A drug discontinued because of: rash, itching, nausea, vomiting?
____Yes ____No

5.5 Difficulty in swallowing tablets or capsules? ____Yes ____No

5.6 Or been told that you've had a reaction to a drug, shot, or medicine?
____Yes ____No

5.7 Have you been in a hospital in the last year? ____Yes ____No

If yes, which hospital _____

6. Please return this form to your health care practitioner as soon as possible.

cations found that 81 percent had symptoms that might be considered to represent adverse reactions. Similar findings were reported in 58 percent of healthy volunteers taking placebos.[19]

The older patient taking drugs, who complains of symptoms, should be taken seriously until thorough evaluation of the problem has been completed. Several studies have shown clinicians to be reluctant to believe that their drug therapy may have compounded the patient's problems.

The most common potential adverse drug interactions found in a nursing home have been described.[10] The most significant drug interactions involving older patients seem to involve digitalis with diuretics, anticoagulants, anti-infectives, and multiple CNS depressant and anticholinergic use. A paradoxical finding in one study of elderly patients is that more neuroactive CNS depressants (analgesics, major tranquilizers, and sedative–hypnotics)

were prescribed for those patients with superior mentation and minimal physical disability; that is, the least mentally impaired were the most heavily drugged or chemically restrained.[11] There are manual systems for detecting potentially significant interactions.[20]

PATIENT ERRORS, COMPLIANCE, AND EDUCATION

Elders have difficulties with drugs because of factors that relate to both the prescriber and patient. Assuming that a rational approach to drug therapy is undertaken, the prescriber must then turn to patient knowledge and capability to follow the therapeutic plan.

PERSONAL DRUG INFORMATION CHECKLIST

Patient's name ——————————

Date ——————————————

Pharmacist ————————————

Pharmacy —————————————

Pharmacy telephone ———————

Physician ——————————————

Physician's telephone ——————

To the pharmacist: Use this form in counseling the patient about his or her medications.
To the patient: Use this form to assist in asking for information about your medications.

Prescription No. ————————————

Name of drug ————————————

Purpose for
taking this drug is ————————

Prescription can be renewed ————
times
Take ——————— every ————
(Amount)   (How Often)

By ——————— for ————
(Route or Method)   (How Long)

Circle hours the drug is to be taken.

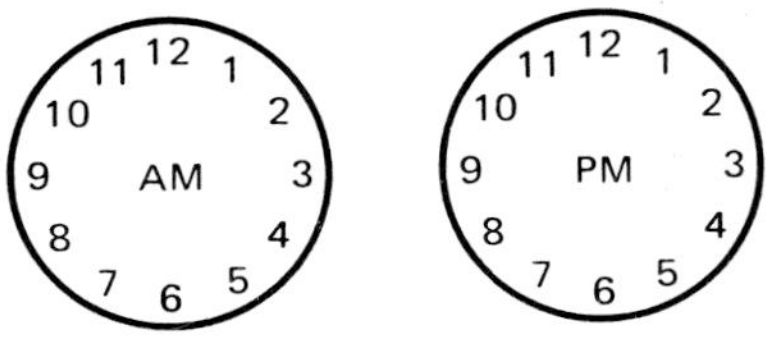

[Clock face: AM — 12 1 2 3 4 5 6 7 8 9 10 11] [Clock face: PM — 12 1 2 3 4 5 6 7 8 9 10 11]

Physical description of the drug —————

This drug should
not be taken with ————————

This drug
should be taken with ————————

Possible side effects ————————

Contact your physician or
pharmacist if the following side effects occur ——

Special instructions ————————

Prescription No. ————————————

Name of drug ————————————

Purpose for
taking this drug is ————————

Prescription can be renewed ————
times
Take ——————— every ————
(Amount)   (How Often)

By ——————— for ————
(Route or Method)   (How Long)

Circle hours the drug is to be taken.

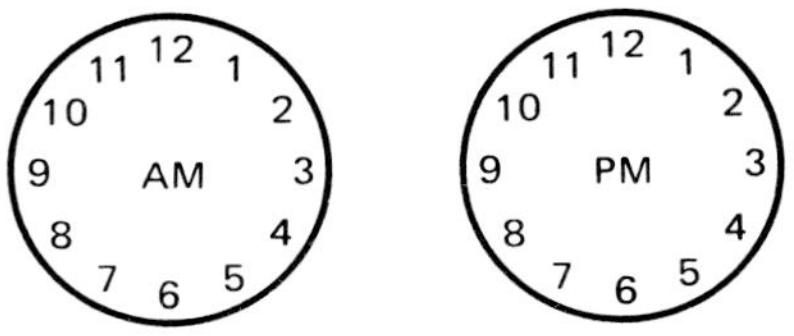

[Clock face: AM — 12 1 2 3 4 5 6 7 8 9 10 11] [Clock face: PM — 12 1 2 3 4 5 6 7 8 9 10 11]

Physical description of the drug —————

This drug should
not be taken with ————————

This drug
should be taken with ————————

Possible side effects ————————

Contact your physician or
pharmacist if the following side effects occur ——

Special instructions ————————

Fig. 6-2. Personal drug information checklist

(Front Side)

DRUG ALERT CARD ————————————

Patient name ——————————————————

Home address ——————————————————

Business address —————————————————

Home telephone —————————————————

Business telephone ————————————————

Home telephone —————————————————

Business telephone ————————————————

In case of emergency notify:(NAME) ——————————— (PHONE) ——————————

PATIENT PHYSICAL DATA

Height———————————— Weight———————— Birthdate—————————

Special Problems:

——————— Hearing ————————Vision ————————Speech ————————Internal organ

————————Other (explain): ————————————————

(Reverse Side)

R_x
Drug   MEDICATIONS
                                        Pharmacy/Dr.   Directions
——————————————————————————————————
——————————————————————————————————
——————————————————————————————————

OTCS ——————————————————————————

Allergies (food, drugs) ——————————————————

Immunizations
——————— Tetanus ———————— Flu ———————— Other
——————— Date ———————— Date ———————— Date

Fig. 6-3 Drug Alert Card

Table 6-4

A 16-Point Health Team Approach to Elder Patient Education

The geriatric patient should:

1. Understand why he or she is taking the medication and why the drug is needed. Patients tend to comply with the physician's instructions more closely if they understand the reason for taking the medication.

2. Understand the dosing schedule, so the medications will be taken on time and properly sequenced. Doses should be keyed to activities of daily living (brushing teeth, meals, bedtime).

3. Get medication refilled on time, so therapy will not be interrupted.

4. Know that there may be some side effects caused by drugs and understand the relative importance of these effects. This is to prevent unnecessary concern over minor side effects and to prevent unwarranted discontinuance of the drug because of these effects.

5. Know any special storage requirements for the drug (e.g., refrigeration, etc.) to prevent deterioration of the drug. Never store drugs in bathroom medicine cabinet due to high humidity.

6. Know any special directions for using the drug (i.e., Can it be taken with food or milk? Will it increase the skin's sensitivity to sunlight?) to promote safe and effective utilization of drugs by the patient.

7. Have the ability to monitor his or her own therapy including the reporting of any untoward or suspicious effects to guard against drug-induced disease, allergy and to ascertain that the drug is doing what it was intended to do.

8. Understand that the prescription is tailored for one person only and should, therefore, not be shared or offered to friends to prevent abuse and misuse of prescription drugs and prevent possibly fatal or serious accidents.

9. Know that the pharmacist can give useful advice about nonprescription and prescription medication. This is a readily available but underused resource for the geriatric patient to help in preventing drug interactions and the irrational use of medications.

10. Know that all health care practitioners need to know and *care* about the drug(s) being taken.

11. Know that easy-to-open closures on prescription bottles are available for the asking to avoid the frustrations of opening safety caps.

12. Be able to develop a medication calendar to aid in proper dosing, an important aid-to-memory for patients on multiple medications.

13. Have respect for medications. Drugs are effective when used properly but dangerous when misused.

14. Prepare and carry a wallet drug profile card on which the following information would be printed. See Fig. 6-3.

15. Know that many over-the-counter drug products should not be used by the elderly and/or may interfere with the action of some prescription drugs. This is to avoid unexpected drug-induced problems and to assure the proper action of prescribed drugs.

16. Should have special labels for impaired vision.

Patient errors of commission and/or omission in the self-administration of drugs in ambulatory elderly patients are common.[16,21] One report found that 59 percent of an elderly outpatient population with chronic illnesses made errors in the self-administration of prescribed medications and more than 25 percent committed potentially serious errors.[22] In another study of ambulatory patients who self-administered drugs in a skilled nursing facility (SNF) and in a hospital, a 60 percent error rate was seen in those who received drugs without instructions, whereas only 2.3 percent error rate was seen in instructed patients.[23]

The need for supervision of the elderly patients receiving long-term drug therapy was recently re-emphasized in a study in which 20 percent of randomly selected elder patients taking medications had no recorded contact with their physician for six months or longer.[24] Another survey[8] of elderly patients (conducted in their homes) found that many stored their drugs improperly, tended to hoard drugs, and did not have enough explicit instructions regarding indications for taking the drugs. In the study of drug-related problems[9] influencing the need for admission, lack of patients' knowledge of cations found that 81 percent had symptoms that might be considered to represent adverse reactions. Similar findings were reported in 58 percent of healthy volunteers taking placebos.[19]

In the elderly patient who has a number of needed medications and has impaired memory or thought processes, the clinician should be willing to help ensure proper drug usage by continuously reinforcing instructions verbally and with drug profile and memory aids such as those found in Figs. 6-2 and 6-3.

Discussion of pertinent instructions with the patient is essential in order to insure success of such patient education. The simple question, "What do you know about the use of this medication?" often helps reinforce this information. Table 6-4 presents a guideline for clinicians.

REFERENCES

1. Miller DB, Lowenstein R, Winston R: Physicians attitudes toward the ill aged and nursing homes. J Am Ger Soc 24:498, 1976
2. Rabin DL: Use of medicine, USPHSDEW Pub, HSM-73-3012, 1972
3. Long-Term Care Facility Improvement Study, USPHSDEW-Office of Nursing Home Affairs, Stock No 017-001-00397-2, 1974
4. Laventurier MF, Talley RB: The incidence of drug-drug interactions in a medi-cal population. Calif Pharm 20:18, 1977
5. Law R, Chalmers C: Medicines and elderly people: A general practice survey. Bri Med J 1:565, 1976
6. Bergman HD: Prescribing of drugs in a nursing home. Drug Intell Cl Pharm 9:365–368, 1975
7. Melmon KI: Preventable drug reactions. New Engl J Med 284:1261–1270, 1971
8. Hurwitz N: Adverse drug reactions and hospitalization. Bri Med J i:539–540, 1969
9. Frisk P: Patient profiles link community and hospital practice. Masters' thesis, University of Rhode Island, 1975
10. Cooper JW et al: A seven nursing home study of potential drug interactions. JAPhA NS:15–24, 1975
11. Ingman SR et al: A survey of the prescribing and administration of drugs in a long-term care facility for the elderly. J Am Ger Soc 23:309–314, 1975
12. Miller MB, Elliott DF: Errors and omissions in diagnostic records on admission of patients to a nursing home. J Am Ger Soc 25:108–112, 1977
13. Hoyumpa AM: Disposition and elimination of minor tranquilizers in the aged and patients with liver disease. Sou Med J 71:23–28, 1978
14. Jeliffew RW: Creatinine clearance: Bedside estimate. Ann Int Med 79:604–605, 1973
15. Bennett W, Singer MD, Coggins CH: A practical guide to drug usage in adult patients with impaired renal function. JAMA 214:1468–1475, 1970; 233:991–997, 1973
16. Hayflick L: The cell biology of human aging. New Engl J Med 295:1302–1308, 1976
17. Caird FI, Andrews GR, Kennedy RD: Effect of posture on blood pressures in the elderly. Br Heart J 35:327, 1973
18. Exton-Smith AN: Accidental hypothermia. Bri Med J 4:727, 1973
19. Cooper JW: Implications of drug reactions-recognitions, incidence and prevention. RI Med J 59:274–280, 1975
20. Fish KH, Cooper JW: A manual system for drug-drug interaction detection. JAPhA, NS:15 28–31, 1975

21. Stewart RB, Cluff LE: A review of medication errors and compliance in ambulant patients. Cl Pharmacol Ther 13:463–470, 1972

22. Schwartz D et al: Medication errors made by the elderly chronically ill patient. Am J Pub Health 52:2018–2027, 1962

23. Libow LS, Mehl B: Self administration of medications by patients in hospitals or extended care facilities. J Am Ger Soc 18:81–84, 1970

24. Shaw SM, Opit LJ: Need for supervision in the elderly receiving long-term prescribed medication. Bri Med J 1:507–508, 1976

7

Psychological Changes

Berthold E. Umland, M.D.
Darlene Jelinek, R.N., F.N.P.
John Santos, Ph.D.

There has been a steady growth in the theory and practice of psychological/psychiatric treatment of the elderly. This chapter emphasizes the importance of active management of psychological problems and the capacity for renewal and restoration of mental health with proper treatment. It also emphasizes the need to avoid the sharp conceptual dichotomy between mind and body, which is so thoroughly ingrained in our culture and professions influencing our diagnosis and treatment of aged and other patients.

Psychological aspects of aging are being viewed less in terms of an "inevitable process of decline" and more from the perspective of emerging and elicited changes across the entire life span. Coping mechanisms used in the past can provide valuable clues to the problems and functioning in old age. Personality traits that were effective during the younger years may be maladaptive when they are not counterbalanced by other characteristics and new coping mechanisms in the elderly. A very aggressive approach to life's problems may make an individual successful in the working world but may cause unnecessary problems in the day-to-day life of a "retirement home."

There may, however, be potential advantages even to abrasive personality styles as suggested in the delightful report by Morton Lieberman on "Grouchiness: A Survival Asset."[1] Based on a number of investigations, he proposes that:

… the most important characteristic of the aged and their ability to adapt to crisis is a personality quality that is almost the polar opposite of the gracious elderly. Those who were aggressive, irritating, narcissistic, demanding, were the individuals … most likely to survive major life crises intact. They certainly were not the most likable elderly. Being a good guy—passive acceptance—were qualities … found in people most likely *not* to survive.

Thus, he suggests that "growing old gracefully may be an invention of poets rather than an adequate guide to survival." Needless to say, Lieberman's observations provide some important clues and thoughts for all service providers who must deal with the elderly and particularly those "survivors" that he describes with an almost grudging admiration.

Regardless of popular misconceptions, most do not see themselves as living in their "golden years" after the age of 65. They remember and value their past achievements. When they become restive or aggressive about current failures and limitations, the health care provider has an obligation to respect the feelings of the older person and not acquiesce to demands of the "custodians" to prescribe inappropriate sedatives or tranquilizers to make them more "manageable." The needs and best interests of the elder must always come first.

INCIDENCE OF PSYCHOLOGICAL PROBLEMS IN THE ELDERLY

For a variety of reasons, the mental health needs of the aging and the aged continue to remain largely ignored. In addition to the predictable physical and social losses that the individual experiences with time, there are additional problems and burdens bred by prejudice, isolation, and societal ignorance regarding the process of aging. Facts such as the following cannot be ignored:

- Mental illness appears to be more prevalent among elders than in younger adults; even conservative estimates suggest that 15–25 percent of elders have significant symptoms of mental illness.[2,3]
- Psychopathology of various types increase with age. There are 2.3 new cases per 100,000 of serious psychiatric disorders under age 15, but over age 65 the number rises to 236.1 per 100,000.[4]
- The incidence of depression for those over 65+ living in the community is in the range of 10 percent.[5]
- While persons over 65 represent only 10 percent of our population, they account for just slightly less than 20 percent of the nation's reported suicides.[6]
- Organic brain syndromes, in mild and severe forms, affect three million elderly. The prevalence of these disorders increases with age.[7]

Elders are subject to multiple life stresses which contribute to their emotional problems:

- 86 percent (more than 18 million) have chronic health problems.[8]
- Decreased mobility leads to reduced social interaction.[8]
- Multiple personal losses exist for the 50 percent of women who by age 65 are widowed and for 70 percent of those who by age 75 have lost their spouses.[9]

Responses in the form of programs from government and private agencies to urgent needs and problems of the elderly have been inadequate:

- Access to outpatient care services is limited. Only 4 percent of persons seen at community mental health centers are over 65, and this drops to 2 percent in private practice.[10,11]
- Adequate institutional care is also lacking. Approximately 50–70 percent of nursing home residents have been estimated to have symptoms of mental illness but few mental health professionals are available to assist these patients.[12]
- "Deinstitutionalization" of the nation's mental hospitals has resulted in an extensive relocation to nursing homes with less adequate treatment for most of the elderly involved.[13,14]

COMMON PSYCHOLOGICAL PROBLEMS

Elders tend to have virtually all of the functional psychological disorders that appear in younger age groups with some of these problems occurring in greater frequency at the older age levels. Depression and paranoia are more commonly diagnosed in elderly patients, although classic bipolar depression (manic-depressive psychosis) is seldom seen in the aged.

Hypochondriasis and other preoccupations with the body and its functions are more prevalent. According to Butler and Lewis[17] and others, schizophrenia seldom has its initial onset in old age, although persons with this disorder may live to be old. Misuse and abuse of prescription and nonprescription drugs is very common though not always intentional.

STRESS

Many of the common mental problems of the elderly are related to the life stresses connected with growing old. Changes in lifestyle with concomitant losses and attendant grief states may precipitate debilitating emotional states or reactions, such as: grief, guilt, loneliness, depression, anxiety, rage, and a sense of impotence and helplessness.

In dealing with such powerful emotions, the elder will often revert to coping mechanisms that have been developed and strongly established over a lifetime. Adaptive techniques common among elder people are: denial, humor, projection, fixation, regression, displacement, idealization, rigidity, and selective memory.

Obviously at certain times and under certain circumstances these mechanisms, if taken to extremes, may be more maladaptive than adaptive.

Clinical Presentations

The following may be seen as clinical indicators of stress and therefore are cues to potential psychological problems in the elderly.

1. Alterations of homeostasis: Change in circumstances (financial, marital, living arrangements); death or impending death of a loved one or an anniversary of such a death; and new serious medical diagnoses or exacerbation of chronic symptoms.

2. Symptoms caused by or aggravated by stress: Insomnia–hypersomnia; malaise; anorexia–weight loss; vague, poorly defined pain; and loss of ability to concentrate.
3. Signs of loss of coping ability: Seeking more medical attention for trivial complaints; poor compliance with previously established medical therapies; requests for excessive or inappropriate psychoactive drugs; and confusion and disorientation.

When clinical intuition and clues in the patient's manner and behavior suggest that stress and its psychological consequences are a major problem, the elder may better be served by talking than by carrying out an exhaustive physical examination and laboratory work-up. (See Table 7-1.)

Management of Stress-related Problems

The patient should be told when psychological stress appears to be causally related to the symptoms or illness for which the patient is being evaluated. Virtually everyone understands that some symptoms can be caused by stress and that all symptoms may be worsened by stress. Whether or not the stress is the obvious cause, it must be considered. The patient must be made to recognize that he or she is not being told that "it's all in your head" and therefore of no consequence.

Once the causes or conditions producing the stress are identified, every effort should be made to alleviate or eliminate them. This often requires an interdisciplinary management of medical, psychological, and environmental factors. For example, when an elderly woman develops severe muscle tension headaches that appear to be related to

Table 7-1
Questions to Identify Stress Situations in Elders

Ask about:
1. Recent changes in life situations: retirement, divorce, decrease in income, moving from the family home, loss of independence
2. Death of significant others: spouse, child, friend
3. Chronic changes of mood: feeling "blue," feeling angry or frustrated
4. Sleep patterns: less than usual, more than usual, early morning awakening
5. Inability to make decisions
6. Inability to see options available

difficulties in managing her invalid husband, it will probably be ineffective simply to prescribe analgesics or to tell her to relax. More likely she will need appropriate psychosocial support and active intervention.

It should also be remembered that diagnostic interventions can be as (or more) stressful than the disease itself. Older persons should be spared exposure to unnecessarily traumatic or invasive procedures. When this is not feasible, they should be informed of the likely discomforts and told of the results as soon as possible.

PROBLEMS COMMONLY MISDIAGNOSED OR OVERLOOKED

Due to the multiplicity of symptoms and alterations of response patterns in the aged, a number of conditions require special diagnostic evaluation. The following conditions are treatable and are commonly overlooked[4]:

1. Reversible brain syndromes that occur alone or are superimposed upon chronic brain syndromes. (See Chapter 9.)
2. Drug reactions. (See Chapter 6.)
3. Depressive reactions simulating organic brain disorders.
4. Paranoid states without organic brain disease: generalized or circumscribed; chronic paranoid state with reversible crisis.
5. Subdural hematomas. (See Chapter 9.)

GUIDELINES FOR CLINICAL EVALUATION

The vast majority of people try to take care of their problems by themselves before they seek professional help. When individuals do seek assistance, it is important to look for precipitating event(s) that overcame the individual's or the family's ability to cope and that caused them to look to outside help. The primary care clinician can play a key role in assisting the elder and family in sorting out the sources of stress and in helping to alleviate them.

Collecting the Data

It would seem to be elaborating the obvious to point out that if the clinician does not ask about psychological health or dysfunction, or at least maintain an openness to discuss this area, nothing will be learned. Unfortunately, all too often during a "routine office visit," blood pressure is measured and discussed or an arthritic joint is examined and treated, but no concern is shown for the overall functioning of the individual in his or her life situation. Though it would be convenient if patients would announce at the outset of an office visit that "I am having a pathological grief reaction to the death of my spouse" or "my paranoid ideation is getting out of hand," this is unlikely.

The necessity of using open-ended questions to elicit information and evoke reactions pertaining to highly charged emotional problems cannot be overemphasized. The following questions are suggested as examples of statements that may be effective in letting the patient know that you are interested in more than the blood pressure or the sore joint:

- How are things going for you at home since you retired?
- Can you tell me more about how your (medical diagnosis) affects your daily living?
- Do you have any concerns about your health that we haven't been able to talk about before?

Responses to these questions may be monosyllables ("fine" or "not at all") that effectively close the discussion, but the interviewer must also be aware of nonverbal cues, such as foot or finger tapping, facial gestures or whole body posture, which suggest that there really is concern about some problem. It must also be kept in mind that the older client may also react to nonverbal cues from the clinician, so care must be taken to insure that interest in these areas are not feigned. Probing questions should not be asked while flipping through lab reports if a reasonable answer is to be expected. Such questions should be given when the clinician is prepared and able to listen. In general, the quality of the patient–clinician relationship should determine whether or not it is safe to pursue the subtle cues that may trigger intuition about problem areas without making the patient hostile. The quality of this relationship with the patient is or can be a most important therapeutic tool.

Patient Counseling

The following are some of the common problems for which the health care professional can offer important therapeutic intervention[15]:

- Adjustments to sensory changes
- Maintaining orientation for time and place
- Development and maintenance of communication skills
- Promoting self-knowledge and understanding of aging
- Developing satisfaction with the present life situation
- Suggestions relating to the enrichment of social life

Approaches and Pitfalls

In expanding the therapeutic relationship with older patients, some simple approaches may provide considerable advantages[16]:

- *Make yourself "gently" available.* Older persons generally respond well to clinicians who make themselves "gently" available—giving the elder and other family members time to talk—and who hear the whole story.
- *Be compassionately realistic.* Encouraging overly optimistic expectations often inhibits the expression of the patient's real feelings and sets the stage for frustration and failure.
- *Taking care of yourself.* Avoid the trap of replying to "What do you suggest . . . ?" with specific answers. Encourage the elder and those that make up the significant members of his or her support system to develop their own plan.
- *Take one problem at a time.* Hear out the entire list of problems, then choose one to focus on. See Herr and Weakland[16] for further suggestions.

Family Involvement

Research indicates that most elders are not alienated from their families: Therefore, it will often be the case that any problem involving an older person will also have an impact on his or her family. Family research has identified the impact of an elder's problems on the entire family network. On the other hand, an elderly patient may simply be reflecting what may be a family-wide pathology. Important issues in family therapy may include decisions about institutionalizing the older person, feelings of guilt and abandonment, old family conflicts, and the need for continuous care.[17]

The family's well-being is often central to the concerns and well-being of the older patient. A family that provides ongoing care for the elderly parent or relative is often in need of "respite" services. This may involve help from friends or obtaining help from a service agency to care for the patient in the home so the family can be free on weekends and vacations. In particularly stressful times, it should be possible to admit the frail older person into an institution for a brief stay to give the family an opportunity to rest and recover. These respite services, which are based on English models, are not yet fully developed or generally available in most locations in the United States.[17]

The Role of the Health Care Professional

It is incumbent upon the primary care provider to recognize the early signs of psychological problems. Being aware that an aged person who has sustained the loss of a loved one and who is likely to develop a severe depressive reaction may, for instance, help to avert suicide. Knowing that an elder, recently admitted to a nursing home because of physical infirmity, will probably feel isolated and dependent should help us in making efforts to forestall withdrawal and even avoid psychotic reactions in some cases. Asking the older man with a fragile sense of self-esteem if his antihypertensive medication has compromised his sexual potency may help to save a marital relationship.

Education of elders, along with their families and/or caretakers, regarding the early signs of psychological dysfunction will certainly make possible earlier intervention. An explanation of potential adverse side effects of newly prescribed medication before it is taken may prevent patients from developing the anxiety that they are "losing their minds." Finally, it must be kept in mind that strange behavior in an elderly person does not necessarily reflect irreversible brain damage or senility, and the family must be informed and reassured about this.

AFFECTIVE DISORDERS (DEPRESSION/MANIA)

Many common psychological disorders have as their principal manifestation a disturbance in mood, either in the direction of depression or, more rarely, in the direction of elation. Even in a relatively healthy population of elders living in the community, depressive episodes lasting from a few hours to a few days is common. The prevalence of such reactions in old age is not surprising in view of the many losses, traumas, and stresses that often are experienced during this phase of the life span. Also of particular importance is the fact that these devastating events often occur at a time when physical, psychological, social, and even financial resources are wanting. This may predispose to feelings of helplessness and hopelessness that tend to facilitate depressive reactions.

The Relationship Between Physical Illness and Depression

Loss of physical ability may be closely related to certain depressive reactions in the aged. It has been shown that elders can tolerate the loss of loved ones and prestige better than the decline in their own physical health.[16] When a new and particularly anxiety-producing medical diagnosis is made and the facts are communicated, it is wise to be alert for clues of possible episodes of depression that may follow.

The Path to Depression

The clinical manifestations of depression may vary a great deal. There is often a group of psychological symptoms that manifest themselves with the usual individual variations.[18] These include:

- Abject and painful sadness—"I feel so low and sad all the time"
- Generalized withdrawal—"He or she wants to sleep all the time and won't eat"
- Pervasive pessimism—"Nothing is ever going to go right again"
- Lowered self-esteem—"I'm just not worth anything anymore"

The physiological aspects of depression may be manifested in the following symptoms:

- Sleeplessness
- Loss of appetite/weight loss
- Fatigue
- Constipation or diarrhea
- Psychomotor retardation
- Agitation
- Daily repeated mood swings

Many older individuals consult a primary care clinician as they become aware of these somatic manifestations. Generally, it is only secondarily, if at all, that they become aware of or complain about the psychological manifestations. These persons may be described as having "depressive equivalents."[19,20]

Depressive Equivalents

Although pain perception and expression may be diminished in the elderly, depression may be manifested in pain symptoms. This presentation may be demonstrated in a typical middle-aged patient who complains of severe pain, usually located in the head, neck or back. The pain has developed gradually and may often be present for weeks or months. The patient has been in good health and has been successful in social and/or business activities. It often becomes apparent from physical expression and posture that the patient is depressed; however, when the clinician asks about depression, its existence is usually denied. At this point, it is often helpful to inquire about other biological signs previously mentioned. If these are present, the patient generally attributes them to the fact that he or she is experiencing pain. It is only when asked about the feelings directly associated with the pain that the patient can express discouragement and depression.

The treatment for people experiencing depressive equivalents is similar to that for other forms of depression. Why some people develop such symptoms rather than overt depressive reactions is not entirely clear. Often these individuals hold high expectations of themselves and are unable to admit to any personal failures or psychological symptoms. In a sort of "choice-of-illness" sense, they seem to have "chosen" to be in physical pain rather than emotional pain. This in turn may well inhibit or retard the full-blown development of the psychological disorder.

Treatment of Depression

A vigorous approach to the management of depression is necessary. Patience and continuous involvement with the patient and family are cornerstones of therapy. Since much of the elder's depression may be associated with various types of losses, supportive counseling and reconnections to the social network are essential.

Depressive episodes may respond to one or a combination of the following approaches:

- *People therapy—(psychotherapy, counseling, social interaction)*. Almost everyone with depression needs at least some short-term counseling. The clinician can use the first three or four sessions to establish rapport with the older client, define the problem, determine the course of further therapy, and identify family and social contacts that will be helpful in ameliorating the problem. The restoration of social relationships that have been lost can be accomplished through individual counseling or group therapy.[21] The patient can also be encouraged to join social groups, clubs, etc., in order to help reestablish these associations.

- *Exercise*. A regular program of exercise and activity often may serve to lessen overt symptoms and also help to alleviate the underlying depression. While jogging is inappropriate for many elders—walking, bicycling, swimming, and dancing are good alternatives in providing physical stimulation. There is also the added benefit of increased social interaction in group programs. For more information on exercise see Chapter 17: Alternative Therapies.

- *Drug therapy*. It is important to distinguish between medications that only treat symptoms (sedative–hypnotics for insomnia or tranquilizers for agitation) and drugs that treat the depression itself. All too often an elderly person who complains of sleeplessness is given a prescription for a potent sedative that may produce further depression. See Table 7-2.

The milder sedative–hypnotics can be used for very brief therapy (two weeks or less) in *mild* depression, but tolerance develops rapidly and habituation may occur. See Table 7-3.

Several classes of drugs are used to treat the depression itself. Some are more effective than others in a particular patient and a trial and error approach may be indicated.

Geriatric patients, in general, respond well to tricyclic antidepressants (TCAs) but the use of monoamine oxidase inhibitors (MAOIs) in the elderly is not advisable, except in the hospital, due to

Table 7-2
Drugs to Avoid in Depressed Elders

1. Barbiturates: rapid development of tolerance and habituation; potentiate anticoagulants and other CNS depressants
2. Glutethimide (Doriden): tolerance, addicting with high lethality potential in overdose
3. Methaqualone (Quaalude): same as 2
4. Ethchlorvynol (Placidyl): same as 2

Table 7-3
Dosage of Milder Sedatives

1. Diphenhydramine (Benadryl): an antihistamine which may cause drowsiness in a dose of 25–50 mg at bedtime.
2. Hydroxizine (Atarax or Vistaril): a mild tranquilizer–antihistamine which may induce sleep at a dose of 50–100 mg but the effect lasts only a few days.
3. Benzodiazepines (Dalmane, Valium, others) are highly promoted and do induce sleep at relatively safe doses but tolerance and habituation occur fairly rapidly. Rarely cause frank addiction.
4. Chloral hydrate in a dose of 500–1000 mg induces sleep fairly consistently but tolerance and addiction are fairly rapidly developed. Will potentiate anticoagulants and other CNS depressants.

multiple interactions with drugs and other substances.[22]

Lithium salts have been very effective in patients of all ages with manic-depressive illness and occasionally in unipolar depression as well. Maintenance dosage is usually 300 mg tid or qid and serum levels must be carefully monitored (maintain below 1–1.5 mEq/liter). Unfortunately, there are increasing numbers of reports of irreversible renal and other organ system damage even when serum levels are in the "safe" range, especially in the elderly.

Amphetamines and methylphenidate (Ritalin) are occasionally used as antidepressants. This practice is to be deplored as these drugs (especially amphetamines) are highly addictive and potentially very dangerous, causing hypertension acutely and central nervous system dysfunction with chronic use.

In summary, when drug therapy is absolutely necessary for moderate to severe depression, the TCAs are the durgs of choice. They generally are fairly sedating and can, therefore, be used to help treat the insomnia and agitation that may accompany depression. Maximal antidepressant effects

may take up to six weeks to develop so an adequate trial is necessary before trying other alternatives. Common side effects that may cause problems are dry mouth, constipation, and urinary retention. Some tolerance for these side effects may develop with time. See Table 7-4.

Combination therapy is strongly promoted by drug manufacturers and combinations of a TCA and benzodiazepine (Limbitrol) or TCA and phenothiazine (Triavil) are available. They are advertised as promoting "tranquility" while the TCA is becoming effective. In general, however, they are more expensive than the TCA alone and are often continued long after the effect of the "extra ingredient" is needed.

Electroconvulsive Therapy (ECT)

When all the therapies suggested above are ineffective and severe depression continues unabated, ECT may be an effective alternative. It is potentially dangerous, but the effects are frequently very dramatic.[4] Psychiatric consultation is mandatory before it is used.

Table 7-4
Dosage of Various TCAs

1. Amitriptyline (Elavil, Endep): for mild depression, start with 10–25 mg tid and 50 mg at bedtime. For more severe depression, start with 25–50 mg tid and 50–100 mg at bedtime. Moderately sedating.
2. Protriptyline (Vivactil): usual dose is 5 mg tid. Not particularly sedating, so bedtime dose not helpful when insomnia present. May have slightly more rapid onset of effect than amitriptyline and imipramine (2–4 weeks).
3. Imipramine (Tofranil and others): start with 10 mg qid. Quite sedating and entire dose of 30–50 mg may be given at bedtime. In severe depression may need 75–100 mg total daily dose.
4. Doxepin (Sinequan, Adapin): a dose of 50–75 mg at bedtime generally induces sleep, and daytime sedation is minimized. Theoretically it has less cardiovascular side effects than other TCAs.

MANIA

Manic psychosis does occur in the elderly, although it is not common.[23] With the introduction of lithium therapy, the prognosis has improved remarkably. When lithium is contraindicated due to cardiac, renal, or electrolyte abnormalities, the phenothiazines may be of help.[17] Psychiatric consultation is always indicated, especially in the case of acute manic episodes.

LOSS, DEATH AND DYING, SUICIDE

Most elderly patients have suffered many losses throughout their lives. In the later years, however, such losses occur with increasing frequency. It is common for the elderly to lose a mate, other family members and friends as well as their job, prestige, and much of their personal and economic independence.

Clinical Presentation

The response to these losses may be to overreact and to generalize that, for example, losing one's job means one does not need to work. Multiple losses may cumulate to an unbearable level and cause much grief. Some patients, on the other hand, may rationalize (deny) the significance of the losses, suppress the feelings of grief, and adjust by becoming withdrawn, depressed, or hostile.

Management Strategies

The provider can help the patient adjust, work through the feelings, and come to understand that it is normal to grieve over losses. If a move from the home is required, there must be adequate time to decide where to go and to prepare for the move and the changes related to it. At the same time, it is important to be alert to crisis situations and intervene in case of loss of control or autonomy.

Death and Dying

Often it is found that the elderly have reconciled themselves to the fact of personal death. This usually is not true of younger patients or providers.

Elizabeth Kubler-Ross describes dying, if properly handled, as providing an opportunity for growth in which those who understand and are able to face this event can learn from the experience to deal productively with other traumatic changes that life may present.[24]

The elderly in many cases are better prepared for their own death and have less fear of it than other age groups, perhaps because they have already lived a long and eventful life.[25] In fact, much work by developmental researchers and theorists suggests that acceptance of death in later life is predictable. During the middle years, findings suggest a shifting orientation toward the end of life[26] and the later years appear to bring an increased frequency of death thoughts with a general decrease in death fears. For younger groups, on the other hand, death fears are high, but the occurrence of death thoughts are low.[25]

It is of great importance to the elderly to retain some degree of control over what is done to them as they approach the time of death. For this reason, many indicate that they do not want to die in a hospital connected to tubes and lingering when there is no hope of survival. Recently, the "Living Will" has gained popularity in allowing patients to improve the possibility of having a dignified death in spite of the fact that the document may not necessarily be legally binding.

STAGES OF DEATH

Kubler-Ross describes "five psychological stages of dying" through which patients and those around them may progress when dying or learning of a terminal illness or following the sudden death of a loved one.[24,27] These usually involve denial and isolation, anger, bargaining, depression, and acceptance as the salient components when the person comes to deal with the harsh realities of death. In coping with these experiences in a mature and adequate fashion, the individual may well die or may emerge more psychologically stable than he or she was before.

In arriving at the realization that they are going to die, patients may spend considerable time involved with thoughts or *tasks* that are largely inner-directed.[17] This often requires much energy and is frequently misunderstood by the family and providers. Withdrawing may be necessary in order to deal effectively with the emotions, to organize thoughts, attitudes and outlook without interruption or distractions. Providers must help the patient through this difficult time with understanding and support and by working with the family.

TEAM APPROACH TO MANAGEMENT

Members of the health care team often forget the most important team member—the patient. In the case of a dying patient, there is a great need for some member(s) of the team to help the older person and his or her family work toward a stage of acceptance. The ability to work through this sort of problem is a necessary and useful skill for all team members. However, the primary care provider may not necessarily have the ability or interest to be the best supporting person for the patient. In this case, it may be wise to allow others with better capabilities to deal with the problem. Nevertheless, the primary care provider is the one who must be sure that *someone* is assisting the patient in this respect at this crucial time. It must not be left to chance.

Ideally, everyone in the health field should have some academic as well as practical experience with death and dying to gain better perspectives and skills that help a patient work through the difficult task and "stages of dying." Kubler-Ross offers considerable guidance and expertise that can be very helpful in clinical and therapeutic work of this type.[24,27]

Suicide

Suicide occurs with high frequency among elders (see Fig. 7-1). As already pointed out, the elderly, with advancing years, face increased stress from multiple losses, changes in job status (retirement), less financial security, etc. The roles that contribute to feelings of self-worth are lost, diminished or changed. Physical symptoms of sleeplessness, weakness, apathy, and fatigue may approximate the psychological symptoms of despair, hopelessness, and despondency that lead to depression. Not recognizing the problem of depression or not correctly differentiating it from existential sadness (appropriate sadness concerning a loss) may lead to consequences as serious as suicide. Suicide behavior in the elderly differs from that in younger adults in a number of significant ways:

- An exceptionally high proportion of older suicide attempts are successful.[28]

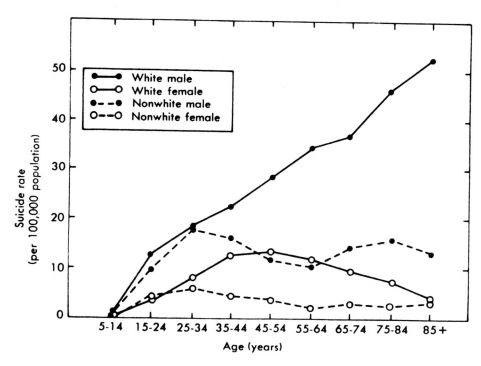

Fig. 7-1. Suicide rates by age, sex, and color in the United States, 1969. (Data from United States Department of Health, Education, and Welfare: Vital statistics of the United States, 1969, vol. II. A. Mortality, Rockville, Md., 1974, National Center for Health Statistics.)

- The suicide rate for the elderly (65+ years) is 1.7 times that found in young adults (15–24 years).[6]
- The elderly most often attempt suicide because of severe psychological problems rather than physical pain or illness.

The rate of suicide among widows and widowers in the first years following the death of a spouse is alarmingly high,[28] and it is even higher among persons divorced or separated. The aged individual is at high suicide risk up to five years following the loss of loved ones. In the first four years following loss of a spouse, the suicide rate is higher than at any other time in life.

Some other important descriptive data about elders and suicide are:

- The suicide rate is higher among those persons from high rather than low socioeconomic status.[25]
- The rates of successful suicides are almost five times greater in elderly males than in females.[6]
- Men more frequently choose violent, irreversible means of suicide such as shooting themselves, while women choose less active approaches such as barbiturate overdose and poisons. However, recent data show increasing numbers of women to be choosing more active methods.[6]
- Divorced men commit suicide more often than divorced women.
- The risk of suicide is greater in persons who drink excessively and/or present evidence of organicity and, in particular, impaired judgment.

The provider must remember that a patient who is suicidal tends in that direction because no other solution may be apparent to him or her. Threats to commit suicide are relatively uncommon in older age groups. They simply tend to kill themselves

Table 7-5
Suggestions for Identifying Suicide Risks

---

1. Be alert to feelings of guilt and hopelessness in the patient.
2. Recognize an increased risk following the death of a loved one.
3. Ask questions about sleep patterns and how they've changed.
4. Remember a suicidal patient feels there's "no other solution."
5. Know that confusion and disorientation may reflect physical disorders rather than psychological problems.

---

without notable warnings or fanfare. Because so many disengaged and depressed elderly live in relative isolation and may be in poor physical health, they are likely to show an exceptionally high attempt to success ratio.

Sometimes open discussion with the provider will help to identify problems and ventilate emotions. Contrary to the belief that asking a patient about suicide thoughts and intentions may give them the idea, it is actually the only way to assess the tendency. If there is confirmation, then steps to counteract it can be taken.[29] See Table 7-5.

MANAGEMENT STRATEGIES

The treatment of a patient with suicidal tendencies requires that, if possible, the cause of the depression or other problem be identified and alleviated. Treating a physical problem that caused depression or discontinuing a medication that stimulates depression may be fairly straightforward, but alleviating emotional problems that predispose a patient to self-destruction will certainly prove to be more difficult and challenging. Allowing the patient to ventilate grief and anger may help in dealing with or accepting the reality of the situation. Helping the elderly person to develop new interests and friendships may facilitate an adaptation to changing status. In addition, the provider may need to encourage the patient to give up potentially dangerous activities (e.g., driving a car).

Ideally, the provider should maintain care and contact with the patient after the peak period of suicidal attempts has apparently passed. Available data suggests an increased incidence of suicide for six months to a year following discharge from a psychiatric hospital.[29]

When a depressed patient is improving, the provider should be particularly alert to symptoms that would suggest a renewal intention to commit suicide. This sometimes occurs during an intermediate phase of recovery when the person regains enough energy to carry out an earlier suicidal plan.

As much as possible, the provider should continue to follow the patient in a supportive role even after the person has made "satisfactory adjustments" in his or her life situation.

PARANOID REACTIONS

Paranoid states are psychotic reactions that may involve delusions along with persecutory or grandiose ideation. These symptoms of course may occur throughout the life span but are more frequent in old age.[30] They tend to occur more frequently under conditions that cause isolation from human contact, visual and hearing loss being the most important with elders.[17] The anxiety produced by loss of sensory information can cause the external environment to be perceived as more threatening than it is.

Treatment

The immediate goal of treatment is to reduce the conditions and anxiety that tend to encourage the development of paranoid ideation. Any or all of the following techniques might be employed:

- Psychotherapeutic intervention—involving an attempt to establish clearer and more appropriate contacts with persons in the environment that may reduce anxiety and have a calming effect.
- Reducing the threat of the external environment—arranging for the patient to be in a familiar and uncomplicated environment with adequate correction of visual and hearing defects. Other community resources may also be needed for support (companionship, housekeeping, etc.)[18]
- Anxiety-alleviating drugs—(discussed in the section on Anxiety, below).

HYPOCHONDRIASIS

Hypochondriasis involves a morbid preoccupation with one's own body and is frequent among older patients.[30,32,34] The use of the sick role is an acceptable one in our society for gaining attention and is frequently used by the elderly.[33] In old age, the additional factors of isolation and impoverishment of the social environment along with whatever "disengagement" tendencies are involved may be expected to exaggerate existing trends toward oversensitivity toward internal rather than external sources of stimulation. With less interesting and attractive events in the external (social) environment internal "aches and pains" are likely to receive increasing emphasis and therefore may be used as a means to get attention and sympathy from friends, relatives, and health care personnel, particularly when and if other methods fail.

Thousands of elders have been living together in common law arrangements to preserve their pen-

Table 7-6
Management Strategies for Hypochondriasis

1.	Avoid the extremely complex diagnostic work-up to rule out a very rare disorder.
2.	Avoid potentially addictive drugs (analgesics and tranquilizers).
3.	Avoid the trap of reassurance—it will not help.
4.	Educate the family that the "real problem" involves a preoccupation with illness that produces consequent secondary gains.
5.	Do not get angry or try to avoid the patient. Be supportive. Hear him or her out.

used to defend against anxiety and to solicit sympathy, forgiveness, and help from others.[18] See Table 7-6.

ANXIETY

When the elderly are subjected to stresses of any type, it is likely that anxiety reactions will result. Under such circumstances, a certain amount of anxiety is normal and the patient should be reassured about this. Anxiety is not always clinically apparent and sometimes it is uncovered only when the patient is directly questioned by the provider.

Verwoerdt identifies five types of anxiety in the elderly based on their origins. These include depletion anxiety, helplessness, chronic neurotic anxiety, acute anxiety, and anxiety associated with psychoses.[35] Frequently anxiety and its expression are incorrectly diagnosed as senility and as such are wrongly considered to be untreatable.[17] Anxiety can also be a manifestation of depression (see Depression in this chapter).

Common Clinical Presentations

Some of the common symptoms of anxiety include insomnia, nightmares, restlessness, sweating, dry mouth, frequent urination, lightheadedness, tachycardia, shortness of breath, and vague aches and pains (compare with symptoms of depression). The patient may report feelings of fearfulness without apparent cause.[36]

Physiologically, anxiety affects the patient by accelerating autonomically controlled body processes and sometimes increasing the tonus of voluntary muscles. The body reacts to fear by accelerating bodily processes (to facilitate flight or defense). With anxiety a similar process occurs as if the person were mobilizing for an emergency. In a normal situation, however, the speeded-up physical processes slow down after a few moments while in chronic anxiety these processes may remain accelerated for a long period of time producing tenseness, a depletion of resources, and eventually a feeling of fatigue and exhaustion.[37]

Treatment of Anxiety

Psychotherapeutic and environmental intervention can help to alleviate many of the conditions and concerns that may trigger anxiety reactions by:

- Providing a calmer, quieter environment
- Educating the patient to use deep muscle relaxation techniques
- Initiating the use of mild analgesics or alcohol before bed
- Suggesting mental imagery to reduce anxiety-producing thoughts
- Bringing the family in to help in learning ways to support the anxious elder

- Suggesting regular exercise to produce more natural fatigue and encourage subsequent relaxation

Occasionally, the only relationship the patient has that does not promote severe anxiety is the one with the provider. However, the older person may feel the provider does not have the time or the interest to talk about the problems if the provider seems insistent only on prescribing a medication. It is crucial to establish a long-term supportive relationship that will encourage the patient to return as needed.

Drug Therapy

Tranquilizing drugs may be used along with supportive therapy if other interventions do not alleviate symptoms of anxiety (see Fig. 7-2). Since many elders may have minimal organic brain disease, drugs in the barbiturate family and other central nervous system depressants are generally contrain-

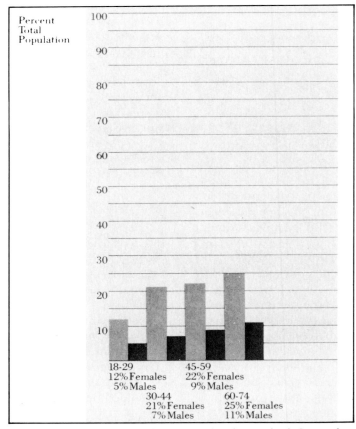

Fig. 7-2. Prevalence of minor tranquilizer use in the United States by sex and age. [Reprinted from Parry HJ, Balter MB, Mellinger GD, et al: National patterns of psychotherapeutic drug use. Arch Gen Psych 28:769–783, 1973. Copyright 1973, American Medical Association.]

Table 7-7
Dosages of Minor Antianxiety Drugs

1. Benzodiazepines: Safest of these drugs; habituating; rarely addicting; rarely lethal in overdose; may cause sedation and confusional states.
   a. Diazepam (Valium): 2–5 mg twice or 3 times a day. Frequently used for muscle tension though not demonstrably better than other benzodiazepines.
   b. Chlordiazepoxide (Librium): start with 5 mg twice a day, up to maximum 30 mg in 24 hours.
   c. Oxazepam (Serax): 10 mg tid initially; up to 60 mg in 24 hours.
2. Meprobamate (Equanil, Miltown) is not superior to phenobarbital, is habituating. Start with 200 mg qid, maximum dose 1600 mg in 24 hours.
3. Short acting barbiturates such as phenobarbital are occasionally used but are sedating rather than tranquilizing and they are addicting. Occasionally cause excitation rather than sedation.

dicated. Elders are also far more sensitive to usual doses of psychoactive drugs, so that the lowest possible doses should be used.[18] These drugs are classified as minor and major tranquilizers and are used for anxiety and major thought disorders respectively. See Table 7-7.

The major tranquilizers are also called antipsychotic medications. They must be used very cautiously for simple anxiety states and in very low doses. They are appropriate in higher dosage for true psychoses and paranoid states, but in those cases they should be used in consultation with a psychiatrist. Unfortunately, they are often "abused" by the elder's caretakers, especially in institutional settings. See Table 7-8.

Table 7-8
Dosages of Major Tranquilizers

1. Thioridazine (Mellaril) is one of the less sedating phenothiazines. It has the potential to cause many serious side effects. Start with 10–25 mg tid. It is seldom necessary to exceed 300 mg/24 hours.
2. Haloperidol (Haldol) is a butyrophenone but has similar side effects to the phenothiazines. Initial dose is 0.5–2.0 mg bid. Occasionally a very resistant patient will require up to 100 mg/24 hours.
3. Other phenothiazines and butyrophenones are available but all have approximately the same side effects.

Measures of serum levels of many of the psychotropic drugs are now available. If an older patient appears to be exhibiting unusual behavior or side effects, the drug should be stopped and the serum level checked to be sure that a concomitant medical condition is not compromising the patient's ability to metabolize and excrete the drug.

DRUG ABUSE AND ALCOHOLISM

Elderly Americans do not have a unique problem with drug abuse. The problem involves all generations, although there are differences in the drugs that are involved. Currently the use of "street drugs" is almot nonexistent beyond the 45–50 year age groups. Similarly, a large proportion of those elders who have overindulged in alcohol usage in years past can be expected to become abstainers in old age. However, there are two groups of medications that are frequently used improperly by the elderly: over-the-counter (OTC) preparations and prescribed, controlled drugs.

OTC Medications

Many patients do not report what OTC drugs they are taking because they do not realize that some are *real* medications which can interact with each other and with prescribed drugs. When obtaining a medication history, it is essential to ask specifically about the use of nonprescription drugs and home remedies. (See Chapter 6.)

Prescribed Medications

Family members or institution staff members may use sedatives or tranquilizers to make their charges easier to manage. Clinicians may also employ these drugs to "get the old fogey off my hands," and avoid having to spend time listening and caring. Patients, of course, may take medications as a means of escaping the realities of being old, lonely, and poor. Finally, confused patients may be at risk for inadvertent overdoses.

Alcohol

Alcohol is the only "tranquilizer" available without a prescription. Concurrent use of alcohol, sedatives, tranquilizers, and even antihistamines potentiate the central nervous system effects of each. Just as stress may cause increased use of other drugs, it may cause increased alcohol consumption. It is important to warn patients about potentially dangerous interactions of alcohol and the drugs that may be prescribed.

Signs of Drug Abuse

1. Requests for drug refills that indicate use out of proportion with objective signs and symptoms or more rapid use than the directions would require.
2. Requests for refills of controlled drugs prescribed by another provider, especially if several drugs are involved.
3. Requests for refills before the original prescription is finished (to avoid withdrawal symptoms).
4. Requests for specific, usually very potent drugs, especially when other drugs in the same class are said to be ineffective or cause adverse reactions.
5. Undue familiarity with many potent psychoactive drugs, their appearances, side effects, and formulations.

Signs of Alcohol Abuse

Although the following examples are not pathognomonic of alcohol abuse, they should raise the suspicion of a problem in this area:

1. Multiple somatic complaints (not unlike those of hypochondriasis or depression).
2. Insomnia and lack of energy, an inability to get up in the morning to face the day.
3. Increasingly constricted social contacts and interactions.
4. Accident-proneness, neglected injuries, and injuries more severe than would be expected based on the history of the traumatic event.
5. Increasing family and personal disorganization. See Table 7-9.

Management Strategies

Obviously, there are as many strategies as there are varieties of drug problems. See Table 7-10 for a diagnostic and therapeutic plan of management strategies. Overprescribing of sedatives and tranquilizers by physicians is a professional problem. Establishing an internal or external audit of patients receiving these medications is a sound approach.

"Unhooking" a drug or alcohol abuser is an impossible task for the health provider alone. It is significant that Alcoholics Anonymous has a much higher success rate than physicians. One reason is that AA does not try to "do it alone." Specialty consultation is mandatory when withdrawal of high levels of drugs is to be achieved. There are many

Table 7-9

Subjective and Objective Evaluation of Patient Drug History

1. Subjective: What medications and drugs are taken regularly? What are the patient's indications for taking any particular preparation? What symptoms seem to need the most attention?
   a. "Do you find that you need to take more (specific medication) than you used to in order to get relief from (specific symptom)?"
   b. "How do you use alcohol?" "Has your use of alcohol changed?"
   c. "Have you ever worried or has your spouse or child ever told you that you have a problem with the use of alcohol/tranquilizers/sleeping pills?"
2. Objective findings with drug or alcohol abuse:
   a. Complete list of drugs being used.
   b. Change in level of function from previous encounters.
   c. Depressed affect, lack of spontaneity.
   d. Intellectual disorganization, slowing of cognitive ability.
   e. Slurring of speech.
   f. Occurrence of nystagmus not present previously.
   g. Deterioration of fine motor coordination.

Any or all of these signs may occur in a patient who does not otherwise fit the sterotype of a "drunk" or drug abuser.

Table 7-10
Diagnostic and Therapeutic Plan or Management Strategies

1. Diagnostic plan
   a. Get a complete list of drugs being used. May need to have a family member empty the bedside stand and the medicine chest or send a public health nurse to the home to survey medicines.
   b. Lab tests
      (i) Blood alcohol and serum levels of drugs being taken (salicylate, barbiturates, tranquilizers, etc.)
      (ii) CBC with special attention to red cell indices (MCHC falls with iron loss, MCV rises in alcoholism)
      (iii) liver enzymes to diagnose toxic hepatitis
      (iv) renal function tests (BUN and serum creatinine) to examine whether drug excretion might be decreased
   c. Specialized x-ray or nuclear medicine scans if end organ damage is suspected
2. Therapeutic plan: It is common for health professionals and the lay public alike to feel that "drug abusers" and "alcoholics" are not worth trying to salvage because "cure rates" are too low. Such pessimism is not justified, particularly since the same attitude is not as widespread concerning other "uncurable" chronic disease (e.g., arthritis, heart disease, COPD, etc.)
   a. The abused drug must be removed fairly rapidly without provoking severe withdrawal syndrome. When drug levels are very high, this needs to be done in a hospital.
   b. If chronic pain is an issue, there may be a need to provide alternate analgesic methods (acupuncture, physical therapy, antidepressants, relaxation, hypnosis, etc.).
   c. Disulfiram (Antabuse) may be a helpful adjunct for treatment of alcoholism.
   d. Supportive psychotherapy (formal or informal) will be necessary during and after withdrawal of the drug(s).

program resources available, some of which have been specifically designed for elders. City and county programs, as well as private facilities, can be of great assistance in this respect.

SEXUALITY

Sexuality is a crucial factor in the personality configuration of any individual. From primitive times to the present, the loss of sexual performance has been equated with death. Consequently, various remedies including magic, potions, tissue implants, and drugs have been used to try to correct sexual dysfunction. To many, becoming elderly means a loss of sexuality and consequently, a loss of womanliness or manliness.

The elderly are not asexual; in fact, the need for intimacy and love may be more critical in later life than ever before because of losses of mate, job, friends and family as well as prestige, confidence, and power. It is vital for the elderly to have an opportunity for sexual activity in order to provide needed physiological and psychological outlets and satisfactions in their later years. Unfortunately, most of our hospitals and long-term care institutions are arranged to prevent this. Studies indicate that 70 percent of men over 65 are sexually active.[38] Figures are much more difficult to obtain for women since many deny sexual expression unless they are married. The double standard is obvious in this age group so that an older man who has a relationship or marries a younger woman is thought to be "really alive" while an older woman who does the same is often ridiculed. This results in a situation where many older women regard their sexual feelings as undignified and slip into a neutered, sexual oblivion. Increasing female longevity has created a situation in which many women do not have partners and have not been encouraged to explore extra-marital affairs, masturbation, and homosexual options.

Thousands of elders have been living together in common law arrangements to preserve their pensions, because of restrictive and unrealistic Social Security regulations. Recent changes in regulations now allow a widow to retain her previous benefits or choose her new husband's benefits, whichever is preferred.

Primary care clinicians must play an important role in encouraging sexual activity for elders. Their opinion is often valued, and the encouragement of sexual expression can have broad therapeutic ramifications and benefits.

Sexual Myths

Elders and health care professionals share a number of myths about sexuality that often interfere with optimal sexual expression[17]:

- "Older people do not have sexual desires"
- "They could not make love even if they wanted to"
- "They might hurt themselves or die"
- "They are physically unattractive and undesirable"
- "In old age it's shameful and perverse"

Physiological Changes

Age-related physiological and anatomical changes related to sexual functioning affect older men as follows:

1. It takes an older man longer to achieve a full erection and to reach a climax.
2. He experiences fewer genital spasms and there is a reduction in both the force and amount of his ejaculation.
3. It takes him longer before he can have another erection.

Older women are affected also[39]:

1. There is less lubrication and elasticity of the vagina.
2. The tissue lining of the vagina is more easily irritated.
3. The uterine contractions that accompany orgasm may become spastic and painful.

Many of these symptoms can be dealt with through appropriate treatments and should not detract from the pleasures of sexual activity in later life.

Organic Basis for Dysfunction

Many elders are concerned that their general physical ability will significantly influence their sexual performance, and there are a number of specific conditions which do have an effect on sexual functioning. However, psychological aspects are a very important factor in continued performance, and these are often neglected in lieu of more "strictly" physical concerns.

Cardiac Disease

After congestive heart failure or a myocardial infarction, many elders are concerned about resuming sexual activities. With the exception of those who are severely impaired (see Chapter 11), most people can resume normal activity within four to six weeks. Studies have shown that the cardiac expenditure during intercourse is approximately equal to climbing two flights of stairs.[40] For severely ill patients, other less strenuous activities, such as touching, stroking, and embracing should be encouraged.

Diabetes

Long-standing diabetes may interfere with functioning of both the peripheral and autonomic nervous systems. In addition to running a glucose tolerance test on older men with recent impotence, it is wise to check for neurogenic impairment of the bladder as well as other signs of neuropathy.

Alcohol, Tobacco, and Drugs

Alcohol, tobacco, and other drugs impair potency and libido rather than increase them. Chronic alcoholism in males impairs hepatic function so that endogenous estrogens are not conjugated and metabolized properly. Full doses of barbiturates and phenothiazines may also reduce libido. Several studies have shown that heavy cigarette smoking can produce similar effects.

Hypothyroidism

Hypothyroidism is slowly progressive and diminishes energy and libido, but thyroid replacement can help to alleviate these problems. Unfortunately, when there is pre-existing atherosclerotic heart disease, the thyroid replacement therapy may bring on angina and even sudden death.

Arthritis

Joint pains may certainly cause the elderly to diminish or avoid sexual activity. However, there is good evidence that such activity may actually help to alleviate pain and even decrease the need for analgesics.

Senile Vaginitis, Vulvitis, and Perineal Pruritis

Senile vaginitis, vulvitis, and perineal pruritis are low-grade inflammations that cause a great deal of discomfort and itching, both of which tend to decrease sexual pleasure. They may be caused by hormonal deficiencies, vitamin deficiency or sugar in the urine. This problem can be resolved with appropriate therapy (see Chapter 12).

Pelvic Relaxation

Pelvic relaxation, leading to uterine prolapse, cystocele, and/or rectocele, may also interfere with sexual function. The uterus may be surgically removed or, if this is medically contraindicated, a pessary may be used, though it will complicate sexual intercourse. A cystocele and rectocele are able to be surgically corrected.

Hysterectomy

Hysterectomy with or without ovariectomy in the postmenopausal woman does not produce any physiological changes in sexual desire or performance, but may cause psychological complications. Mastectomy causes similar fears related to loss of desirability.

Ileostomies and Colostomies

Ileostomies and colostomies can also lead to sexual dysfunction in men and women. There are some very good patient education materials which address these problems and concerns (see Chapter 12).

Prostatectomy

Transurethreal prostatectomy may cause sexual dysfunction. Nevertheless, some *70 percent of patients* subjected to the operation remain potent. The perineal and suprapubic approach are more likely to cause organic impotence. Following surgery, the structure of the bladder neck is changed so that the semen may be ejaculated into the bladder. The impotence that frequently follows usually is related to psychological problems.

Impotence is not synonymous with sterility, but some patients feel these terms mean the same thing. Impotence may be complete or partial, permanent or temporary. The provider's attitude is extremely important in helping the patient work through the problem of real or perceived impotence. In cases where impotency is organically based and irreversible, a penile prosthesis sometimes offers a satisfactory solution. Both rigid and inflatable prosthetic devices are available.[41]

Treatment Modalities

With both elderly males and females, the influence of the past is very strong. An enjoyable, active sex life in earlier years increases the likelihood of continued positive sexual expression in later years.

It has been pointed out that older people need not maintain the sexual behavior of their youth in order to enjoy sexual experiences. Sex is qualitatively different in later years. It is recreative rather than procreative. Sexual arousal and behavior need not necessarily be aimed at achieving orgasm. Most importantly, sexual activity in the later years may fulfill the human need for the warmth of physical nearness and the intimacy of companionship. Old people should be encouraged to seek this fulfillment.[39]

A simple model for the health care professional in approaching sexual concerns is the PLISSIT model. This acronym stands for Permission, Limited Information, Specific Suggestions, Intensive Therapy.[42] A large percentage of sexual problems and concerns in later life can be dramatically helped just by giving permission (P) and basic information (LI) to dispel myths.

The primary care provider should consider sexuality a vital component of any patient's life. It is important to get a sexual history on the elderly patient. Appropriate support will include ascertaining any concern on the part of the patient for his or her ability to function sexually. This should be followed by explaining normal physiological changes in aging relevant to sexual performance, and by supporting the patient's need to be sexually active. The elderly patient should be reassured that masturbation is okay and will not cause brain damage or insanity. Individuals should be allowed the opportunity to experience their sexuality and sensuality regardless of age.

SUMMARY

The present chapter has dealt with various aspects of psychological changes in the elderly that may be encountered in clinical settings by primary care providers. These have included a consideration of stress, anxiety, hypochondriasis, drug abuse and alcoholism, sexual problems, bereavement, death and dying, paranoid reactions, depression and suicide. The problems have been looked at in terms of clinical aspects and the development of data relating to the problem in the patient, as well as from the point of view of management and therapeutic strategies.

In general, the approach has been practical and has strongly emphasized the need to be aware of, and prepared to deal with, psychological and social as well as medical dimensions of the problems that elderly clients bring to health care providers. Further, the interaction of these factors in the production of illness and health has been emphasized throughout. Where relevant, factual information is provided on the extent and the seriousness of various problems that affect the elderly, and the findings of significant scientific studies have been cited.

Perhaps most important, the challenges of dealing adequately and sensitively with the psychological, social, and medical problems of the aged is presented as a complicated enterprise requiring the concerted efforts of physicians and nurses as well as other health care providers, psychologists, and social workers.

Practical and everyday examples of relevant problems are offered, specific questions and guidelines for obtaining information are provided, and solutions are proposed with straightforward indications of expected outcomes and limitations.

REFERENCES

1. Lieberman M: Grouchiness: A survival asset. University of Chicago Magazine, 1973
2. Lowenthal M, Berkman P: Aging and Mental Disorders in San Francisco. San Francisco, Jossey-Bass, 1977
3. Cohen GD: Mental health and the elderly. Unpublished issues paper, Rockville, Maryland, NIMH, Center for Studies of the Mental Health of the Aging, February 28, 1977
4. Ugdin G, Lewis JM: Psychiatry in general medical practice. New York, McGraw-Hill Book Company, 1979
5. Gurland B: The comparative frequency of depression in various adult age groups. J Gerontol 31:283–292, 1979
6. McIntosh J, Santos J: Unpublished analyses. Chicago, 1979
7. Roth SM: The psychiatric disorders of later life. Psychiat Ann, 6:9, 1976
8. National Center of Health Statistics: Advance Report, Final Mortality Statistics, 1975. Washington, DC, US Government Printing Office, February 11, 1977
9. Bureau of Census: Demographic aspects of aging and the older population in the United States. Current Population Reports: Special Studies. Series 23, No. 59, Washington, DC, Supt of Documents, US Government Printing Office, 1976
10. Redick RW, Kramer M, Taube CA: Epidemiology of mental illness and utilization of psychiatric facilities among older persons, in Busse RW, Pfeiffer E (eds): Mental Illness in Later Life. New York, American Psychiatric Association, 1972, p 231
11. National Institute of Mental Health, Division of Biometry and Epidemiology: Provisional Data on Federally Funded Community Mental Health Centers. 1975–1976, April 1977
12. National Institute of Mental Health: Patterns of Use of Nursing Homes by the Aged Mentally Ill. Statistical Note No. 107, Washington, DC, Division of Biometry, 1974
13. National Institute of Mental Health: Referral of Discontinuations of Inpatient Services of State and County Mental Hospitals. U.S. 1969, Biometry Branch, Statistical Note No. 57, Washington, DC, US Government Printing Office, 1971
14. Kahn RL: The mental health system and the future aged. Gerontol 15:24–31, 1975
15. Glasscote PM, Sussex JJ, Cumming E, Smith LR: The Community Mental Health Center: An Interim Appraisal. Washington, DC, The Joint Information Services of the American Psychiatric Association and the National Association for Mental Health, 1969
16. Herr JJ, Weakland JH: Counseling Elders and Their Families, Practical Techniques for Applied Gerontology. New York, Springer Publishing Co, 1979
17. Butler RN, Lewis MI: Aging and mental health, ed 2. St Louis, CV Mosby Co, 1977
18. Busse EW: The mental health of the elderly. Internat Ment Heal Res News 10:13–16, 1968
19. Pfeiffer E: Treating the patient with confirmed functional pain. Hosp Phys, XX:68–71, 91–92, 1971

20. Kennedy F, Wiesel B: The clinical nature of "manic-depressive equivalents" and their treatment. Trans Am Neurol Assoc 71:96–101, 1946

21. Altholz J: Group therapy with elderly patients. Alternatives to Institutional Care for Older Americans: Practicing and Planning. Durham, NC, Duke University, 1973, pp 172–177

22. Lehman HE: The use of medication to prevent custodial care, in Eisdorfer C, Friedel RO: Cognative and Emotional Disturbances in the Elderly: Clinitest Issues. Chicago, Year Book Medical Publishers, 1977

23. Roth M: The natural history of mental disorders in old age. J of Ment Sci 101:281, 1955

24. Kubler-Ross E: Death the Final Stage of Growth. Englewood Cliffs, New Jersey, Prentice-Hall, Inc, 1975

25. Kastenbaum R, Aisenberg R: Psychology of Death. New York, Springer Verlag, 1972, p 271

26. Neugarten B: Middle Age and Aging. Chicago, University of Chicago Press, 1968

27. Kubler-Ross E: On Death and Dying. New York, The MacMillan Co, 1970

28. Riley M, Johnson M, Foner A: Aging and Society, vol 3. New York, Russell Sage Foundation, 1972

29. Shneidman ES, Farberow NL: Cry for Help. New York, McGraw-Hill Book Co, 1961

30. Fish FJ: Senile paranoid states. Gerontol Clinica 1:127–131, 1959

31. Busse EW: The treatment of hypochondriasis. Tri-State Med J 2:7–12, 1954

32. Earley LW, Von Mering O: Growing old the outpatient way. Am J Psychiatry 125:963–967, 1969

33. Parsons T: The Social System. Glencoe, Ill, The Free Press, 1951, pp 436–437

34. Busse EW, Pfeiffer E (eds): Mental Illness in Later Life. Washington, DC, American Psychiatric Association, 1973

35. Verwoerdt A: Clinical Geropsychiatry. Baltimore, The Williams & Wilkins Co, 1976

36. Strain J: Psychological Interventions in Medical Practice. New York, Appleton-Century-Crofts, 1978

37. Steinberg FU (ed): Cowdry's—The Care of the Geriatric Patient, ed 5. St. Louis, CV Mosby Co, 1976

38. McCarthy P: Geriatric sexuality: Capacity, interest and opportunity. J Gerontol Nurs 5:20–24, 1979

39. Kart CS, Metress ES, Metress JF: Aging and health: Biologic and social perspectives. Menlo Park, Calif., Addison-Wesley, 1978

40. Busse E, Pfeiffer E: Behavior and Adaptation in Later Life, ed 2. Boston, Little, Brown, 1977

41. Furlow WL: Surgical treatment of erectile impotence using the inflatable penile prothesis. Sexuality and Disability 1:299–306, 1978

42. Robinson CH, Reich L, Pion G, et al: The office management of sexual problems: Brief therapy approaches. J Rep Med 15: 127–144, 1975

8

Dentistry

James Bennett, D.D.S., M.S.
Howard Creamer, Ph.D.
Donna J. Fontana-Smith, R.D.H.

Problems of the oral cavity are prevalent in elders. The primary care clinician is often the initial source of oral assessment and therefore an important link to further dental services. Dentistry has a special preventive role with elders, both in direct care and in education of primary care clinicians.[1] Routine assessment and maintenance, nutritional counseling, home care instruction, and application of fluoride are mainstays of a preventative program. Many elderly have spent a lifetime attempting to maintain their mouths.

Dental care for the elderly should focus on the removal of unsalvageable teeth, replacing lost structures with fillings, crowns, bridges, and dentures in a basic and conservative mode.

For elders, many situations can be temporized indefinitely; for an extremely ill person, temporary dental treatment may be both an ideal and a final form of treatment. It is important to stage any dental care so that it best fits the patient's needs and circumstances. In a few communities, portable and mobile dental equipment enables dental care wherever the patient is located.

There are a number of basic assessment procedures that can be performed to assist elders in maintaining their oral health. The following set of standards can be used as a guiding framework for oral health care: (1) a thorough evaluation of oral status will be part of the physical exam; (2) oral health promotion and maintenance is a joint effort between dentistry and primary care clinicians; (3) significant dental problems will be given priority along with physical and emotional problems for treatment in planning care; (4) team members will be responsible for the coordination and resolution of dental problems.

See Table 8-1 for a Glossary of Terms used in this chapter.

INCIDENCE OF DENTAL PROBLEMS IN THE ELDERLY

Elders do not suffer from unique, isolated dental problems. Significant problems usually do not have simple etiologies or end points. See Fig. 8-1. Dental problems usually begin at an earlier age and continue to be endemic throughout life.[2] The chapter's major perspective emphasizes the importance of prevention and ongoing maintenance—teeth are meant to last a lifetime. One prevalent myth is that loss of teeth is an inevitable result of aging; an understandable myth since virtually 100 percent of the 23 million people over 65 years of age have had one or more oral disease problems. About 60 percent of elderly have one or more natural teeth remaining, and we can predict that the majority of that group will have mild to severe problems related to dental plaque control.[3] Dental caries in both the tooth crown and root areas are common. About 45 percent of elders have full dentures, while about 25 percent have partial dentures.[4] About 30 percent of denture wearers require adjustments and repairs.[2,3] The mere presence of natural teeth and/or prostheses does not assure either adequate function or acceptability.

Oral cancer occurs in about 4 percent of the elderly; it is more frequent in the male and is often

Table 8-1
Glossary of Common Terms

Dental plaque: tenacious, organized masses of bacteria and their products associated with the teeth. *Materia alba:* whitish deposits of bacteria, food, and cellular debris which accumulate about the teeth and gingiva when oral hygiene is poor. Plaque enhances the formation of *calculus* (tartar), decay, periodontitis, and fetor oris (bad breath). The primary goal of brushing and flossing is the removal of the above materials from the mouth.

Dental decay: (cavities), the destruction of enamel and dentin by microorganisms of plaque.

Periodontitis: (gum disease—pyorrhea), inflammation and destruction of the periodontium primarily by dental plaque. *Gingiva:* gums; early inflammation (*gingivitis*) precedes periodontitis.

Prosthodontics: dentures or prosthesis or false teeth. Maxillary denture is the upper denture, mandibular denture is the lower denture. *Full* dentures are plates; cover the entire edentulous ridge while *partial* dentures cover the alveolar ridge where teeth are missing, and attach to natural teeth (abutment teeth) by clasps. *Temporary* and/or *treatment* dentures are used to provide dental function on a short-term basis. *Overdentures* may gain more stability from having healthy tooth roots remaining in the alveolar bone beneath.

Crowns: caps or jackets. Porcelain, gold, and other metals are used to cover most or all of a tooth crown. Crowns and *pontics* (dummy teeth) are fused together to form bridges across edentulous spaces; *abutment* natural teeth hold the bridge in place.

Hyperkeratoses: keratoses or white patch or leukoplakia, an unusual buildup of keratin of the epithelium in areas of chronic irritation. Dysplasia of the cells may lead to a premalignant state and finally carcinoma-in-situ and/or squamous cell carcinoma; the latter is the most common malignancy of the mouth.

associated with individuals who experience high levels of irritation to the lips and mouth (e.g., sunlight on the lower lip; smoking, especially pipes and cigars; high alcoholic intake).[5]

The Aging Mouth

Aging of the mouth is the result of normal physiological changes, environmental stress, and disease. Some common changes in the mouth associated with aging can be summarized in this way (see Figs. 8-2, 8-3, 8-4, and 8-5A and B)[5]:

- Progressive wear (attrition) with loss of tooth anatomy
- Atrophy and regression of tooth pulp with diminished sensory levels
- Masticating efficacy decreases
- Ability to withstand local disease diminishes
- Oral epithelium atrophies
- Supereruption of teeth due to loss of opposing teeth
- Intermaxillary space decreases
- Diminished taste sensation
- Diminished neuromuscular activity
- Decreased salivary flow

Immunocompetency of the Mouth

The oral cavity appears to have a remarkable resistance to invasion by most pathogens. Primary, *invasive* infections of nondental, oral tissues are

COMMON PROBLEMS

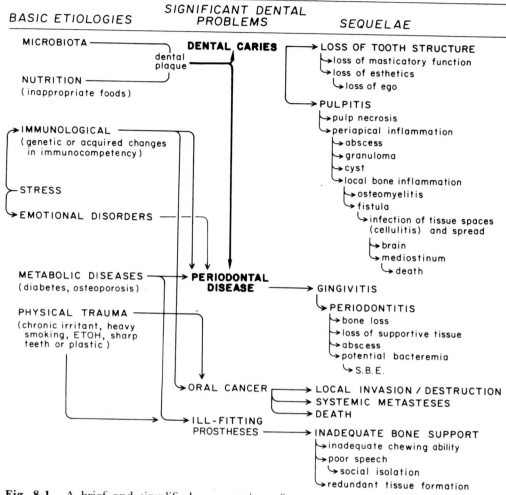

Fig. 8-1. A brief and simplified presentation of some common dental problems, factors related to etiology, and some possible sequelae if not treated. As in most other health problems, the etiologies are often more complex than presented. The iatrogenic sequelae are not shown; treatment effects can be especially pronounced in oral cancer.

relatively rare and are caused by a limited number of viruses (e.g., primary herpes) and bacteria (e.g., primary syphilis). Most other invasive infections of oral soft tissues appear to be caused by opportunistic organisms during periods of lowered host resistance. Such "opportunistic" infections include candidiasis (thrush),[6] oral actinomycosis[6] and noma (cancrum oris).[7]

This remarkable level of resistance is not yet thoroughly understood but the following have been cited as possible factors[8]:

- Oral epithelium is a barrier to direct penetration

- Cleansing effect of exfoliation of surface epithelium
- Flushing effect of saliva
- Antimicrobial substances in saliva
- Antimicrobial effect of established flora
- Immune system secretion of antibody class IgA
- Richly endowed blood supply and lymphatic drainage

In spite of the above, dental decay (an invasive disease of the teeth) and periodontal disease (an infectious, progressive but noninvasive disease of the gums and supporting bone) are rampant in our society.[9]

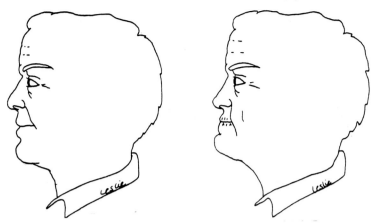

Fig. 8-2. Decrease in intermaxillary space. The chin tends to move towards the nose when there is uncompensated loss of tooth structure (or teeth) and/or of the alveolar bone.

PROBLEMS OF THE ORAL CAVITY

Although there are other problems of the oral cavity apart from purely dental problems, the prevention and treatment of dental decay and periodontal disease is a large and important part of elder dental care. The mouth is also a frequent site of minor trauma, ulcerations, immunological reactions, and variations of normal structure and function. Long-standing irritations and chronic dysplasias of the soft tissues may result in excess keratin formation (callus-like keratoses), formation of re-

dundant tissues, fibromas, and vascular enlargements (varices). Chronic inflammation of the teeth, periodontium, and jawbones commonly results in formations of granulation tissue, cysts, or sclerosis of bone (See Fig. 8-6.)[5] It is far more rational to prevent and/or intercept such problems at an early stage.

Lips

Cracking, drying, and chapping of the lips is very common; angular cheilosis or cracking of the corners of the mouth is often seen in debilitated patients or persons with moniliasis, malnutrition and/

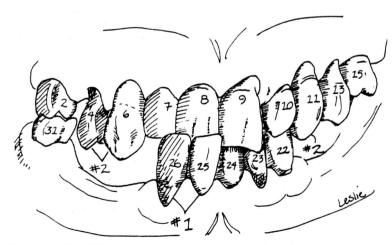

Fig. 8-3. An example of inadequate masticatory function due to missing teeth with no prosthetic replacement. Note the following: (1) anterior crossbite with two mandibular teeth lying in front of maxillary teeth; (2) extrusion of teeth #4, #6, #11, #13 due to lack of opposing teeth; and (3) only two areas of chewing function, #2 on #31 and #8–#10 on #22–#25.

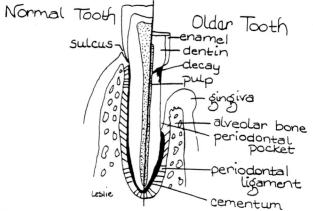

Fig. 8-4. Comparison of a younger tooth (left) with an older tooth (right). The main features are: (1) reduced periodontium, which includes losses of alveolar bone, periodontal ligament, and root surface attachment; (2) increased cementum thickness; (3) marked decrease in pulp size with obliteration of root canal at its coronal juncture; (4) dental caries attacking root surface (below enamel); and (5) marked abrasion resulting in loss of incisal height. "Lung-in-tooth" refers to increased clinical length of teeth where the gingiva and periodontium have receded.

or severe loss of intermaxillary space. Keratoses of the lower lip is common in individuals who have spent a lot of time outdoors; it should be considered a premalignant condition if it does not respond to emollient treatment.

Cheeks and Vestibules

These areas are subject to biting and chewing trauma. The vestibules are subject to aphthous ulcerations and keratoses that may be associated with long-term snuff holding. Lichen planus is a common keratoses of the cheek; it is a lacy-white keratotic process that should be monitored on a routine basis. It tends to cycle and some clinicians feel it has a premalignant potential.[5]

Teeth and Periodontium

Abrasion and erosion of the incisal and root areas of teeth are common to elders with natural teeth. (See Fig. 8-6.) They are caused by excessive grinding (bruxism), excessive acidic agents in the mouth, and by improper toothbrushing and toothbrushes. Overly stiff brushes may also contribute to the marked recession of the gingiva (and periodontium) found in individuals who have been extremely conscientious about oral care. Fractured enamel is common to teeth with large fillings and/or deep cavities.

Palate and Soft Palate

These areas are quite subject to trauma from hot foods and mechanical injury. A normal bony protuberance in the midline of the hard palate (torus palatinus) may be mistaken for an exophytic tumor.

Tongue and Floor of the Mouth

The tongue has been called the barometer of the body; the papillae (or lack of) often seem to reflect systemic conditions such as fever, nutritional changes, and drug responses. Malnutrition and pernicious anemia are often reflected by a sore, red, and smooth tongue. Hyperplasia of the filiform papillae may cause a "hairy" appearance of the tongue; brown to black staining of the papillae is common.

Varicosities, keratoses, and ulcerations are some of the main problems seen in the floor of the mouth and underside of the tongue.

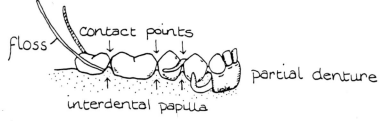

Fig. 8-5A. Concepts in oral health maintenance: (1) metal clasps hold a partial denture to the natural teeth. There is high risk for dental decay in the area underneath the clasps and the interdental spaces; (2) contact points help stabilize the natural teeth and protect the interdental areas; the latter are often sites for trapping and stagnation of plaque, food and cellular debris; and (3) dental floss is used to clean interdental space. It should be carried into the dental sulcus on each side of the interdental papillae.

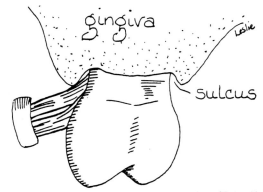

Fig. 8-5B. Tooth brush bristle placement. The soft bristles of the tooth brush should traverse as far into the sulcus (or periodontal pocket) as possible without undue trauma.

Jawbones and Temporomandibular (TM) Joint

The TM joint may be afflicted by "going out of joint" (subluxation), osteoarthritis, and the TM-joint pain-dysfunction syndrome. The process is characterized by tenderness (myofascial pain), clicking, and difficulty with chewing; the etiology is often related to stress and improper articulation of the teeth. Problems in managing this syndrome has led to multiple referrals to a wide variety of medical specialists.[5]

The jawbones are frequent sites of chronic inflammatory problems associated with the teeth and periodontium. Frank tumors of the bones are less common; however, odontogenic tumors such as the ameloblastoma may still occur in older persons. Paget's disease, commonly affecting alveolar bone, is more common in persons over 40 years of age. It has a high predilection for malignant transformation.[5]

Salivary Glands

The major glands may be affected by infectious autoimmune problems such as Sjögren's disease, by tumors such as the pleomorphic adenoma, by certain drugs such as antihistamines, which decrease saliva productions, or by atrophic loss of functioning acinar units, which can change the amount and consistency of saliva produced.[5] The minor salivary glands may suffer the same problems. It may not, however, be as clinically obvious. Duct stones (sialolithiasis) may cause duct obstruction and swelling of the glandular unit.[5] Heavy diuretic medication may lead to severe dehydration; salivary ducts may

become infected (retrograde) with blockage of the duct.[10]

DIAGNOSIS AND TREATMENT OF COMMON DENTAL PROBLEMS

Dental Caries

Dental caries is one of the most common disease entities of mankind. It afflicts all ages, resulting in astronomical loss of tooth structure and teeth. Elderly with any natural teeth are at high risk to develop caries, particularly of root surfaces which have been exposed due to recession of the gingiva and/or loss of periodontium.[9] Caries are primarily attributed to indigenous oral flora (dental plaque), which colonizes the teeth (and tissues). The destruction of the enamel and dentin are attributed to the production of acidic metabolities produced by the colonies when readily fermentable carbohydrates are available for metabolism. The softer root structure of the tooth is especially vulnerable to decay.[3]

The diminished size of the tooth pulp (nerve) often allows fillings to placed without anesthesia. Also, dental caries can be insidious, silent, and hidden in the early stages. In elders, they often occur between the teeth, on the roots, and/or beneath fillings, crowns, or clasps; the loss of enamel segments may be the first evidence of significant disease. Repair of the caries in crucial teeth is an important service to elders, particularly for esthetics, chewing, and preserving remaining teeth to serve as carriers for bridges and partial dentures. Control of caries is accomplished by good oral hygiene, appropriate nutrition, and routine application of fluoride preparations.

Periodontal Disease

Inflammatory disease of the gingiva and periodontium is as widespread in the elder patient's mouth (with natural teeth) as are dental caries in the population below age 40.[8] Periodontal disease usually commences in childhood or in young adults and continues until the supporting structures of the teeth are lost or until control is initiated. The pathogenesis is keyed to the chronic presence of dental plaque initiating inflammatory disease of the gingiva. Without adequate plaque control, the inflammatory process extends deeper into the periodontal structures, resulting in the loss of sulcular nonkeratinizing epithelium, connective tissues, and,

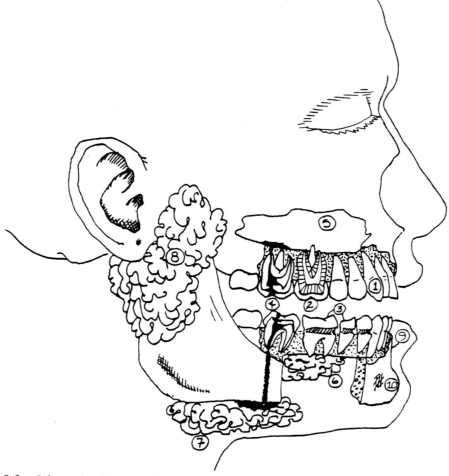

Fig. 8-6. Schematic diagram of the jaws. Note the following: (1) normal teeth held in jawbones by the periodontium and alveolar bone, (2) Cross-section of tooth: the crown is made up of enamel enclosing dentin, the latter constitutes the greater part of the crown and roots. The pulp chambers are often filled-in more than shown. (3) Teeth showing faceting of chewing surfaces; there is erosion and/or decay at the neck of the tooth. (4) Decay of molar teeth with pulp necrosis and fistulation into the maxillary sinus and submandibular space. (6,7,8) Major salivary glands, which should be palpated during oral assessment. (9) Alveolar ridge supports teeth and/or dentures. (10) Basal bone of the mandible; this bone is more stable than alveolar bone.

finally, alveolar bone. As the destructive process proceeds, the tooth loses its support and is lost.

Control of dental plaque is basic to the management of periodontal disease. Steps to periodontal disease control are:[10,11]

- Frequent assessment by dentist or dental hygienist.
- Proper toothbrushing, use of dental floss, and mouthrinsing as part of daily regimen.
- Maintain sound nutritional balance for the op-

timal health of the periodontal tissues and immunocompetence of this system.
- Ensure adequate stress management. Stress affects nutritional uptake, assimilation, and immunocompetency. Some antecedent affects are oral hygiene performance, alcoholic intake, and heavy smoking.
- Monitor drug intake and drug interactions, especially tranquilizers and immunosuppressants.
- Check masticatory habits and malocclusions.

Ill-fitting Dentures

Ill-fitting dentures are a very common problem among elders. Several factors contributing to this problem are: (1) loss of weight, (2) loss of alveolar bone, and (3) diuretic drugs or exacerbation of metabolic problems (e.g., diabetes). Sometimes a denture may not have been fitted properly at the outset. It is, however, more common to find that there has been some change in the elder's health. The patient's usual complaints are dentures that move around too much when eating or talking, or that fall free of the alveolar ridge.

One common treatment is to reline (rebase) the denture. If the patient has had the prostheses for a long time, remaking the appliance may be more ideal. Often the oral tissues supporting the denture are inflamed, and there may be a concomitant monilial infection. New plastics have been developed that stay softer and more resilient than the cured, hard plastics traditionally used in most dentures. Such softliners are used while treating inflamed oral tissues and must be monitored frequently. Soft plastic liners may be the final, ideal treatment for a terminal (or very ill) person.[1]

Keys to denture maintenance: (1) urge the patient to clean the dentures and the soft tissues at least once a day; (2) dentures should be left out at night in a container of clean water; and (3) encourage the patient to seek dental help when the dentures become loose or do not function properly.

Oral Cancer

Oral cancer occurs in about 4 percent of the adult population and commonly presents as a squamous cell carcinoma.[5] The lower lip is the most common site, while the lateral border of the tongue is a common intraoral site. In the early stages, the process involves epithelium, and the early clinical findings are often white patches (keratoses); less common is the red velvety plaque on the oral mucosa. The keratotic areas may be interspersed with reddened, inflamed portions. Once the process has proceeded from the epithelium into the underlying connective tissues, the areas of involvement can become thickened and quite firm to palpation (induration). The process is usually painless until underlying nerves become involved, at which time there is a fair chance the tumor cells have entered local lymphatics and/or local lymph nodes. True neoplasia does not respond to topical emollient therapy.

Given the above characteristics of squamous cell carcinoma, and also the potential for other types of tumors to occur (especially in the salivary glands), it is extremely important for the mouths of elders to be routinely examined and palpated. The high risk individual for lip cancer is usually a male who is blue-eyed, fair-haired, and has been chronically exposed to actinic radiation, hot pipe stems, or cigars and cigarettes.

Intraoral cancers can occur in any soft tissue area and often are preceeded by a premalignant and/or early epithelial developmental stage (carcinoma-in-situ). The sites of occurrence often appear to lie where varying types of epithelial tissues abut (e.g., keratinizing epithelium versus nonkeratinizing epithelium versus gland duct epithelium). Sites of occurrence also seem to favor areas of chronic, frequent irritation such as from cigarettes, cigars and pipes. In one 60-year-old male with an extremely heavy smoking habit (eight cigars a day), five separate oral cancers were detected over a period of about three years (field cancerization).

The task of the primary care team is to assure that elders have thorough oral assessments on a routine basis. Counsel the patient in regards to nutrition, oral habits, sun screens, and follow-up. Lesions that persist longer than two weeks after stimuli have been removed should be biopsied; if nonkeratonic, Papanicolaou's smears may precede biopsy. The early oral cancer can be innocuous in appearance and painless.

Once the diagnosis has been established, the patient should be referred to a head and neck specialist who can provide a well-balanced judgment for further management, e.g., surgery, radiation, chemotherapy, or combinations thereof. The oral cancer patient should be closely followed by the primary care team since they may need continual supportive therapies such as daily topical fluorides, artificial saliva, frequent oral prophylaxis, etc.

ORAL HEALTH MAINTENANCE

Oral health maintenance includes procedures done by and for an individual that will result in an optimum level of oral health. It should be carried out on a routine basis. There are three steps to oral health maintenance; oral assessment procedures, oral hygiene, and oral health counseling.

Oral Assessment

REVIEW OF THE MEDICAL HISTORY

Health Conditions. Take into account those that might affect the ability of the individual to perform his or her own oral care (arthritis, multiple sclerosis, or paralysis of the upper extremities).

Medications (prescribed and over-the-counter medications). Some medicines have the potential to influence oral health directly by causing excessively dry oral tissues or uncontrolled mouth and tongue movements (phenothiazine derivatives such as Mellaril and Thorazine). These conditions often influence the success of the denture or partial denture wearer's ability to wear the appliance(s). Other drugs that affect oral tissues include Dilantin (causes gingival hyperplasia), antihistamines (xerostomia), and diuretics (dehydration of tissue).

Metabolic Problems. Such problems, especially diabetes, may cause xerostomia or contribute to the inability or slowness of tissues to heal following dental procedures. Diabetes can also influence the rate of dental caries or periodontal disease.

Epilepsy and Other Seizure Disorders. These often indicate that the patient may be taking Dilantin which can cause gingival enlargment (hyperplasis).

Diet. Some oral manifestations are a result of nutritional deficiencies. Poor nutrition, including high-candy intake, is frequent and contributes to caries and periodontal disease. Burning tongue, angular cheilosis, and atrophic glossitis can be the result of or related to vitamin B complex deficiencies.[5]

DENTAL HISTORY

1. The patient's dentist; date of last exam
2. Chief complaints
3. Denture history (e.g., how long have dentures been worn, how many sets of dentures)
4. Oral habits (e.g., teeth-clenching, smoking, etc.)
5. Oral hygiene practices (denture cleaning, etc.)

ORAL SCREENING EXAMINATION

Inspection and palpation are essential to assess the mouth. See Fig. 8-7.

Extraoral Examination. The shape of the face: Are both sides of the face symmetrical? Is there swelling over jawbone, below the eyes, or in the submandibular region? Palpate the structures of the face and neck with particular attention to the lymphatic and salivary gland regions. See Fig. 8-6. Check lips and corners of the mouth.

Intraoral Examination. (Use a flashlight, tongue blade, and mouth mirror.) Occasionally a patient will have such poor oral hygiene that it will be necessary to debride the mouth of the accumulations of debris just to check the soft tissues and teeth thoroughly. This can be done by using either a gauze sponge wrapped around an index finger or a soft bristled toothbrush to remove the soft debris from the tissues and teeth. The examiner might also use this as an opportunity to assess the capability of the patient in performing oral care procedures. This is easily done by giving patients a soft-bristled toothbrush and asking them to brush their teeth.

Inspect the mouth in a systematic fashion: Labial and buccal mucosa, vestibular areas, floor of mouth, and hard and soft palates (Fig. 8-7). Check for color changes, traumatic lesions, irritations, swellings, and lumps.

Tongue: Check the lateral borders, dorsal and under surfaces. Have the patient stick out the tongue so that the examiner can hold it with a gauze square. Gently pull the tongue first to one side and then to the other to visually check and palpate manually the posterior lateral borders. Check the entire tongue for lesions, swellings, or changes in color. Check the dorsal surface for accumulations of soft debris.

Gingiva: Check for color, bleeding, lesions, and swellings.

Teeth: Check the teeth for caries, fractures or sharp edges, mobility, and root tips (teeth broken off at the gumline).

Dentures and partial dentures: Check the denture for sharp edges, fractures or cracks that the patient might not be aware of. In general, the patient is perhaps the best judge of how his or her dentures or partials are fitting or functioning. What might appear (to the examiner) as an extremely loose or worn denture will be (to the patient) very adequate.

Type of dentition: Several types of dentition are possible, and it is important with respect to oral hygiene measures and oral health counseling to determine what type of dentition each patient has.

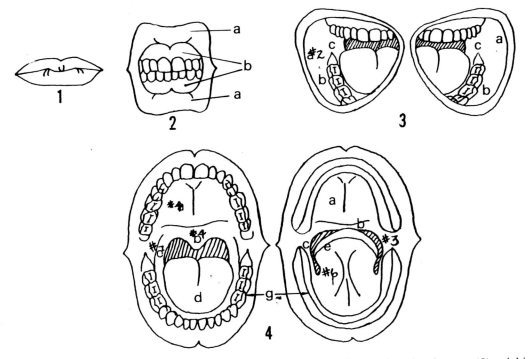

Fig. 8-7. Areas of the mouth to be routinely assessed: (1) lips and perioral areas; (2) *a.* labial mucosa and *b.* gingiva; (3) *a.* buccal mucosa, *b.* vestibules, and *c.* retromolar areas; (4) *a.* hard palate, *b.* soft palate, *c.* tonsils and oropharynx, *d.* dorsal surface of the tongue, *e.* laterial borders of the tongue, *f.* undersurface of the tongue and floor of the mouth, and *g.* teeth or alveolar ridges.

1. *Natural*—patient does not have any appliances and has some or all of own teeth. This patient may have fixed bridge work.
2. *Mixed*—patient has some natural teeth plus one or more appliances such as a full upper denture or one or more removable partial dentures.
3. *Edentulous*—this patient has no remaining natural teeth and may or may not have full upper and lower denture replacement.

SELF-CARE ABILITY

Elders vary in ability or inability to perform daily oral care. Some general guidelines to help establish this are a necessary part of any oral assessment.

1. *Completely capable.* The individual is able to do all of his or her own oral care, does not need to be reminded or assisted.
2. *Partially capable.* The individual can do the basic oral care procedures, but may need to be reminded or perhaps given supplies. (This applies to the individual who is somewhat confused, bedridden, or immobile.)

3. *Moderately capable.* The individual can perform a minimal amount of his or her own oral care but the result is usually an inadequate level of oral hygiene. Such an individual will require additional assistance.
4. *Completely incapable.* This individual will require complete assistance with oral hygiene procedures.

Oral Hygiene Measures

Instruction and supervision of oral hygiene can be the responsibility of a variety of primary care team members depending on the problem. The nurse, nurse's aide, and physical or occupational therapist can all be instrumental in the instruction and supervision of proper hygiene.

BASIC PROCEDURES

The basic supplies include, but are not limited to, a soft-bristled toothbrush, dental floss, and/or denture brush. We refer the reader to the many excellent resources listed in the references for exact detail and techniques[2,5-11] and to Fig. 8-5B for a guide to toothbrush placement.

An often neglected or forgotten aspect of oral care is brushing the tongue and other soft tissues of the mouth (gingiva, vestibule and edentulous ridges and palate). This is to clean away any excess soft debris and food particles that the patients are no longer capable of removing through the actions of their tongue and cheek muscles. The stimulating and massaging effect of this will also help promote a more healthy tissue tone and improve the capacity for taste sensation. Use a soft-bristled toothbrush that has been moistened with some water, and brush the tongue from the posterior and middle sections to the outer edges by using a gentle rolling motion of the brush. The gingiva, edentulous ridges, and palates can be brushed in a circular motion.

Oral Health Counseling

This component of oral health maintenance begins with informing the patient of assessment findings and of what is necessary to improve and/or maintain an optimum level of oral health. A specific patient education plan and dental referral are important.

NONPRESCRIPTION PREPARATIONS

Elders often use over-the-counter preparations for home treatment of dental problems; some of the more common are described below.

Aspirin is a common analgesic. It is, however, sometimes placed on tissues and teeth to relieve pain. Although the pain may be temporarily relieved, severe chemical burns may ensue. Tyelenol may be a preferred short-term analgesic.

Hydrogen Peroxide (1.5–3 percent) is often used for oral ulcerations, erosions, and postsurgical care, particularly if the patient should not use stronger ionic mouthwashes such as NaCl. Long-term use of

H_2O_2 can stimulate hypertrophy of the filiform papillae on the tongue causing a hairy appearance. Peroxide is not recommended for wounds healing by granulation.[12]

Mild Fluoride Mouth Rinses (anticariogenic) are now available for over-the-counter use; elderly are also well advised to receive stronger fluoride applications following cleaning of the natural teeth. For patients with decreased or mucinous salivary flow due to radiation (or from other causes), daily fluoride applications may be essential to control decay in the remaining natural teeth.

Artificial Saliva (with or without fluoride) can be obtained for patients with dry mouth (xerostomia). Dehydration can be related to diuretic drug therapy with an accompanying xerostomia.

Emollients for sore mouths are constituted of such items as milk of magnesia, sodium bicarbonate (baking soda) and Kaopectate.[12]

SUMMARY

The primary health care team can assist patients in optimizing their oral health. A plan to achieve this goal includes: (1) assessment of the mouth; (2) incorporating standards and protocols for oral health maintenance into the practice; (3) assisting and training the patient in oral hygiene; (4) educating the patient in the principles of disease control; and (5) providing the encouragement and follow-through to obtain dental care.

Primary care health professionals play an important role in providing and advocating preventive and restorative dental care. The articulation of the dental team—composed of dentists, dental assistants, hygienists and technicians—with the primary care team can be a very important part of maintaining the health and social well-being of elders.

REFERENCES

1. Bennett J: Oral health maintenance, in Carnavali D, Patrick M, (eds): Nursing Management for the Elderly. Philadelphia, JB Lippincott Co, 1979

2. Dummet C: Dental health problems of the geriatric population. J Nat Med Assoc 71:182–185, 1979
3. Bennett JS: Final Report on Model Dental Program.

Grant '90-A-307. HEW Office of Research, Demonstration and Manpower Resources, 1976

4. Gift HC: Attitudes and dental health status of the elderly. Paper presented at the International Association for Dental Research, March 1979

5. Lynch M (ed): Burket's Oral Medicine, ed 7. Philadelphia, JB Lippincott Co, 1977

6. Burnett GW, Scherp HW, Schuster GS: Oral Microbiology and Infectious Disease, ed 4. Baltimore, Williams & Wilkins, 1976

7. Grant DA, Stern IB, Everett FG: Periodontics, ed 5. St. Louis, CV Mosby, 1979, p 171

8. Creamer HR, Line SE, Wright WW: Study of periodontal status of the elderly. Paper presented at the International Association for Dental Research, March 1979

9. Jordan HV, Sumney DL: Root surface caries: Review of the literature and significance of the problem. J Periodontol 44:158–163, 1973

10. Caldwell RC, Stallard RE: A Textbook for Preventive Dentistry. Philadelphia, WB Saunders Co, 1977

11. Maurer J: Providing optimal oral health. Nurs Clin NA 12:4, 1977

12. American Dental Association: Accepted Dental Therapeutics, ed. 211 East Chicago Avenue, Chicago, Illinois 60611, 1977

RECOMMENDED RESOURCES

A Manual of Oral Hygiene for Handicapped and Chronically Ill Patients. Oregon State Health Division, Dental Health Section, PO Box 231, Portland, Oregon 97207

American Cancer Society, Oregon Division, Inc, 1530 SW Taylor Street, Portland, Oregon 97205

American Dental Association: Accepted Dental Therapeutics ed 37. 211 East Chicago Avenue, Chicago, Illinois 60611, 1977

Bennett JS: Final Report on Interdisciplinary Training Program in Gerontology. Contract 'RX-74-12. HEW, 1976

Bennett JS: Final Report on Model Dental Program. Grant '90-A-307. HEW Office of Research, Demonstration and Manpower Resources, 1976

Creamer HR, Line SE, Wright WW: Study of periodontal status of the elderly. Paper presented at the International Association for Dental Research, March 1979

Davidoff H, Winkler, Lee WHM: Dentistry for the Special Patient: The Aged, Chronically Ill and Handicapped. Philadelphia, WB Saunders Co, 1977

DP-2, VA Central Office Film Library, 810 Vermont Avenue, NW, Washington, DC 20420

Educational resource catalogues and brochures. American Dental Association, 211 East Chicago Avenue, Chicago, Illinois

Franks AST, Hedgegard B: Geriatric Dentistry. Oxford, England, Blackwell Scientific Publications, 1973

Gift HC: Attitudes and dental health status of the elderly. Paper presented at the International Association for Dental Research, March 1979

Nizel AE: Role of nutrition in the oral health of the aging patient, in Alfano MC, De Paola DP (eds): Symposium on Nutrition. Dent Clin of NA 20:3, 1976

O'Malley K, Judge TG, Crooks J: in Avery, GS (ed): Geriatric Clinical Pharmacology and Therapeutics in Drug Treatment. Sidney, Australia, Adis Press, and Littleton, Mass, Publishing Sciences Group, Inc, 1976

Patient education pamphlets. Colgate-Palmolive Co, PO Box 518, Chicago, Illinois 60677

Price JH: Oral health care for the geriatric patient. J Geront Nur 5:25–29, 1979

Sharawy AM, Sabhoreval K, Socransky SS, et al: A quantitiative study of plaque and calculus formation in normal and periodontally involved mouths. J Peridontol 37:495–501, 1966

Swoope CC, Smith DE, Lukens EM: Geriatric dentistry, in JW Clark (ed): Clinical Dentistry, Haggerstown, Maryland, Harper & Row, 1979

9

Neurology

Michael Podlone, M.D.
Clark H. Millikan, M.D.

Much of what we identify as normal aging reflects changes in the nervous system. The most readily recognized features are slowing of responses, weakening of muscle power, and loss of agility. The most poignant changes involve the subtle decline in mental abilities, creativity, and memory.

Under clinical scrutiny, additional changes are found to correlate with senescence. These include diminution of vibratory sense in the lower extremities, decreased sensory acuity in general, restriction of upward gaze, and loss of fine coordination.

These patterns, however, are not uniformly predictable, as there are sufficient individual differences. It is likely that genetic factors play a role in the degree to which the usual senescent changes are expressed. Underlying the clinical manifestations are a variety of physiologic changes that occur in the aged: there is a 20 percent decrease in cerebral blood flow and a 10 percent reduction in weight of the brain. Microscopically, one finds a loss of neurons and increasing numbers of neuritic (previously senile) plaques and neurofibrillary tangles. Biochemically, there are diminished and imbalanced levels of neurotransmitters.

The diseases that will be discussed in this chapter are not part of the normal aging process. They represent pathologic entities superimposed on an involuting nervous system.

INCIDENCE OF NEUROLOGICAL PROBLEMS IN ELDERS

The most frequent neurologic diseases the practitioner will encounter are cerebrovascular conditions (stroke and TIA), dementia, and parkinsonism. Often patients will have specific complaints for which an underlying etiology must be sought. Dizziness, headaches, and parethesia are among the most common neurologic symptoms in the elderly.

When an elder patient experiences a headache, a number of disorders not commonly found in younger persons needs to be considered. Cervical osteoarthritis may often cause neck pain and headaches in this age group. Tension headaches and migraines are not common in an older population, but headaches in association with depression is a more prominent diagnosis. Occasionally, new onset of headaches may signal a dangerous disorder such as temporal arteritis or a space-occupying intracerebral mass.

Cerebrovascular disease is the third most common cause of death in the nation. There is a direct correlation with age: under aged 50, cerebrovascular disease is rare; from 50–59, the incidence is about three per 1,000 population/year; then there is a steady increase to 20 per 1,000/year in the age range of 75–79. At least 200,000 deaths/year are attributed to these conditions. Recently a decline in the incidence of stroke, particularly in the oldest ages, has been documented.[1] The factors responsible for this decrease have not yet been elucidated.

Parkinsonism has affected one in 100 persons over the age of 55. This high occurrence is probably due to the viral encephalitis epidemic of 1918. As the persons affected are now in their 70s and 80s, it is likely that the incidence of Parkinsonism is decreasing.

The prevalence of severe chronic dementia is estimated at 4 percent. Mild dementia probably afflicts 10–14 percent of persons over aged 65. Although not usually listed as a prime cause of death, studies have pointed out a marked reduction in the life expectancy of these patients.[2]

UNCOMMON PROBLEMS

There are many neurologic processes that are not often seen in the primary care of elders. When encountered, e.g., seizure or meningitis, prompt specialty consultation should be obtained. Chronic subdural hematomas can often occur, secondary to falls, in elders. Elders can forget falls or head trauma. The history is often only a recent but slow and gradual deterioration of personality, confusion, forgetfulness, and loss of judgment. Headaches, although not often present, dementia, and focal neurologic signs are all consistent with a diagnosis of chronic subdural hematoma.

Temporal arteritis is a rare disorder that is confined to older patients. Classic findings include headaches, visual disturbances, and a tender temporal artery. The erythrocyte sedimentation rate is markedly elevated. If needed, a temporal artery biopsy may help to confirm the diagnosis but may be falsely negative in one-third of patients. It is important to recognize this disease because, untreated, it may cause blindness and a stroke-like picture. The arteritis usually responds to treatment with corticosteroids.

Dementia

Becoming demented is not a normal consequence of aging changes in the brain. Dementia has a broad definition: a deterioration in mental or intellectual ability. Organic brain syndrome and encephalopathy describe the same clinical problem. Categorization of illnesses with mental impairment is ham-

pered by a lack of precision in terminology. Dementia is often defined as a chronic process. As used in this section, dementia means no more than a diminished intellectual ability. Thus, we will discuss both acute-onset dementia and chronic, insidious-onset dementia.

Acute-onset Dementia

Patients, especially the elderly who may mistakenly be diagnosed as demented, include those with dysphasia, dysarthria, and benign memory loss. The mode of onset of a dementing disease is a critical clinical feature. Acute-onset dementias are dramatic and life-threatening events. The precipitating cause is usually a disorder outside the central nervous system that interferes with brain metabolism. Pneumonia, myocardial infarction, hepatic or renal failure, hypnotic and anticholinergic drugs are all common causes of acute dementia in the elderly. Others are listed in Table 9-1. In practice, most acute dementias are reversible.[2b] They have as their key feature a sudden deterioration in mental function. In contrast to the chronic dementias, there is often impairment not only of higher functions (calculation, judgment, orientation, etc.), but also of general alertness and perception. Acute dementias tend to cause more global impairment of cerebral activities. Delirium is characterized by agitation, delusions, hallucinations, and confusion.

Table 9-1
Some Causes of Acute Dementia

Process	Disease or Problem
Hypoxia	Pneumonia, pulmonary embolus, respiratory failure, CO poisoning
Ischemia	Myocardial infarction, CHF, CVA, hypertension
Metabolic disturbance	Hypoglycemia, dehydration, hypercalcemia
Drugs	Sedatives, anticholinergics, cimetidine, L-dopa, phenytoin, phenothiazines, amantadine, corticosteroids, alcohol, etc.
Infections	Fever, septicemia, meningitis, urinary tract infection
Other diseases	Diabetes, hyperthyroidism, seizures, head trauma, subdural hematoma

MANAGEMENT

Patients who present with an acutely altered mental state should be hospitalized. A thorough history, physical, and basic diagnostic tests will usually uncover the precipitating cause, and treatment can be initiated. (See Data Base section under Chronic Dementia for mental states exam, below.) Admission diagnostic studies of UA, CBC, CXR, ECG, electrolytes, and a screening chemistry panel are sufficient to pinpoint most of the processes listed in Table 9-2 as causes of acute dementia. The prognosis is variable and depends on the underlying condition, e.g., acute myocardial infarction as opposed to drug-induced hyponatremia. There should be full recovery to the baseline mental state once the precipitating cause has been resolved.

Chronic Dementia

Dementia may be defined as chronic when the disease has been present for at least six months. A few chronic dementias have an acute onset, e.g., anoxic encephalopathy postcardiac arrest or carbon monoxide poisoning. However, the problem that more often faces the primary care practitioner is the patient who has quietly and subtly become demented.

There is no one area of the cerebrum where intellectual ability is localized. Chronic dementia results from diffuse cerebral dysfunction in most cases. Recent studies suggest that about 20 percent of these patients may have treatable conditions. The diseases that cause chronic dementia are quite different from those causing the acute disorder. The major causes of untreatable chronic dementia are Alzheimer's disease and multi-infarct dementia. Also, the Parkinson's dementia complex is common (see page 125).

There is no longer a distinction between senile dementia, and Alzheimer's disease (presenile dementia), which accounts for 50–60 percent of all chronic dementias. Its cause is unknown. Pathologically, it is characterized by cerebral atrophy and accumulation of neurofibrillary tangles and neuritic (senile) plaques in the cerebral cortex. One clinical clue to the presence of Alzheimer's disease is the

Table 9-2
Clues to Treatable Causes of Chronic Dementia

Disease	Findings	Diagnostic Test
Normal pressure hydrocephalus	Gait disorder Sphincter incontinence	CAT scan Radionuclide Cisternography
Neoplasm or subdural hematomas	Focal neurologic signs	CAT scan
Depression	Depressed affect Psychomotor retardation	History Neuropsychiatric test
Drug toxicity	Depends on the drug: Anticholinergic effects or ataxia and nystagmus from sedatives and antiepileptic agents	Drug levels Trial off drugs
Hepatic encephalopathy	Asterixis Signs of hepatic failure History of cirrhosis or portacaval shunt	Liver function tests Arterial ammonia EEG
B_{12} deficiency	Positive Romberg Diminished proprioception Glossitis	B_{12} Assay
Hypothyroidism	Signs of myxedema	TSH, T_4
Syphilis	Argyll-Robertson pupils and positive Romberg	VDRL, FTA on CSF

dissociation between perservation of social skills and impairment of memory and ratiocination.

Many clinicians have the misconception that the most common dementia in old age is due to cerebral arteriosclerosis. Multi-infarct dementia accounts for approximately 10–20 percent of cases of chronic dementia. These patients have a history and neurologic evidence of previous strokes. They often have findings of systemic arteriosclerosis as well. In Alzheimer's disease, arteriosclerosis is not a significant feature.

A number of uncommon degenerative cerebral conditions also cause irreversible dementia. These include Pick's disease, Huntington's chorea, and Creutzfeldt-Jakob's disease.

Treatable etiologies of dementia may be found in about one out of every six patients. Clues to the presence of a reversible cause are provided in Table 9-2.

Although not a cause of dementia in the true sense, depression is listed because it is clinically difficult to separate from chronic dementia. Those features that may help separate depression from dementia include a sharper onset, a more consistent depressed affect, somatic symptoms (anorexia, weight loss, psychomotor retardation), and little intellectual impairment if testing can be accomplished. The presence of frontal lobe disease signs, particularly mild grasp and the snout reflex, may help differentiate the two diseases. Although some authors have suggested empiric trials of antidepressants for many patients with dementia, we feel that careful interviewing and clinical judgment should allow proper diagnosis of depression and the selective use of drugs.

Drug-induced dementia should always be considered. Although drugs more often produce an acute syndrome, they not infrequently contribute to a chronic dementia. Bromides are less available as over-the-counter drugs, and cases are often now due to prescribed medications. Agents most frequently at fault include sedatives, tranquilizers, anticholinergic agents, phenytoin, and others. Clinicians must be alert to the potentially hazardous effects of these drugs in the elderly.

Normal pressure hydrocephalus is a disease characterized by dilitation of the ventricles, stasis of CSF, and a normal spinal fluid pressure. The pathophysiology of the disorder is not well known. NPH may be an idiopathic or secondary condition. Subarachnoid hemorrhage is the most common and trauma the next likely underlying disorder in the secondary cases.

Clinically, these patients demonstrate a triad of dementia, gait disturbance (variable, ataxia or apraxia) and incontinence. Ventricular shunting has been a valuable mode of therapy for some patients—about 40 percent. The response to shunting is more likely in secondary NPH than in idiopathic cases. At this time, there is no way of selecting those patients most likely to benefit from the procedure.

The most frequent causes of reversible dementia in addition to depression are drug toxicity, normal pressure hydrocephalus, and intracranial masses (chronic subdural hematoma and tumors). Less common causes include vitamin B_{12} deficiency and hypothyroidism.

DATA BASE

Family and close friends are the first to note changes in the patient, but usually the earliest signs are often ignored or glossed over. The initial changes of chronic dementia include forgetfulness, loss of initiative, and inability to concentrate. (These nonspecific symptoms are also found in depression and astute clinicians may be hard pressed to distinguish the two diseases.) Patients with dementia also manifest impaired judgment, poor calculating and verbal ability. Later in the course of the disease, a variety of behaviors may emerge—emotional lability, perseveration in speech, disorientation, and paranoia. The pattern of symptoms and manifestations vary among patients. Ultimately, if the disease progresses, the patient enters a vegetative existence where mobility is extremely limited and consciousness is significantly impaired.

Patients may present to clinicians at any stage. Early on, practitioners frequently neglect to test intellectual abilities and the disease goes undiagnosed. At a later phase, the family may bring the patient to the practice because of behavioral problems. At times, when patients cannot care for themselves and the family can no longer cope with the situation, then what has been a slowly developing home problem presents in the office as an acute social catastrophe.

Frequently, patients with mild chronic dementia experience a sudden deterioration in their mental state. This is especially prone to happen in hospital and postoperatively. Patients become completely disoriented, experience visual hallucinations, and are often combative. The cause is said to be sensory deprivation, and the condition is labeled "sundowning" as it most often occurs at night. When any patient with chronic dementia experiences a sudden deterioration, those disorders which cause acute dementia should be sought. See Table 9-1.

A thorough and careful history and physical exam are the cornerstones to a diagnosis of the patient. Areas to emphasize are: duration, progression, and mode of onset of symptoms, history of head trauma, past medical history (anemia, liver disease, CVA, syphilis, neoplasm, thyroid disease, etc.), medications including over-the-counter drugs, prior level of intellectual function, and history of alcohol abuse. It is vital to explore symptoms that may suggest depression.

The signs listed in Table 9-2 may suggest a treatable cause but the high incidence of associated and possibly contributing physical illnesses in the elderly dictates that all systems be examined in detail.

A complete mental status exam is one of the most important tools used to diagnose dementia. While moderate and severe degrees of dementia are easily uncovered, mild dementia is difficult to diagnose. Many of the available brief mental screening tests will miss dementia in its early phases when potential therapeutic intervention is most beneficial.

A standard mental status exam includes assessment of recent and remote memory, orientation, calculation, judgment, abstraction, and graphic ability. Evaluation of overall level of consciousness is a critical part of every neurologic exam. Quantification of errors and the degree of deficit measured by mental status exams has not been standardized. The severity of dementia is proportional to the number of errors made overall. It is only in the severest dementias that orientation to person and place is lost. Some questions, e.g., calculating ability, listing past presidents, or ability to abstract, may depend on the cultural as well as educational background of the patient. It is usually stated that in dementia remote memory is preserved to a greater extent than recent memory. (When testing orientation, it is advisable to warn patients that you are going to ask some very simple questions and that this is routine.)

A variety of neurologic signs correlate with the presence of diffuse cerebral dysfunction. See Table 9-3. These neurologic findings are most representative of bilateral cortical disease; however, some primitive reflexes, especially grasp, may be found with frontal lobe lesions and motor impersistence with right parietal lesions.

For diagnosis of bilateral cerebral dysfunction, Jenkyn, Walsh, and Culver have suggested a screening battery of tests that relies more on testing for neurologic signs than on assessing intellectual ability. Although this may lead to greater accuracy, it is unlikely to lead to earlier diagnosis.[3]

The findings of dysphasia or focal neurologic signs suggests either multi-infarct dementia, a focal or space occupying process, or one of the uncommon progressive degenerative cerebral disorders.

Patients who have chronic dementia merit a thorough diagnostic study to rule out reversible causes. The studies as a group suggested by Table 9-2 include CBC, B_{12} level, TSH, T_4, liver function tests, LP especially for FTA, VDRL, and CAT scan. These should not be ordered shotgun fashion for all patients. Data from history and physical guide the diagnostic workup. These patients may not need hospitalization for diagnosis if an outpatient workup can be done adequately. Alzheimer's disease is a diagnosis of exclusion. The finding of cerebral atrophy on CAT scan corroborates a suspicion of this disease and excludes space-occupying lesions.

In many instances, an etiologic diagnosis of dementia may contribute to management. Patients who have Huntington's chorea will need genetic counseling for their family. Multi-infarct dementia often has hypertension as a predisposing condition and continued blood pressure elevation may warrant treatment.

The development of computer assisted tomographic (CAT) scans of the brain has greatly facilitated the diagnostic process. A computer is used to synthesize multiple x-ray density measurements and create images of the cerebrum at different levels and in different planes. Total radiation is less than two rads, less than for a skull series. Diagnostic accuracy is excellent and has obviated the need for arteriography and pneumoencephalography in many instances.

The goals of managing patients with chronic dementia are maintaining and maximizing current functional abilities and limiting situations requiring skills they lack. It is necessary first to define the patient's deficits and the social/family problems that are on-going. It may be very helpful to visit the patient's home to assess the extent to which a patient has deteriorated, e.g., uneaten meals, signs of incontinence, evidence of paranoia, etc. The family

Table 9-3
Neurologic Signs Correlated With the Presence of Diffuse Cerebral Dysfunction

Suck reflex	Elicited by placing an object between the lips. A positive response is a puckering or sucking motion.
Snout reflex	Elicited by brief pressure on the lips. A positive response is puckering movement.
Grasp reflex	Elicited by stroking the palm (it may be necessary to tell the patient not to hold on). A positive response is grasping or closing the hand.
Palmomental	Elicited by firm stimulation (like eliciting a Babinski's) of the thenar eminence. A positive response is nonfatiguing contraction of the ipsilateral mentalis muscle.
Glabellar blink	Elicited by light tapping on the glabellar region approaching the patient from above. A positive response is nonfatiguing blinking.
Nuchocephalic reflex	Elicited by briskly turning the shoulders of a patient to the right or left while standing. A positive response is the head keeping its original position (normal response is for the head to turn in the direction of the shoulders).
Paratonia (gegenhalten)	An inconsistent and irregular resistance to passive movements of the limbs (instructions to relax are given first).
Motor impersistence	An inability to sustain certain positions, e.g., keeping the eyes closed for 15 seconds.

will require support throughout this process, especially if the patient is to remain with them.

Once detected, dementia does not conscript patients into becoming institutionalized. Some will be found to have curable etiologies. Many will be able to maintain a functional life at home with families. Others with milder deficits may be able to live independently with the support of visiting nurses, home health aides, and community facilities.

Some patients with dementia can improve or progression can be delayed by providing on-going stimulation. This may take many forms—occupational or recreational therapy, senior citizen organizations, and group interactions. Patients who are disoriented benefit from reminders of day and time. This can be done at home by using signs and by reminding the patient of the date, etc. Reality orientation sessions have been shown to be of value. The willingness of the physician to work with and coordinate social workers, physical and occupational therapists, and nurses is crucial to maintaining the stability of the patient and family.

DRUG TREATMENTS

Pharmacologic therapy, especially in the elderly demented person, is hazardous. The most frequently employed agents are minor and major tranquilizers and antidepressants. Much of the time these are given inappropriately. Many of the minor tranquilizers have long half-lives and tend to accumulate, especially in the aged with diminished metabolic and excretory capacities. Phenothiazines and related compounds have hypotensive and extrapyramidal side effects. Their anticholinergic side effects are additive with other medications, especially the antidepressants. Excessive sedation and anticholinergic toxicity can readily bring out or exacerbate dementia. Elders often react paradoxically to barbiturates. The decision to use these agents must be carefully made, weighing specific indications and potential benefits against the hazards. Drugs with the least sedative effect should be considered. Specific indications may include depression, uncontrollable belligerence, paranoid ideation, and insomnia. The nonsedating phenothiazines, such as low-dose thioridazine and haloperidol are the most effective for agitation, belligerence, or paranoia.

A number of drugs have been recommended to improve memory capacity and overall intellectual function, e.g., cerebral vasodilators. Investigations are currently ongoing into increasing levels of neurotransmitters (acetylcholine) by using physostigmine and lecithin. To date, there is not sufficient evidence to recommend any of these agents.

Dementia is a cruel and crippling condition. Many ethical issues are raised in caring for demented patients. Initially, these patients deserve a one-time evaluation to rule out curable etiologies. Once an irreversible condition is diagnosed, there are still interventions that may make the patient and his or her family more comfortable and more functional. Any decision to withhold treatment or to take a nihilistic approach must take the patient's quality of life, the family's concerns, and the adequacy of prior management into account.

Dizziness

Dizziness is one of the most frequent symptoms in old age. Dizziness has a multitude of meanings and, consequently, of sources in a multitude of body systems: the ear, central nervous system, peripheral nerves, the heart, etc. It is the task of the practitioner first to determine the precise sensation experienced by the patient and then to trace through the labyrinth of differential diagnoses to the cause.

Some elderly patients complain of dizziness when they mean they are afraid of falling and do not have dizziness as defined in Table 9-4.

The genesis of vertigo, dysequilibrium, and some types of lightheadedness is found in body systems which create an awareness of spatial orientation. These systems are: the eyes, providing visual information; the proprioceptive sensors and tracts, pro-

Table 9-4
Interpretation of Dizziness

Symptom	Sensation
True vertigo	There is a spinning or rotatory sensation. Either the patient or the environment seems to be moving, and there is a sense of impulsion as if falling. Occasionally the complaint is of the environment wavering back and forth—oscillopsia.
Faintness	This is a sensation of impending loss of consciousness. Patients may experience brief grey outs (presyncope) with dimming of vision, blunting of perceptions and consciousness, weakness, and diaphoresis. It may presage frank syncope or blackout.
Lightheadedness, giddiness	All ill-defined sensations of wooziness, fuzziness, or feeling not quite right.
Dysequilibrium	A sensation of impaired balance.

viding kinesthetic data from muscles and joints; the vestibular system and labyrinth, providing information on changes in velocity and position; and the nuclei and integration circuits involving the brainstem, cerebellum, and cortex. Faintness, as opposed to other types of dizziness, is due to hypoperfusion of the brainstem and cerebral cortex.

A key clinical dictum is that dizziness of the faintness type may well be due to life-threatening cardiovascular disorders, while dizziness of other categories is only rarely life-threatening. Since at times it is impossible to distinguish the types of dizziness, especially in the elderly, it is imperative first to rule out dangerous etiologies—particularly cardia arrhythmias and hypovolemia.

TRUE VERTIGO

In general, most cases of true vertigo are due to disease of the labyrinth and less commonly to central nervous system disorders. In the elderly, however, there is a shift to degenerative and vascular etiologies. Table 9-5 lists the causes of vertigo.

Perhaps the most common cause of dizziness in the elderly is the multiple sensory deficits syndrome.[4] Patients with this disorder complain of difficulty walking, especially when making turns. The sensation may be of mild vertigo or of lightheadedness. The typical combination of deficits includes peripheral neuropathy, cervical spine disease, and vestibular dysfunction. Often there is diminished vision and hearing as well. It is known that disease of the cervical spine and neck muscles can cause vertigo. The extent to which this cervicogenic vertigo contributes to the multiple sensory deficits

syndrome is not clear. This syndrome is more likely to occur in diabetic patients.

Vertebrobasilar artery disease is found primarily in the older population. Episodes of ischemia to the brainstem cause true vertigo but not as an isolated symptom. There are associated, neighboring neurologic symptoms and signs. Circumoral paresthesiae, bilateral paresis, diplopia and ataxia are the most specific concomitants. The problem is usually one of ischemic attacks involving the posterior circulation, but frank infarction may occur as well as result in severe vertigo and permanent deficits (e.g., occlusion of the posterior inferior cerebellar artery). (See the section on TIA for further discussion of

Table 9-5
Causes of Vertigo

Site	Disease	Diagnosis
Labyrinth	Benign positional vertigo	+ Nylen-Barany maneuver with fatiguing response
	Labyrinthitis/vestibular neuronitis	Patients are acutely ill with vomiting; often unilateral hypoactive caloric response
	Meniere's disease	Confirmed by audiologic studies; 90 percent have unilateral hearing loss
Middle ear	Rare causes: impacted cerumen, otitis media, cholesteatoma, fistula	Otoscopic exam
Eighth nerve	Acoustic neuroma	Prolonged history, No discrete attacks, Unilateral sensorineural hearing loss and cranial nerve palsies
	Drugs: aminoglycosides, aspirin	Drug levels, history of recent use
Peripheral nerves* Cervical spine* Eyes	Multiple sensory deficits syndrome	Symptoms present when walking, peripheral neuropathy
Brainstem*	Vertebrobasilar ischemia Multiple sclerosis Cerebellopontine tumor	Associated neurologic symptoms or signs
Cerebellum	Hemorrhage Tumor	Headache, vomiting Ataxia, gaze palsy

*Most common cause in elders.

diagnosis and treatment.) The subclavian steal syndrome is a rare cause of vertebrobasilar insufficiency.

When there is hearing loss that occurs in association with vertigo, a different group of diagnoses needs to be considered. While presbycusis is common in the aged, the onset of vertigo with *recent* hearing impairment should direct the clinician's focus to the ear and the eighth nerve. In the older ages, impacted cerumen, eustachian tube dysfunction, cholesteatoma, and otitis media all may induce vertigo. It is particularly important to rule out a drug-induced cause. Drugs known to be ototoxic are listed in Table 17-2 of Chapter 17. Aminoglycosides may be quite hazardous in the elderly in whom renal function is diminished. Less common causes of hearing loss and vertigo in the elderly are hypothyroidism, Meniere's disease, and acoustic neuroma. The latter two diseases are suggested by the finding of unilateral hearing loss.

Benign positional vertigo is a common cause of vertiginous symptoms. It is a self-limiting disorder of unknown etiology. Episodes of vertigo are induced only by specific changes in head position, e.g., turning the head and looking up. The condition persists for a variable period, then resolves. Positional vertigo may occur with central lesions as well. Diagnosis is confirmed by the Nylen-Barany maneuver described in the next section.

Acute labyrinthitis is a dramatic illness associated with inflammation in the middle ear. The exact cause is usually unknown, although infection of viral etiology is postulated. Patients are acutely ill; they tend to lie still and minimize any head movement which exacerbates the vertigo, nausea, and vomiting they experience. The attack lasts days to weeks and slowly resolves. Acute labyrinthitis is differentiated from brainstem ischemia by the lack of accompanying neurologic symptoms or signs. Occasionally, patients have recurrences that may be brought on by fever, viral syndromes, or stress. A most uncommon cause of vertigo is acute cerebellar hemorrhage. These patients require emergency neurosurgery. They present with sudden onset nausea, vomiting, and headaches. Ataxia, gaze palsy, and peripheral facial palsy are often present.

PATIENTS WHO DO *NOT* HAVE TRUE VERTIGO

Within this heterogenous category, the causes of dizziness are legion. When the dizziness is actually a sense of faintness, cardiovascular disease must be sought. Cerebral hypoperfusion is the mechanism

by which multiple disease processes cause faintness. Syncope or actual loss of consciousness may occur if the cerebral hypoperfusion is prolonged. There are three key mechanisms that underlie cerebral hypoperfusion: cardiac disorders, hypovolemia, and impaired cardiovascular reflexes. See Chapter 11 for discussion.

When a patient complains of lightheadedness, it must be kept in mind that this may represent mild forms of vertigo or faintness. The lightheadedness or giddiness due to hyperventillation, which is frequently seen in younger patients, is unusual in older patients. Multiple sensory deficits may also cause lightheadedness. Dysequilibrium is not a common symptom and when present suggests drug toxicity (e.g., phenytoin, alcohol, or aminoglycosides) or cerebellar disease.

DATA BASE

A thorough history and physical are of paramount importance in focusing on the potential cause of dizziness. Descriptors of the symptom should be sought in all cases: character of the dizziness; onset; duration of episodes; frequency; precipitating factors—change in position (i.e., is it orthostatic), turning the head, turns while walking, straining, exercise, cough, micturition; relieving factors; syncope; medications—especially regarding ototoxic drugs and antihypertensive agents; and past medical history. Symptoms associated with specific causes can then be pursued. See Table 9-6.

Table 9-6
Focused Data Base for Dizziness

True vertigo	Expect nausea, vomiting, diaphoresis, a reluctance to move about
Ear diseases	Tinnitus, hearing loss, prior ear disease or surgery, pain, discharge
CV disease	Chest pain, palpitations, dyspnea on exertion, edema, history of myocardial disease, heart murmur
Hypovolemia	Diarrhea, persistent vomiting, hematemesis, melena, overt bleeding, anticoagulant use.
Neurologic diseases	Headache, diplopia, ataxia, paresthesia, paresis
Psychiatric diseases	Acral paresthesia, anxiety, breathlessness, recent life crisis

During the physical exam, it is possible to clarify the patient's symptom by performing dizziness simulation maneuvers. It is important to be careful of the safety and comfort of elders during these exams. These are:

1. Have the patient stand for three minutes after a period of recumbency. Check blood pressure and pulse in both positions. This will detect orthostatic hypotension and should be performed in all patients.
2. Valsalva maneuver.
3. Sudden turns while walking.
4. A Nylen-Barany maneuver—this is performed by moving the patient suddenly from a sitting position to a supine position with his head extending over the examining table, tipped 45 degrees back and 45 degrees to one side.
5. Carotid sinus massage has been included in dizziness simulation batteries. This, however, may be hazardous especially in the elderly and should not be considered routine. If it is done, the patient should be monitored by ECG and precautions taken in case of syncope.

The degree to which the physical exam can be focused depends on the specificity of symptoms. The following areas may need evaluation:

1. *True vertigo or dysequilibrium* Check for nystagmus; ear exam; neurologic testing including gait, pinprick sensation, Romberg, cerebellar testing; auscultate for carotid and subclavian bruits; check BP in both arms, if you are considering the subclavian steal syndrome.
2. *Faintness.* Orthostatic BP and pulse; cardiac exam; stool guiac; abdominal exam.
3. *Lightheadedness.* Sensory testing; eye exam; depending on the patient's age and his or her symptoms, it may be necessary to do all of the above.

DIAGNOSTIC TESTS FOR VERTIGO

Nystagmus. Careful observation of nystagmus may provide evidence of the origin of vertigo. Clues to a central nervous system cause of vertigo include: vertical nystagmus, unilateral nystagmus, nystagmus without vertigo, associated cranial nerve palsies, and focal neurologic signs. Rotatory nystagmus is mostly seen with labyrinthine system disease.

Nylen-Barany Maneuver. Proper interpretation of this test is necessary to distinguish central causes from the benign positional form of vertigo.

In benign positional vertigo, when the patient's head is tilted, there is a *latent* period before vertigo and nystagmus occur. The response is not sustained and fatigues on repetition. The direction of the nystagmus is fixed and severe vertigo and nausea usually occur.

In central causes of positional vertigo, there is no latent period, the response is nonfatiguing, the direction of the nystagmus may change, and accompanying vertigo and nausea are usually mild.

Calorics. Irrigation of the external auditory canals with iced or tepid water provides data on the function of the labyrinth and vestibular system. This test is used to detect a hypofunctioning labyrinth. In the office, it rarely helps to distinguish the different causes of vertigo.

Electronystagmography (ENG). This is a procedure used to record direction and speed of nystagmus. Visual fixation may abolish nystagmus, but this technique allows recording of nystagmus with the eyes closed. It therefore allows more accurate and precise determinations of nystagmus and is useful to distinguish peripheral from central forms of vertigo.

Audiometric Studies. These tests are indicated when patients have audiologic symptoms or hearing loss in association with dizziness. They are used to help differentiate Meniere's disease from acoustic neuroma and central lesions. If acoustic neuroma is suspected, x-rays of the internal auditory canal and a CAT scan are indicated. They are also of value in monitoring patients on ototoxic drugs.

DIAGNOSTIC TESTS FOR FAINTNESS

Where a cardiovascular etiology is sought, an ECG and rhythm strip are indicated. In addition, you may monitor the patient's pulse during the history to detect infrequent irregularities. Twenty-four-hour Holter monitoring is indicated for faintness of undetermined etiology and when paroxymal arrhythmia is suspected.

TREATMENT

Specific therapy depends on defining the cause of dizziness. Patients with multiple sensory deficits may be difficult to treat. Efforts should be made to improve correctible problems. Since the dizziness is often manifest when walking, support with a cane may lead to improvement. Cataract extraction may be considered if the problem with mobility is a severe one. The role of cervical spondylosis is unclear, but some have advocated use of a soft cervical collar.

If the patient has benign positional vertigo, treatment is: (1) reassurance and explanation; (2) avoidance of specific positions that initiate vertigo; and (3) at times a soft cervical collar may be helpful.

When labyrinthitis is diagnosed, treatment includes bedrest and cautious use of antiemetic, antivertiginous agents. Drugs used to attenuate symptoms are antihistamines (e.g., meclizine, dimenhydrinate, diphenhydramine) or phenergan. Other antichlorinergic drugs—scopalamine and atropine—are also useful. Anticholinergic side effects may be significant in the elderly, and these medications should be used judiciously. Some authorities recommend minor tranquilizers as valuable adjuncts to treatment, particularly low-dose diazepam, 1–2 mg, three to four per day.

When the problem is medication-related, then ototoxic drugs should be discontinued, and measurement of drug levels may help document toxicity.

Where faintness or syncope is the problem, the emphasis is on cardiovascular etiologies. Often these patients will require hospitalization. Recently, there has been controversy as to the management of patients who have dizziness and bifasicular block on ECG. The latest recommendations are against prophylactic pacemaker insertion unless there is documentation of a symptom inducing arrhythmia.[5]

In summary, dizziness is a common complaint of the elderly. Within the multiplicity of causes are many potentially life-threatening cardiovascular disorders. This is especially true when the dizzy sensation is faintness. Drug-related dizziness is especially common in the aged. The antihypertensive drugs may lead to orthostatic hypotension, while aminoglycosides and sedatives affect the neuro-otologic organs that induce vertigo. True vertigo is usually a peripheral labyrinthine disorder but in the geriatric group ischemia must be considered as well.

Parkinsonism

Parkinsonism is the third most common neurologic problem in elders. The syndrome, characterized by tremor, rigidity of muscles, and a paucity and slowness of voluntary movements, affects one in 100 persons over the age of 55. Idiopathic Parkinson's disease (paralysis agitans) is the most common cause of this syndrome. Drugs (phenothiazines, butyrophenones, and reserpine) can induce a similar constellation of findings. Less common etiologies

include a postencephalitic form and an arteriosclerotic form (the existence of this latter entity is debatable). Patients who have parkinsonism as a result of the viral encephalitis epidemic in 1918 may have a milder and more slowly progressive disease than the idiopathic cases.

Pathologically, there is loss of pigmented cells in the substantia nigra and, biochemically, there is depletion of the neurotransmitter dopamine. This imbalance of neurotransmitters, dopamine lack, and cholinergic excess can be modified by drug therapy with L-dopa, the precursor of dopamine, or with anticholinergic agents.

DATA BASE

Elders with paralysis agitans have a clinical presentation similar to younger adults. The most common presentation in elders is imbalance and mild rigidity, and there is often a history of frequent falling. Early in the course of the disease, the tremor affects the distal extremities, especially the hands. Typically this is a pill-rolling tremor that is present at rest and temporarily lessens on voluntary movement. Usually the tremor disappears with sleep. It progresses with the disease and can involve the entire extremity and head and neck. The findings of parkinsonism may begin unilaterally.

Muscle stiffness and slowness initiating movement are particularly distressing symptoms. These result in interference with activities of daily living and restrict the patient's independence. Many normally minor volitional movements are blunted. These patients sit unusually still; they have fewer eye blinks and a masked, rigid face.

Late in the course of the disease, additional features become evident. Handwriting is small and cramped. The voice becomes hoarse and of low volume. Posture is distorted with the patient assuming a stooped position on standing and impaired ability to balance and walk. The festinating gait is typical of this latter problem. These patients also suffer from seborrheic dermatitis and excessive drooling.

The most problematic symptoms are changes in the emotional state. Depression is common and difficult to manage. Social withdrawal and depression are likely to occur in reaction to this disabling and frustrating disease. Usually the patient and family have difficulty adjusting to parkinsonism.

There is a high frequency of dementia in association with parkinsonism.[6] This appears to be greater than can be explained by simple concurrence of two common diseases of the elderly. Therapy with levodopa may cause mental changes, some of which are reversible with lowering of dosage. Long-term studies on levodopa have shown that the dementia continues and progresses.[7] It is not known if this is due to the underlying disease or to the drug treatment.

TREATMENT

A treatment plan is best begun in concert with a neurologist or internist familiar with levodopa. Levodopa therapy has dramatically changed the management of parkinsonism. The frequent side effects in the elderly, however, require careful attention to details of management.

Except for the mildest cases, levodopa in combination with a dopa decarboxylase inhibitor is the treatment of choice. The addition of the enzyme inhibitor decreases peripheral destruction of the drug and diminishes side effects.

Side effects of levodopa therapy include nausea, vomiting, arrhythmias, and postural hypotension. Later in the treatment course, involuntary movements and mental changes can occur. Many patients experience daily fluctuations in the efficacy of levodopa. These rapid changes in motor performance, called the on–off phenomenon, may be limited by individualizing drug dose and scheduling.

Levodopa is contraindicated in patients with coronary disease, TIAs, and with a history of psychiatric illness.

Anticholinergics still have value, but their role in the elder population is limited by side effects, especially urinary retention, confusion, or exacerbation of glaucoma. Low-dose tricyclic antidepressants may be a valuable adjunct to therapy when depression remains a problem.

Surgery is rarely indicated since the advent of levodopa.

The overall management of the patient may be enhanced by utilization of a physiotherapist to help in the treatment of muscle symptoms and to improve gait and balance. Psychotherapy for both the patient and his or her family also may prove beneficial.

Although there is no cure, the outlook for Parkinson's disease has brightened since the availability of levodopa. Unquestionably patients experience significant functional improvement, and it appears that mortality from the disease is lessened as well.[7]

Stroke

CLINICAL PRESENTATION

A stroke is a sudden onset of focal neurologic deficit due to disruption of vascular function or integrity. The consequence of the interruption of perfusion is ischemia/infarction in the territory of brain supplied by that vessel. Stroke syndromes fall into well-described patterns of clinical abnormalities depending on which area of the cerebrum is involved, e.g., occlusion of the left middle cerebral artery causes right sided sensory loss, right sided hemiparesis, aphasia, and right homonymous hemianopsia. Knowledge of localization of function in the cerebral cortex, cerebellum, etc., allows prediction of which vessel has been affected. These clinical configurations of stroke are detailed in most available medical and neurologic texts.

Within the last two decades, patterns of lacunar strokes (multiple small infarcts) have been delineated. This type of stroke is due to occlusion of small penetrating vascular branches in the brain. The result is often limited, discreet neurologic deficits which have a good prognosis for recovery.

The vascular disruption causing a stroke is most often due to one of three processes: thrombosis, embolism, or hemorrhage. A recent prospective study analyzed the types of stroke frequently seen.[8] Thrombotic events were the most common form— large vessel, 34 percent; lacunar, 19 percent. Thirty-

Table 9-7
Type of Stroke

	Thrombotic	Embolic	Hemorrhagic
Temporal pattern	Sudden complete or stepwise progression	Sudden complete	Smoothly progressive or sudden complete
Hypertension	Common	Common	Very common
Distinguishing features	Evidence of atherosclerosis	Atrial fibrillation; valvular heart disease	Headache, vomiting, bloody CSF

one percent were embolic strokes which were more common than expected. Hemorrhagic events were least common totalling 16 percent. (Ten percent were intracerebral bleeds; 6 percent, subarachnoid hemorrhage.)

Since the management of each type of stroke is different, it is imperative to define the type of vascular occlusion. The clinical history provides valuable clues (see Table 9-7). The temporal pattern of symptom development is strongly suggestive of the mechanism of vascular disruption. However, clinical history alone is an inadequate basis for therapy decisions.[8b]

Thrombotic strokes often occur during the night and announce their presence when the patient awakens. In many cases, there will have been a history of transient ischemic attacks in the same vascular distribution. Many mechanisms may trigger the thrombotic event. It is likely that in the elderly the most notable initiator is hypoperfusion secondary to hypotension or cardiac arrhythmias. The temporal pattern of thrombosis may result in either a sudden complete deficit or stepwise progression of deficits. Some authorities recommend anticoagulation for a progressing *thrombotic* stroke. The controversy regarding this issue is discussed under management.

Embolic strokes occur with precipitous suddenness, especially when of cardiac origin. Patients may have a history of systemic embolization and either chronic atrial fibrillation or recent myocardial infarction. It is difficult to prove absolutely that a stroke has an embolic origin. This diagnosis is made when a sudden complete neurologic deficit occurs in a patient who has an obvious potential source for emboli. Emboli may arise from intra-arterial sources as well. These often present with attacks of transient ischemia for example, from an ulcerated carotid plaque. Clinically it should be emphasized that embolic strokes may occur in a nonsudden fashion— 19 percent in the series previously cited. Also, emboli to the vertebro-basilar system are quite rare, the middle cerebral artery being the most commonly affected.

Hemorrhagic strokes occur as primary intracerebral bleeds or rupture of a berry aneurysm or arteriovenous malformation (these often lead to subarachnoid hemorrhage). The temporal pattern of hemorrhage is either sudden and complete or smoothly progressive. Almost all patients with intracerebral hematomas have hypertension at the onset of symptoms. Nausea, vomiting, and headaches are more characteristic, but not diagnostic of a hemor-

rhagic stroke. Stiff neck is, of course, typical of subarachnoid hemorrhage.

Occasionally, other processes may lead to vascular occlusion. These rare causes of stroke include polycythemia, hyperviscosity syndromes, arteritis, thrombocytosis, bleeding diatheses, fibromuscular hyperplasia, and dissecting aneurysm.

When patients present with focal neurologic deficits, other central nervous system disorders must be considered. Although the chronology of symptom development and associated findings often allow differentiation, some diseases may masquerade as simple vascular occlusion. Subdural hematoma and neoplasm occasionally mimic a stroke picture.[10] Diagnostic confusion is more likely to occur when there is stepwise progression of symptoms. Less common differential entities include brain abscess and granulomatous cerebral infections. A CAT scan may be indicated to rule out these disorders.

RISK FACTORS

Hypertension is the single, paramount risk factor for stroke. The presence of hypertension increases the risk for all types of stroke. The strongest associations are for intracerebral hematomas and lacunar infarcts. The other potentially treatable risk factor is heart disease. Embolic cerebrovascular events become likely when mural or valvular thrombi develop (in chronic atrial fibrillation, myocardial infarction, and valvular heart disease). In fact, Fisher has recommended that anticoagulants be used prophylactically in chronic atrial fibrillation, since waiting for the first embolic event results in a high percentage of death and disability.[9] Other associated conditions and putative risk factors include hyperlipidemia, diabetes, and smoking.

DATA BASE

An extensive history is needed in elderly patients presenting with a stroke-like picture. Evidence as to the type of stroke, potential causes, and associated disease will help guide management. Standard terminology and classification of stroke is essential to good patient records.[8b] Table 9-8 is an outline of areas of importance.

Physical Exam. Since almost all patients with a new stroke are hospitalized, a complete evaluation is needed. Those facets most pertinent include vital signs and BP in both arms.

Cardiovascular Exam. Includes auscultation of vessels for bruits.

Table 9-8
Areas of Importance in the Management of Stroke Patients

I.   Present illness
    A.   Onset
    B.   Precipitating factors: position, exertion, palpitations, recent trauma
    C.   For patients with a neurologic deficit determine or monitor:
        1.   Temporal pattern: sudden maximal deficit; smoothly progressive; stepwise progressive
    D.   For patients with no deficit, i.e., TIA history:
        1.   First occurrence of neurologic manifestations, duration, frequency, change in frequency, character of attack(s).
II.   Symptoms
    A.   Headache, confusion, nausea/vomiting
    B.   Visual disturbance, amaurosis fugax
    C.   Paresis, paresthesia, bowel disturbance
    D.   Ataxia, dysphagia, dysarthria, dysphasia
III.   Associated disease and past history
    A.   Hypertension, coronary artery disease, diabetes
    B.   Valvular heart disease, prior cerebrovascular disease
    C.   TIA, peripheral vascular disease, hyperlipidemia
    D.   Neoplasm, migraine, hematologic diseases
IV.   Current symptoms
    A.   Angina
    B.   Claudication
    C.   Syncope
    D.   Palpitations
V.   Current medications (note recent changes in medications.)
    A.   Especially diuretics
    B.   Antihypertensive agents
    C.   Anticoagulants
VI.   Habits
    A.   Smoking
    B.   Prior level of independence and intellectual activity

Neurologic Exam. Includes level of consciousness, mental status, funduscopic visual fields, cranial nerve testing, reflexes, Babinski, primitive reflexes, muscle strength and tone, gait, if possible, cerebellar testing, sensation, and meningismus.

Data is obtained both as baseline for serial evaluation and as evidence for the etiology of the stroke. Significant hypo- or hypertension will require treatment if detected. A difference of greater than 15 mm in systolic blood pressure of the arms raises the possibility of subclavian stenosis and steal syndrome. Cardiac exam may reveal atrial fibrillation or murmurs suggesting an embolic etiology for the stroke.

Detection of vascular bruits suggests arteriosclerosis and points to further studies in patients with transient ischemia. Bruits should be tracked to the point of maximal intensity and to be certain they do not originate at the heart valves. They should be described as to quality and intensity. Change with

head position should be assessed to rule out a venous hum.

Funduscopy may show retinal emboli. Indications of long-standing hypertension, diabetes, or rarely hyperviscosity may be present. Signs of subarachnoid hemorrhage, e.g., a subhyaloid hemorrhage, may be visualized as well as papilledema.

MANAGEMENT

There is sufficient overlap in the clinical presentation of the different types of stroke that additional diagnostic studies are required to guide therapy decisions. This is especially true when anticoagulation is considered. Diagnostic studies of value include:

1. *Routine chemistry:* CBC, electrolytes, UA, chemistry panel.
2. *ECG:* this should be a routine test in all stroke patients, since the stroke may have been trig-

gered by an acute myocardial infarction or arrhythmia.

3. *Lumbar puncture:* a potentially hazardous procedure; it is indicated to confirm subarachnoid hemorrhage. RBCs are found in only 70 percent of cases of intracerebral hemorrhage and in some cases of embolism. If a mass lesion is suspected, or if there is alteration of consciousness and focal neurologic deficit, a scan should be obtained before lumbar puncture, since herniation is a risk in those circumstances. Papilledema is also a contraindication although if meningitis is suspected, an LP should always be performed.

4. *CAT scan:* in thrombotic occlusion, the scan is positive after one to two days. Lacunar infarcts show no defect. CAT scans are of most value in defining intracerebral hemorrhage. If anticoagulation is to be used for a presumed thrombotic stroke in evolution, a scan should be obtained first to rule out a hemorrhagic stroke. It will also detect brain abscess, neoplasm, and subdural hematomas.

5. *Brain scan:* this has less diagnostic accuracy than the CAT scan. Thrombotic infarcts may not appear for many days. If a CAT scanner is not available, the brain scan and LP or arteriography should be used if anticoagulants are considered.

6. *Arteriography:* in completed stroke, there are few indications for this procedure. They are: when the diagnosis is in doubt after other tests, when a subarachnoid hemorrhage has occurred, occasionally with very mild strokes where extracranial carotid disease is likely and the patient may be considered for surgery.

7. *Echocardiography:* may be of value in defining mural thrombi or valvular lesions.

TREATMENT

Once the vascular insult has been completed, there is no medical intervention at this time that can reverse the deficit. If the patient survives the stroke, then the chances of at least partial functional recovery are good. Impaired consciousness and severe neurologic deficits indicate a relatively poor prognosis. Treatment goals include limiting the extent of infarction, preventing recurrent stroke, avoidance of in-hospital complications, and maximizing the degree of functional adaptation and self-care achieved during rehabilitation.

Agents to control cerebral edema include dexa-methasone, mannitol, and glycerol. Although these may be temporarily needed to control significant cerebral edema or threatened herniation, studies have not shown that they affect the outcome of stroke (death or deficit).

Surgery is indicated as follows:

1. In some cases of stroke where the deficit is mild or has resolved; if extracranial carotid disease is likely and the patient is a candidate for endarterectomy.

2. Cerebellar hemorrhage: when this is recognized, early surgery may be life-saving by preventing herniation.

3. Prevention of recurrent subarachnoid hemorrhage due to aneurysm or arteriovenous malformation. Procedures are usually postponed until one-to-two weeks after the ictus.

4. Intracerebral hemorrhage, in some cases where the clot is accessible and is causing critical cerebral edema.

5. Indications for the new microsurgical anastomoses, e.g., temporal artery to middle cerebral artery, are currently under study.

Anticoagulants. The use of heparin or warfarin in the setting of an acute stroke is very controversial. These agents carry a greater than normal hazard for the elderly patient. In addition, there exists a risk of converting a bland thrombotic infarct into a hemorrhagic infarct. Anticoagulants are most appropriately considered where there is a defined cardiac source of emboli. In some centers, these agents are used for strokes in evolution (i.e., where there is stepwise development of neurologic deficits) *once* hemorrhage has been ruled out.

Antihypertensive Agents. These are primarily used in acute management of subarachnoid hemorrhage. Sodium nitroprusside allows fine control of blood pressure moment-to-moment but needs to be monitored, usually in the setting of a critical care unit and with an intra-arterial pressure gauge.

The details of management of subarachnoid hemorrhage are beyond the scope of this chapter. Treatment should be undertaken in concert with a neurosurgeon or neurologist. Principles include strict bed rest, blood pressure control, use of anti-fibrinolytic agents, and probably drugs to prevent vasospasm.

With intracerebral hemorrhage and other types

of stroke, if antihypertensive agents are used, it is imperative to avoid hypotension.

Rehabilitation. Initial mortality from stroke is high: approximately 35 percent of patients will die in the hospital. This mortality increases with age. The most common causes of death after a stroke are cardiac diseases. The majority of survivors of a stroke will be able to return home. About 80 percent will eventually be ambulatory, and 20 percent will need assistance with mobility.[11]

Rehabilitation should begin as soon as possible; often this is feasible within one-to-two days of the patient's admission to the hospital. Studies have documented the efficacy of rehabilitation to improve functional ability. Simple steps which can begin early in the course of hospitalization include: mobilization (increasing periods of sitting, then standing); and active and passive exercises for paretic limbs.

Ambulation is a prime goal, as well as maximizing the degree of self-care the patient can attain. Physiotherapists and speech therapists may be valuable adjuncts. It is important to include the family in the rehabilitative efforts and to continue therapies into the home-care phase of convalescence.

TIA

CLINICAL PRESENTATION

A transient ischemic attack is defined as a focal cerebral dysfunction lasting less than 24 hours (most attacks last only a few minutes). Clinically, they are important to recognize as they are harbingers of thrombotic strokes. In many instances, correct diagnosis of a transient ischemic attack can lead to treatment which will prevent a stroke. About two thirds of patients with thrombotic strokes will have antecedent TIAs. The incidence of new TIAs is estimated at 1/1000 population per year.

Patients present with a different constellation of symptoms when the anterior, as opposed to the posterior, cerebral circulation is involved. Diagnostic assessment and therapy differ depending on which territory is affected. Table 9-9 lists common presenting symptoms for anterior circulation TIA (e.g., carotid artery, anterior and middle cerebral arteries, retinal artery) and Table 9-10 for the posterior circulation (i.e., vertebrobasilar and posterior cerebral arteries).

The distinction between vertebrobasilar and carotid TIAs is not always easy to make. A study

Table 9-9
Carotid Artery TIA: Presenting Symptoms

Symptoms	Percentage of Patients
Paresis (mono, hemi)	61
Paresthesia (mono, hemi)	57
Monocular visual	32
Paresthesia (facial)	30
Paresis (facial)	22
Dysphasia	17
Dysarthria	16
Headache	12

Genton E, et al: Cerebral ischemia: The role of thrombosis and antithrombotic therapy. Stroke 8:150–175, 1977. With permission.

analyzing differential features found bilateral visual blurring, diplopia, ataxia, and dizziness correlated with vertebrobasilar origin, and ipsilateral monocular visual disturbances, contralateral paresis or paresthesia, and dysphasia correlated with a carotid origin.[12] Bilateral symptoms strongly suggest a posterior circulation episode. Amaurosis fugax due to transient occlusion of the retinal artery is one of the most typical and common features of a carotid episode.

Caution must be exercised in diagnosing TIAs, especially in the elderly, as other disease processes may mimic some aspects of cerebral ischemia. This applies more to vertebrobasilar TIAs in which the symptoms are variable and less characteristic than

Table 9-10
Vertebrobasilar TIA: Presenting Symptoms

Symptom	Percentage of Patients
Binocular visual	57
Vertigo	50
Paresthesia	40
Diplopia	38
Ataxia	33
Paresis	33
Dizziness	20
Headache	18
Nausea/vomiting	14
Dysarthria	14
Loss of consciousness	14
Visual hallucination	7
Tinnitus	5
Mental change	5
Dysphasia	3
Drop attacks	3

Genton E, et al: Cerebral ischemia: The role of thrombosis and antithrombotic therapy. Stroke 8:150–175, 1977. With permission.

in the carotid territory. Symptoms that often suggest a TIA but may well be due to other causes include: loss of consciousness, confusion, bilateral leg weakness, and vertigo (as an isolated symptom). The differential diagnosis for transient ischemic attacks in the elderly includes Stoke-Adams attacks, postural hypotension, focal convulsive disorders, and many diseases which cause vertigo (for example, labyrinthitis).

Extracranial carotid stenosis is the most important etiology to uncover as, in many instances, surgery (endarterectomy) is indicated. Many mechanisms or causes underlie transient cerebral ischemia. Carotid stenosis and ulcerated atherosclerotic plaques have been the most highlighted. Additional causes, many of which are treatable, include emboli from cardiac sources, transient hypotension, external compression of vessels, and subclavian steal syndrome. (Most of the uncommon causes of stroke listed in the previous section can cause TIAs as well.)

A recent study has pointed out that the TIA symptoms associated with tight carotid stenosis last less than five minutes.[13] Tight carotid stenosis correlates with the nonsimultaneous occurrence of transient monocular blindness and hemisphere attacks. Prolonged TIA symptoms were associated with other causes (embolism, ischemia in small penetrating branches, etc.).

DATA BASE

The same history and physical should be obtained as outlined above for patients with stroke. If a patient is seen early in the course, it is not possible to determine if the defect will resolve and therefore be defined as a TIA, or if it will persist or progress.

Patients who have a classic transient ischemic episode will usually have a normal neurologic exam, and the diagnosis will therefore rest with the history. The circumstances surrounding the onset of symptoms should be detailed, looking for precipitating factors: change in position, position of head, preceding palpitations, exertion, new or changed dosage of medications, especially diuretics or antihypertensives.

MANAGEMENT

Transient ischemic attacks are usually diagnosed by history. Subsequent diagnostic maneuvers are designed to discover a cause for the ischemic episode; they corroborate the history but do not prove the diagnosis. A detailed history and description of the attack are crucial before embarking on management forays. Procedures that are used to diagnose vascular stenosis include:

- *Noninvasive measures.* Ophthalmodynamometry has been available for years as a simple office procedure that may provide evidence of carotid stenosis. More sophisticated, accurate, and expensive tests are now used as noninvasive assessments of carotid blood flow. Doppler studies provide a measure of carotid flow that accurately detects significant narrowing with a low false positive rate. There is, however, a substantial false negative rate. More accuracy can be obtained from combination oculoplethysmography and carotid phonangiography, except that these procedures are not widely available. Carson and Blaisdell have recently discussed the new techniques available.[14] The indications for noninvasive measurements in managing carotid bruits and symptomatic transient ischemia are not yet defined. The advent of highly accurate procedures should facilitate selection of patients for angiography.

- *Arteriography.* This is the definitive diagnostic procedure as the noninvasive tests now available cannot detect ulcerated plaques. A typical carotid transient ischemic history is enough to warrant angiography if the patient is not at excessive risk from the procedure and is a candidate for operation. The finding of a bruit at the carotid bifurcation on the appropriate side strengthens a decision to perform arteriography. But the lack of a bruit or Doppler studies showing good perfusion should not deter angiography, as an ulcerated plaque without stenosis may be the cause of the symptoms.

- *Procedures* used to diagnose cardiac sources for TIA: EKG, Holter Monitor. Recent studies have shown a high percentage of arrhythmias when monitoring is done for cerebral symptoms.

- *Echocardiogram.* This may detect valvular lesions and mural thrombi.

TREATMENT MODALITIES

The devil could quote the medical literature to suit his purpose in deciding treatment for a TIA. Neither uniformity of opinion nor unquestioned judgments can be deduced from the studies available. These treatment recommendations assume the patient has sufficient enjoyment in his or her life to benefit from intervention. In the elderly, when multiple diseases coexist and many lifestyles are slowed and restricted, the benefit of *possible* stroke prevention must be cautiously weighed against the risk of aggressive therapy in each individual. Some guidelines for treatment of TIAs are as follows:

Surgery. Almost all vertebrobasilar TIAs are treated medically as the portions of the posterior circulation affected are not accessible to the surgeon. Carotid endarterectomy will reduce the frequency of carotid TIAs and may well prevent stroke. Surgery is indicated when angiography shows a lesion on the side *appropriate* to the patient's symptoms.

In *experienced* hands, operative mortality should not exceed 1 percent. In one study of community hospitals, however, combined morbidity and mortality for carotid endarterectomy was 21 percent. Multiple comorbid conditions increase operative risk. The most common surgical complications are the development of a neurologic deficit, i.e., a TIA or stroke and myocardial infarction.

Antiplatelet Agents. The Canadian Cooperative Study, in a randomized double-blind study, showed that 300 mg of ASA qid reduced the risk of stroke and death (not stroke alone) in men with TIAs.[15] This effect was most pronounced in men who had no history of myocardial infarction at the time of entry in the study. Women were not benefited by ASA. Sulfinpyrazone alone did not significantly reduce risk and dipyridamole was not studied. Additionally, ASA may be of benefit in postcarotid endarterectomy.

Aspirin may work by inhibiting synthesis of certain prostaglandins that result in platelet aggregation and metabolites which cause vasospasm. It is not known why they are ineffective in women.

Anticoagulants. Again controversy abounds regarding use of anticoagulants. The decision to use these agents is not taken lightly in the elderly, in whom they cause a marked increase in the risk of cerebral hemorrhage. An aggressive approach to the treatment of transient ischemic attacks has been advocated by Sandok.[16] Citing studies that the greatest risk of stroke after the first TIA is in the ensuing few months, they advocate hospitalization, treatment with heparin during the diagnostic work-up, then three months of warfarin. After that time

period, ASA is used. There is no study unequivocably showing the value of this aggressive approach.

Summary of recommendations for thrombotic TIA treatment:

1. Carotid TIA and appropriately placed stenosis or ulcerated plaque; endarterectomy, if patient does not have multiple carotid lesions or multiple risk factors.
2. Vertebrobasilar TIA or carotid TIAs, of recent (less than two months) onset where surgery is not done—anticoagulation is controversial but consider *if there is no contraindication.* Anticoagulation may also be considered in women with continuing TIAs.
3. Aspirin is used after completion of the above treatments or where they are contraindicated.

Management of Patients with Asymptomatic Carotid Bruits

The lack of a controlled trial outlining the natural history of asymptomatic carotid bruits vitiates any conclusions regarding their management.

Extracranial carotid bruits must be differentiated from venous hums and transmitted cardiac murmurs. Some of these bruits may originate in the external, not the internal, carotid artery. The problem is that it is not known what percentage of patients will develop strokes or how soon, but it is likely that, in at least 20 percent of patients who will develop strokes, there will be no TIAs as warning.

Although noninvasive measures of carotid flow may help define the hemodynamic significance of a bruit, no management decisions readily follow from these data. A recent editorial argues that surgery is of unproven benefit and progressing lesions may not become symptomatic because of the development of collateral blood supply.[17]

Asymptomatic bruits or asymptomatic carotid lesions found by angiography prior to thoracic or major surgery present an additional facet of the problem. Intraoperative hypotension may precipitate stroke in some of these patients. The value of prior or simultaneous carotid endarterectomy is not yet known.

Possible roles for prophylactic carotid endarterectomy in asymptomatic bruits include:

1. Younger patients with no risk factors who have hemodynamically significant stenosis.

2. When major surgery is to be performed.
3. When bilateral disease exists.
4. When noninvasive studies show progression of a lesion. Until appropriate studies document the value of prophylactic surgery, however, it is advisable, especially in the elderly, to manage these patients conservatively, i.e., control risk factors where possible and use ASA in men. (Meanwhile, a caveat regarding aggressive treatment of an asymptomatic condition in the elderly is necessary—patients over 65 with hypertension and past myocardial infarction have a significant surgical mortality.)

Paresthesias

Paresthesias are not uncommon complaints of elders. The origin of paresthesia may be difficult to locate due to the multiple disease processes that can cause this symptom. Table 9-11 lists the anatomic sites and some causes of this problem. Herpes zoster is one cause that primarily afflicts the elderly. It often results in protracted pain and discomfort. We advocate a short course of high-dose corticosteroids for patients over 60 to reduce the incidence of postherpetic neuralgia. Other etiologies for peripheral neuropathy in the elderly include arterial insufficiency, B_{12} deficiency, and the remote effects of carcinoma. Paresthesia requires a thorough history and physical to pinpoint, if possible, the underlying cause. Treatment depends on the nature of the problem.

Health Maintenance

Effective health maintenance in the elderly population is restricted by chronic vascular and degenerative changes. For maximal impact, interventions and strategies must begin decades before senescence. This especially applies to control of hypertension, which is the single most important aspect of preventing cerebrovascular disease. The incidence of all types of strokes increases proportionally to blood pressure.

Since cardiac disease is a key risk factor for cerebrovascular disease, health maintenance, as it applies to the heart, becomes significant. Again, early application of the principles outlined in Chapter 11 is necessary.

What can be done now for the geriatric patient at risk? First, control of blood pressure is still valuable at this age, although drug therapy must be used

cautiously. Second, identification of existing heart disease—particularly atrial fibrillation and valvular heart disease—will help select those patients whose cardiac condition is treatable or who are candidates for anticoagulation. Third, recognition of transient ischemic attacks as potentially treatable precursors of stroke will lead to appropriate management strategies (aspirin, surgery, etc.) and diminished risk for many patients.

Finally, and most significantly, we as practitioners have a responsibility to counsel and encourage active, as well as stimulating lifestyles for the elderly.

Table 9-11
Causes of Paresthesia

Site	Common Causes
Peripheral nerve	
Polyneuropathy	Diabetes mellitus
	Arterial insufficiency
	Alcoholism
	Cancer
	B_{12} and nutritional deficiencies
	Guillain-Barre
	Toxins and drugs
Mononeuropathy	Entrapment—especially median nerve
	Bell's palsy
	Diabetes mellitus
	Meralgia paresthetica
	Idiopathic trigeminal neuralgia
Mononeuropathy multiplex	Diabetes mellitus
	Vasculitis
Plexus	Thoracic outlet syndrome
	Pancoast tumor
Spinal root	Cervical spondylosis
	Herniated disc
	Herpes zoster
Spinal cord	Cancer
	Vascular occlusion
	Syphilis
	Abscess
Brainstem	Ischemia
	Infarction
	Tumor
Cortex	Ischemia/TIA
	Infarction-hematoma
	Subdural
	Tumor
	Abscess
	Demyelinating diseases

Theoretically this may attenuate or delay decline in some cerebral functions. The blunted sensory stimulations and tendency toward social withdrawal experienced by many older persons can exaggerate the consequences of age-related neurochemical changes in the brain and contribute to depression.

Helping the patient become involved in social and creative processes is facilitated by a team approach including the family and health care personnel (social workers, occupation therapists, etc.). The benefits of maintaining a vital élan are many, the risks few.

REFERENCES

1. Garraway W, Whisnant JP, Furlan AI, et al: The declining incidence of stroke. N Engl J Med 300:449–452, 1979
2. Katzman R: The prevalence and malignancy of Alzheimer's disease. Arch Neurol 33:217–218, 1976
2b. Task Force, National Institute on Aging: Senility Reconsidered. JAMA 244:259–263, 1980
3. Jenkyn LR, Walsh DB, Culver CM, et al: Clinical signs in diffuse cerebral dysfunction. J Neurol Neurosurg Psychiat 40:956–966, 1977
4. Drachman DA, Hart CW: An approach to the dizzy patient. Neurol 22:323–334, 1972
5. McAnulty JH, Rahimtoola SH, Murphy ES, et al: A prospective study of sudden death in 'high risk' bundle-branch block. N Engl J Med 229:209–215, 1978
6. Loranger AW, Goodell H, McDowell SH, et al: Intellectual impairment in parkinson syndrome. Brain 95:405–412, 1972
7. Sweet RD, McDowell FH: Five years' treatment of parkinson's disease with levodopa. Ann Intern Med 83:456–463, 1975
8. Mohr JP, Caplan LR, Melski JW, et al: The Harvard cooperative stroke registry: A prospective registry. Neurol 28:754–762, 1978
8b. A Classification and Outline of Cerebrovascular Diseases, II. Stroke 6:594–603, 1975
9. Fisher CM: Reducing risks of cerebral embolism. Geriatr 34:59–66, 1979
10. Weisberg LA, Nice CN: Intracranial tumors simulating the presentation of cerebrovascular syndromes. Am J Med 63:517–524, 1977
11. Gresham GE, Fitzpatrick TE, Wolf PA, et al: Residual disability in survivors of stroke—the Framingham study. N Engl J Med 293:954–956, 1975
12. Futty DE, Corneally PM, Dyken ML, et al: Cooperative study of hospital frequency and character of TIAs. JAMA 238:2386, 1977
13. Pession MS, Duncan GW, Mohr MP, et al: Clinical and angiographic features of carotid transient ischemic attacks. N Engl J Med 296:358–362, 1977
14. Carson SN, Blaisdell FW: New techniques in the evaluation of cerebrovascular disease. West J Med 131:355–363, 1979
15. The Canadian Cooperative Stroke Study Group: A randomized trial of aspirin and sulfinpyrazone in threatened stroke. N Engl J Med 299:253–259, 1978
16. Sandok BA, Furlan AJ, Whisnant JP, et al: Mayo clinic proceedings. Proc 53:665–674, 1978
17. Mankowitz C, Taylor JM: A modern view of the surgical treatment of peripheral arterial disease—a critical response. JAMA 241:1467–1468, 1979

RECOMMENDED RESOURCES

Roth, Martin: The management of dementia. Psych Clin NA 1:81–99, 1978

Wells CE: Dementia, ed 2. Philadelphia, FA Davis Co., 1977

10

Endocrine and Metabolic

David N. Sundwall, M.D.
JoAnne Rolando, R.N.
George W. Thorn, M.D.

The endocrine glands, more than any other organ system, have been implicated as either causing or at least contributing to the aging process. There are many reasons for this, but perhaps the most obvious one is the mistaken assumption that the female menopause, with its dramatic changes, is a prototype of all endocrine aging.

The relationship of endocrine glands and the aging process has only recently become a topic of considerable research effort among endocrinologists and biochemists.

In spite of the paucity of information linking endocrine senescence or pathology to aging, a considerable amount of knowledge is available and essential to the clinician caring for older patients.

The majority of endocrine diseases result when there is simply too many or too few *normal hormones*. Many other factors or disease states, however, contribute to endocrine pathology, and they likely play a particularly important role in the elderly patient. Examples of such factors include: decreased plasma proteins resulting in an alteration in the balance between "free" and "bound" thyroid hormones; decreased liver function, which alters the conjugation or degradation of steroid hormones; and a failure of, or diminished, end organ response. Also, it is difficult to talk about endocrine diseases as distinct pathology, especially in older people. There is frequent overlap with malfunction in other organ systems, and this is perhaps best illustrated by the strong association between diabetes mellitus and arteriosclerotic vascular disease. It is hoped that the reader will appreciate the unlikelihood of "pure" metabolic disease in the older patient. Finally, the task of differentiating the changes that occur with normal aging from disease processes is yet to be clearly determined.

THE ENDOCRINE SYSTEM

Figure 10-1 illustrates many of the endocrine glands, their primary hormone, and the servoregulating or feedback mechanisms which govern their release (the parathyroid glands and pancreas are not pictured). The entire system is intimately related to the central nervous system and, particularly, to the autonomic nervous system. In fact, the alterations in endocrine metabolism, which do result from the aging process, seem to be secondary to changes in neural metabolism—and decreased target organ responsiveness—more than degenerative changes in the glands themselves.

Male and Female Climacteric

The female menopause has been mistakenly used as an example that many, if not all, of the problems associated with aging are secondary to waning hormonal function. The dramatic decrease in female hormones produced by the ovaries is documented, and resultant changes in the sexual organs are well known. Also, the level of testosterone in men seems to decline gradually with age. The variation among individuals in any decade is, however, so great that the clinical significance of a falling androgen level is unknown. Therefore, although gonads in both sexes produce less hormones and the secondary effects are integrally related to aging, no specific disease entities are related to this hypofunction. Many remedies have been postulated for male and female climacteric, but all are controversial. Refer

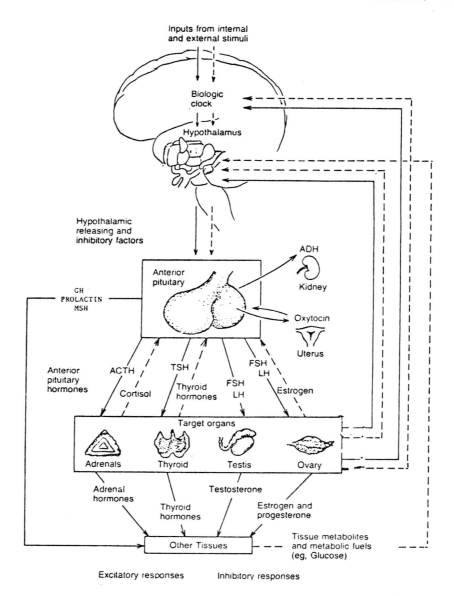

Fig. 10-1. Control of the endocrine system by the nervous system. Note the hypothalamus controls the pituitary through releasing and inhibiting factors. The anterior lobe of the pituitary gland then releases trophic hormones which act on target glands (thyroid, adrenals, and gonads). [Reprinted from Purtile DT: A Survey of Human Diseases. Reading, Addison-Wesley, 1978. By permission.]

to Chapter 8 for a discussion of treatment regarding problems of the sexual organs in the aged.

INCIDENCE OF ENDOCRINE PROBLEMS IN THE ELDERLY

Aging of the endocrine system, with the exception of senescence of the ovaries, cannot be implicated in specific health problems in all older people. However, many people over 60 years of age indeed have pathologic endocrine function. The incidence of such endocrinopathies is difficult to ascertain, but Fig. 10-2 illustrates the results of one study published in *The Geriatric Patient*. The highest incidence of primary endocrine disorders is clearly related to the thyroid, parathyroid, and pancreas glands. The most common problems are diabetes, hypo- and hyperthyroidism.

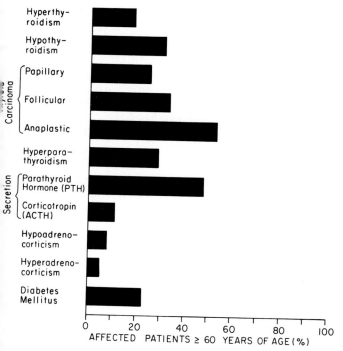

Fig. 10-2. Substantial numbers of patients with endocrinopathies are aged 60 or above, though aging as such does not produce primary alterations in most endocrine glands. [Reprinted from Davis PJ: Endocrines and aging, in Reichel W (ed): The Geriatric Patient. New York, Hospital Practice Publishing Co, 1978, p 87. By permission.]

Uncommon Problems

The primary care practitioner should be aware of the signs and symptoms of more unusual metabolic problems, including hyperadrenalism (Cushing's disease), hypoadrenalism (Addison's disease), hypopituitarism, and acromegaly. This is particularly important for decreased function of the adrenal and pituitary glands because the clinical manifestation of these problems may be mistaken for "normal aging." Consultation with and/or referral to an endocrinologist is appropriate for each of these problems. This is particularly important at the onset of such an illness, or when a problem is suspected, to make a definitive diagnosis and to establish guidelines for optimal medical management. Thereafter, the primary clinician can often manage the problem appropriately, with less expense and inconvenience to the patient. However, periodic consultation or visits with the specialist may be necessary to document progress or change in the disease process and to update recommended therapies. The following must also be considered, particularly when dealing with the elderly patient.

HYPERALDOSTERONISM

Primary aldosteronism is uncommon in elderly patients, but *secondary* hyperaldosteronism, which accompanies cirrhosis, nephrosis, and congestive heart failure, is not unusual in the older patient. The main feature is hypokalemia and hypertension. Potassium deficiency might present as paresthesias, polyuria, weakness, and more rarely tetany. This should be considered when hypertension and a low potassium level are found, particularly when associated with hepatic, renal, and cardiac problems.

ECTOPIC HORMONAL SYNDROMES

The incidence of most malignancies increases with age. Many solid tumors secrete polypeptides that are similar to endocrine hormones, and it is estimated that 10 percent of such tumors produce polypeptides that are clinically significant (i.e., hormonally active). Such polypeptides may be identical with, or at least mimic in their actions, ACTH, ADH, PTH, etc. The importance of this phenomenon in older people is that such hormone production may be clinically significant before the tumor is apparent. Both hypercalcemia and hypokalemia are examples of how this might be manifest. Without other obvious explanations for alterations in these laboratory findings, a tumor source should be sought and appropriate therapy initiated.

DIAGNOSIS AND TREATMENT OF COMMON PROBLEMS

Thyroid Disease

HYPOTHYROIDISM

This is the most common thyroid disease in the older patient and in fact has its peak incidence in the fifth, sixth, and seventh decades of life. The clinician caring for the elderly patient must have a high index of suspicion for this problem because it develops insidiously and so many of its manifestations mimic "normal aging."

The subjective and objective findings of hypothyroidism are listed in Table 10-1. There is great variability among patients, and it is obvious that none of these signs and symptoms is specific to this endocrinopathy. The classical picture of the lethargic, gravel-voiced, edematious, sallow-colored patient is unfortunately atypical, in that most patients with hypothyroidism have more subtle manifestations. Recognizing the extreme variability in pres-

Table 10-1
Hypothyroidism

Subjective	Objective
Weakness	Diastolic hypertension
Fatigability	Skin: dry, coarse, cool, pale and yellow-like
Lethargy	
Cold intolerance	Prominent wrinkles of forehead
Dry skin	
Hair loss	Periorbital edema
Memory impairment	Thinning lateral eyebrows, hair
Voice change	
Constipation	Enlarged tongue
Weight gain	Hyperkeratosis of elbow and knees
Dyspnea	
Anorexia	Goiter (unusual in elderly)
Chest pain	Pseudomyotonia (delay in relaxation phase of deep tendon reflexes)
Edema (facial and peripheral)	
Paraesthesias (hand and foot)	Bradycardia
	Cardiomegaly
Decreased libido, impotence	Pleural and pericardial effusion
Headache/dizziness	Dementia, depression, psychosis

entation and the lack of specific signs and symptoms, it is therefore recommended that all elderly patients be screened periodically for thyroid malfunction. In particular, the patient with altered mental function should be evaluated carefully for decreased thyroid function to rule out a potentially treatable cause of dementia.

Data base. A careful history and physical examination will alert the clinician to the problems in Table 10-1. If the patient is not a good historian, information should be obtained from family or close friends who could be more accurate. Particular attention should be paid to the use of prescription and nonprescription drugs (e.g., the use of saturated solution of potassium iodide as a "mucolytic" agent), associated illnesses, and past medical history (e.g., history of hyperthyroidism or goiter resulting in a thyrodectomy). In addition to the following laboratory tests, a patient should have a chest x-ray to rule out pleural or pericardial effusions and cardiomegaly. An electrocardiogram is often helpful, in that the hypothyroid patient may show low voltage, bradycardia, and flattened or inverted T-waves.

Laboratory findings. All patients suspected of hypothyroidism should have a serum T_4 (thyroxine) concentration measure. This will be low in hypo-

thyroid patients, but it can also be depressed in young and elderly patients with chronic debilitating, nonthyroidal illnesses. Also, it may be spuriously altered by conditions that cause an abnormality in the binding of thyroxine to plasma proteins. These include: hypoproteinemic states (malnutrition, liver disease, renal disease, protein-losing enteropathies); treatment with certain drugs (phenytoin, androgens, aspirin, or glucocorticoids); and familial TBG (thyroid binding globulin) deficiency. These abnormalities can be ruled out by ordering a T_3 resin uptake study. This test will be low or low-normal if hypothyroidism is present, and high or high-normal if there is an abnormality in the thyroid hormone binding as indicated above. A helpful addition to the evaluation of thyroid function is determination of the free thyroxine index. This is calculated from a ratio of the serum T_4 to the T_3 resin uptake, which can be determined by the clinical laboratory upon request. This figure provides a more accurate picture of the thyroid function and helps rule out the spurious causes of a low serum T_4.

Once the diagnosis of hypothyroidism has been made, one must distinguish between primary (thyroid gland disease) and secondary (pituitary or hypothalamic dysfunction) hypothyroidism. A serum TSH (thyroid stimulating hormone) is the next step; it is high in primary hypothyroidism and low in pathology related to the pituitary or hypothalamus. In fact, it is advisable to order the TSH if a low-normal thyroxine value is obtained; if TSH is elevated, the diagnosis of primary hypothyroidism is established. If secondary causes are identified, it would be appropriate for the primary care clinician to consult with or refer the patient to an endocrinologist to determine what further diagnostic tests, if any, would be appropriate and helpful. It would also be important for an endocrinologist to assist the primary care clinician in determining if there are associated multiple endocrine problems. Figure 10-3 shows a schematic diagram of important steps to consider in evaluating the patient with suspected hypothyroidism.

ASSOCIATED NONTHYROID LAB ABNORMALITIES

There are several laboratory tests that might be abnormal when hypothyroidism is present. Table 10-2 lists these possible associated laboratory findings. Other etiologies for these abnormalities must be considered in the hypothyroid patient, particularly if they persist after appropriate therapy has been initiated.

LABORATORY

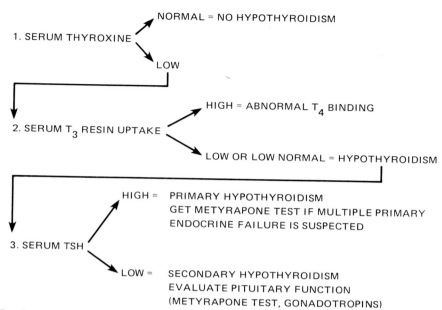

Fig. 10-3. Important steps in the evaluation of patients with hypothyroidism. (Reprinted from The thyroid, in Jubiz W: Endocrinology: A Logical Approach for Clinicians. New York, McGraw-Hill, 1979, p 66. With permission.)

THERAPY

The treatment of mild to moderate hypothyroidism is a relatively simple task, particularly in the absence of other significant health problems. It requires replacement therapy of the deficient hormone, and many endocrinologists recommend synthetic L-thyroxine because of guaranteed bioefficacy. As with any medication in the elderly, the axiom of "start low, go slow" applies. Although younger patients can be started on full replacement therapy (0.15—0.2 mg orally/day), in elderly patients it is advisable to start at 0.025 mg of L-T$_4$ daily and to

increase the dose by this amount at weekly intervals. Such timidity is warranted because of the likelihood that significant arteriosclerotic heart disease may be a concurrent problem. Angina, arrythmias, and congestive heart failure may be precipitated by even the lowest dosage of supplemental thyroid. The combination of a beta blocking agent (e.g., propranolol) with L-T$_4$ can be useful in treating the patient with angina, but is contraindicated in the presence of congestive heart failure. The end point is signaled by a reduction in the TSH level to normal and by remission of signs and symptoms of hypothyroidism.

MYXEDEMA COMA

Profound hypothyroidism occurs almost exclusively in the elderly patient and is a medical emergency requiring prompt and meticulous medical care, preferably in an intensive care unit of a hospital. All of the subjective and objective findings listed in Table 10-1 may be present but the neurological abnormalities predominate (lethargy, stupor, and coma). The crisis is usually precipitated by a concurrent problem, e.g., infections, drugs (especially sedatives and narcotics), cold exposure, myocardial infarction, cerebrovascular accidents, or gastrointestinal bleeding. Those conditions, as well

Table 10-2
Laboratory Abnormalities That May Be Associated With
Hypothyroidism

Anemia: usually normochromic/normocytic
Basophilia
↑ CPK: skeletal muscle origin (MB-iso enzyme)
↑ SGOT
↑ LDH
↑ Cholesterol
↑ Triglyceride
↑ Uric acid
↑ Serum carotene

as the thyroid insufficiency, must be sought out and vigorously treated, if possible. A hallmark of Myxedema coma is hypothermia (temperatures as low as 74° F have been reported), and it occurs in 80 percent of cases. Therapy must be initiated as soon as possible and includes the intravenous administration of large doses of L-thyroxine. However, appropriate management includes support of virtually every organ system (parenteral fluids, ventilatory assistance, corticosteroids, electrolyte balance, etc.); the reader is referred to an endocrinology text for specific recommendations. Unfortunately, the mortality rate for this condition is high—50–70 percent. This figure would in all likelihood be reduced considerably if the primary care clinician caring for the elderly would be more vigorous in screening for hypothyroidism.

HYPERTHYROIDISM

Hyperfunction of the thyroid gland is less common than hypothyroidism, but almost 20 percent of hyperthyroid patients are elderly and approximately one-third of thyrotoxic patients are older than 60 years. It has been estimated that 75 percent of the elderly hyperthyroid patients have "classical" signs as symptoms, which are listed in Table 10-3. The remaining 25 percent of elderly hyperthyroid patients do not have obvious signs and symptoms, and the diagnosis may be much more difficult. Approximately one-third of elderly hyperthyroid patients have no goiter. Of those who do have gland enlargement, half are likely to have a nodular goiter and half diffuse gland enlargement (similar to Graves' disease). In marked contrast to the anxious, tremulous, sweating patient with typical hyperthyroidism, the elderly may appear apathetic and depressed. This is particularly so in the patient with

Table 10-3
Hyperthyroidism

Subjective	Objective
Fatigue	Tachycardia
Weakness	± Arrythmia
Nervousness	Fine tremor
Palpitations	Smooth, warm, moist skin
Sweating	Onycholysis
Diarrhea	Goiter
Weight Loss	Opthalmopathy
Heat intolerance	Hyperreflexia
Decreased libido, impotence	Muscle weakness
	Hair loss
Angina	
Shortness of breath	

concurrent, severe nonthyroidal disease (stroke syndrome, CHF, infections, etc.). Many thyrotoxic elderly patients present with unexplained heart failure and tachyarrhythmias (one-third have atrial fibrillation), which respond poorly to conventional therapy. Others will present with profound muscle weakness (myopathy) or psychiatric disturbances. Surprisingly, one study reported that 15 percent of elderly thyrotoxic patients presented with the triad of weight loss, anorexia, and constipation.

The message to be gleaned from the reports of *atypical* presentation of hyperthyroidism in the elderly is that the primary care practitioner would be well advised to screen *all* elderly patients for thyroid disease. This would be wise on a periodic basis as part of health maintenance. But it should be considered *essential* in the evaluation of ill elderly patients, particularly those presenting with new cardiovascular problems or an alteration in personality or mental function.

Data base. A thorough history and physical examination is required to obtain the necessary subjective and objective information. This should readily alert the clinician to the majority of patients who present with the typical symptoms and signs indicated in Table 10-3. But the astute practitioner will also detect concurrent illnesses that might mask the hyperthyroid state. A chest x-ray and ECG are essential to detect associated cardiovascular disease which may be inapparent clinically.

Laboratory tests. The initial step is to obtain a T_4 and preferably a free T_4, for reasons described in the above section on hypothyroidism. A significant elevation is virtually diagnostic of hyperthyroidism; however, slight elevations of free T_4 may be obtained in euthyroid patients if there is concommitant nonthyroidal disease. This can be excluded by follow-up testing. A more troublesome problem is the occasional occurrence of normal serum T_4 in thyrotoxic elderly patients. The reasons for this are not entirely known but include the occurrence of T_4 toxicosis (hyperthyroidism, which results from isolated overproduction of triiodothyronine). If, however, there is a strong suspicion of hyperthyroidism in a patient with normal or only slightly elevated serum T_4 levels, a radioactive iodine uptake study (131_I) should be obtained. The great majority of elderly patients with hyperthyroidism will have a diagnostically elevated uptake. If there is still confusion regarding diagnosis, consultation and/or referral to an endocrinologist is appropriate. Thyroid suppression tests, biopsies, and other diagnostic procedures are potentially dangerous for the older patient.

ASSOCIATED NONTHYROID LAB ABNORMALITIES

Table 10-4 lists some of the laboratory abnormalities that may be associated with hyperthyroidism. They should resolve with appropriate therapy, and the clinician should be alert to other etiologies for these abnormalities if they are extreme and/or exist.

TREATMENT

Most hyperthyroid elderly people can be successfully treated with radioactive iodine administration (131$_I$). This applies for those with mild to moderate hyperthyroidism. The more severely thyrotoxic elderly patient represents a more serious problem. The reason for this is the frequent association of nonthyroidal disease and, particularly, cardiovascular pathology. As indicated above, patients with thyrotoxicosis may present with cardiac problems, particularly congestive heart failure and tachyarrhythmias, which are refractory to conventional therapy. This requires careful management of the heart failure concurrently with administration of antithyroid agents such as thiourelene drugs (methimazole or propylthiouracil) and iodine. Although the beta blocking agents, such as propranolol, are usually contraindicated with heart failure, patients with a very rapid heart rate (greater than 140 beats/minute) may in fact be most effectively treated with the careful administration of propranolol to block the peripheral effects of the excessive thyroid hormone. This should be used only if conventional therapy with diuretics and digoxin is not successful in managing the heart failure.

The primary care physician should be particularly sensitive to the fact that thyrotoxicosis, or "storm," is often precipitated by concurrent nonthyroidal disease. Often an infection, surgery or systemic drug reactions may either exacerbate mild hyperthyroidism or precipitate thyrotoxicosis in an otherwise asymptomatic patient. Therefore, all hyper-

Table 10-4
Laboratory Abnormalities That May Be Associated With Hyperthyroidism

---

↑ Calcium
↑ Alkaline phosphatase (bone and liver origin)
↓ Cholesterol
Leukopenia, with relative lymphocytosis
↑ Hepatic enzymes (with liver involvement)

---

thyroid patients should be evaluated for such concurrent diseases.

The dosages of methimazole, propylthiouracil, and iodine are similar in older patients as for younger and must be determined according to body weight. It is wise to attempt to render any patient euthyroid with these preparations before referring to an endocrinologist for definitive therapy with ablative radioactive iodine administration. It should be emphasized that surgery is rarely indicated in the older patient; the complications of the radioactive isotope are minimized in the elderly. Nonetheless, the clinician responsible for following these patients must be aware of the potential of gradual development of hypothyroidism with this therapy, and serial thyroid functions must be obtained to detect this.

THYROID NODULES

It is important to recognize that the development of thyroid nodules is apparently a normal aspect of aging. Some postmortem studies indicate that virtually all patients over 80 years of age have multiple micronodules throughout the thyroid gland. Nonetheless, mortality from thyroid malignancy increases with age, regardless of its histological classification. As Fig. 10-2 indicates, almost half of the anaplastic thyroid carcinomas, which have the poorest prognosis, occur in older patients. Therefore, the primary care clinician cannot dismiss a newly identified palpable thyroid nodule as "probably benign." If a nodule(s) has been present for years, feels soft and spongy, seems to decrease in size with suppression therapy (exogenous thyroid hormone), and is not "cold" on radionucleotide scanning, then there is a strong evidence that it is benign. Otherwise, surgical excision is recommended to rule out malignancy or, if a malignancy is found, to facilitate appropriate therapy.

Hyperparathyroidism

This condition is not rare in elderly patients, and one-third of the patients with primary hyperparathyroidism are over 60 years of age. Two or more elevated serum calcium levels should prompt the primary care clinician to confirm a diagnosis by ordering a serum immunoreactive parathyroid hormone level (IPTH). About 90 percent of patients with this problem have one or more benign parathyroid adenomas. Ten percent of these are found in unusual locations such as the mediastinum, intrathyroid, or around the esophagus. Ten percent of patients with primary hyperparathyroidism will have diffuse hyperplasia of the parathyroid glands or, more rarely, malignancy. The subjective and objective findings are similar for old and young patients; they include renal calculi, demineralizing bone disease, general muscular weakness, constipation, anorexia, nausea, abdominal cramps, polyuria, dryness of mouth, and mental confusion. Bone pain and pathological fractures may occur with the specific bone lesion-osteitis fibrosa cystica. It will be apparent to the clinician caring for older people that many of the above symptoms might be overlooked and assumed to be manifestations of aging, particularly if they are insidious. Treatment of this problem in the older patient is determined by symptoms and/or degree of hypercalcemia. Many patients with mild or moderate hypercalcemia are asymptomatic, and surgical exploration for parathyroid adenomas should be avoided because of attendant risks. Some endocrinologists recommend that calcium levels of greater than 11.5 mg percent require at least medical management with oral phosphates or subcutaneous calcitonin. Such therapies are not without side effects and would have to be monitored carefully by medical personnel. An important practical point to be remembered is that thiazide diuretics should be avoided in patients with this diagnosis, since these medications may further elevate serum calcium levels.

Diabetes Mellitus

"Sugar diabetes" is a disease found predominantly in elderly people. The peak age incidence of newly diagnosed diabetics is 60–70 years, and it is estimated that 20 percent of the population over the age of 60 is diabetic or at least has significant "carbohydrate intolerance." This increased incidence of diabetes in the elderly is also reflected in mortality rates. Diabetes mellitus is listed as the sixth leading cause of death in individuals over the age of 65.

Specific definitions of diabetes mellitus vary considerably among diabetologists, but it is manifest as a disorder of carbohydrate, fat, protein, and insulin metabolism affecting the structure and function of blood vessels. The ultimate etiology of the disease is not known, but the derangement in carbohydrate metabolism is due to inadequate physiological effects of endogenous insulin. Insulin production by pancreatic islets may be insufficient or tissues can become less sensitive to the hormone's metabolic effect.

Diabetes is classified into two types: primary insulin deficiency (pancreatic beta cell failure) and primary insulin insensitivity (target organ resistance). Primary insulin deficiency is characterized by low or absent plasma insulin levels. It is usually diagnosed when an abrupt onset of severe ketoacidosis occurs, most often in nonobese young people. The course of the disease is often unstable, and insulin replacement is usually required to control hyperglycemia. In contrast, primary insulin insensitivity occurs frequently in older people who are obese. Decreased sensitivity to insulin of adipose cells, hepatocytes, and muscle cells develops slowly, and plasma insulin levels are often normal or slightly increased. Ketosis is rare; often, a restriction of carbohydrates in the diet and weight reduction are all that is necessary to control hyperglycemia. Although some diabetics who are insulin dependent survive into old age, the majority of diabetics over the age of 60 have the primary insulin insensitivity type of diabetes.

When subjected to the usual glucose load, nonobese elderly persons show a delay in insulin release. The absolute quantity of insulin secreted is reduced, and more of the insulin released may be physiologically "inactive." Therefore, there is an apparent *normal* decreased glucose tolerance with age, and this presents a problem in diagnosing diabetes in the older person. Diagnosis based solely on standards of performance of young subjects may inaccurately define older persons as "diabetic," when their response may be normal for their age. Since diabetes carries the stigma of a chronic illness, caution should be exercised in making the diagnosis.

CLINICAL FEATURES

Symptoms. The elderly diabetic may be entirely asymptomatic. The classical symptoms of excessive thirst, weight loss, polyuria, nausea, and vomiting may occur, although they are often absent. Lethargy and subtle mental changes may predominate.

The undiagnosed elderly diabetic often presents with a variety of symptoms, not due to the metabolic disorder itself, but secondary to frequently associated problems. Examples of such presenting problems include: *decreasing vision* due to hyperglycemia and/or cataracts; *pruritis vulvae* due to monilial vaginitis; *intermittent claudication* due to obliterative peripheral vascular disease; *painless ulcerations* and/or *numbness* of the lower extremities due to peripheral neuropathy; and *weak thigh muscles* due to amyotrophy.

Some elderly diabetics are not diagnosed until they present with diabetic coma. Whereas the younger insulin-deficient diabetic usually develops ketoacidosis, the older diabetic is more likely to develop hyperosmolarity or, more rarely, lactic acidosis as the metabolic derangement leading to coma. This may be manifest in the early stages as simply an alteration in personality and progress to mental confusion, stupor and, eventually, coma. It should be noted that, as in the younger diabetic, such severe metabolic derangements are generally due to severe concurrent illness, e.g., infection, trauma, surgery/anesthesia, or drug reactions.

SIGNS

As indicated above, the elderly diabetic is often asymptomatic. A careful physical examination, however, may reveal signs of frequently associated problems. Table 10-5 lists common findings that may be present on physical examination.

Data base. As with thyroid disease, the primary care clinician should obtain the essential subjective and objective information with a thorough history and physical examination. The diagnosis, however, cannot be made without demonstrating abnormal carbohydrate metabolism. Although urine testing for glucose is helpful as a screening procedure, the threshold for urinary glucose excretion rises with age, and glycosuria may not appear until the plasma glucose exceeds 300 mg percent. Inasmuch as fasting blood glucose levels also rise with age, many endocrinologists recommend that a person not be diagnosed as diabetic unless the fasting blood glucose is consistently greater than 150 mg percent. Perhaps even more significant is a two-hour postprandial blood sugar that is greater than 200 mg percent on two or more occasions. A nomogram developed by Ruben Andres and his colleagues at the National Institute on Aging is helpful in determining which patients are "diabetic," based on two-hour postprandial blood sugar (see Fig. 10-4). It should be emphasized that a 4–6 hour glucose tolerance test is *not* necessary to establish the diagnosis and should be avoided because of the expense and discomfort to the patient.

TREATMENT

The mainstay of treatment of the diabetic patient, whether young or old, is diet. A diabetic diet is well

Table 10-5
Physical Signs Commonly Found in Elderly Diabetics

Skin:	Monilial infections (groin, axillae, inframammary region)
	Skin spots (brown, iron-containing substance that remains after small hemorrhages)
	Necrobiosis lipoidica (irregular shiny patches with a reddish-yellow discoloration over extremities)
Mouth:	Pyorrhea
Eyes:	↓ visual acuity
	Cataracts
	Chronic "simple" glaucoma
	Retinopathy (microaneurysms, hemorrhages, "hard" exudates, tortuous vessels), retinitis proliferans
Peripheral Vascular Occlusion:	↓, or absent pulses in lower extremities
	Dependent rubor
	Shiny, cool, hairless skin over lower legs
	Ulcerations/"dry gangrene" lesions on feet
	Atrophine changes in nails
Neuropathy:	Absent deep tendon reflex in ankles (diminished or about DTRs in knees)
	↓ temperature/vibratory sensation
	Urinary retention (significant residual urine in bladder after voiding)
Myopathy:	Atrophy of small muscles in hands
	Atrophy of thigh muscles

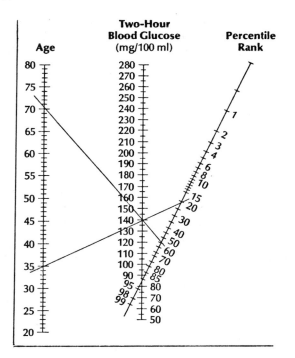

Fig. 10-4. Nomogram for evaluating oral glucose-tolerance test (dose 1.75 g/kg body weight) was developed by Andres et al. It is utilized by ruling line from age scale through test result and continuing it to percentile scale. At age 70, a subject with glucose concentration of 140 is about average; at age 35, same concentration ranks individual in 20th percentile, so 80% of age peers outperform him or her. (Reprinted from Davis PJ: Endocrines and aging, in Reichel W (ed): The Geriatric Patient. New York, Hospital Practice Publishing Co., 1978, p 89. By permission.)

balanced, with an emphasis on limiting carbohydrate intake as compared with the "typical American diet." Such a diet would consist of 40 percent of the calories coming from carbohydrate, and the remaining calories being divided equally between fat and protein. The American Diabetes Association provides printed diet materials, e.g., exchange lists and sample menus, at a nominal charge.

When an older person is diagnosed as being diabetic, it may seem overwhelming to change the dietary habits of a lifetime. However, with appropriate dietary counseling, and particularly with the assistance of a dietician, a remarkably varied and palatable diabetic diet can be provided. If this dietary plan includes foods that are peculiar to the patient's ethnic and cultural background, the likelihood of compliance improves considerably. Also, the diet must take into consideration realities of economic limitations. The older person on a fixed income simply may not be able to afford the fresh

fruits and vegetables so frequently recommended for optimal nutrition. Problems with dentition must also be considered in making a dietary program. Additional problems might include the restriction of cholesterol in the patient with Type II hyperlipoproteinemia, sodium restriction in the patient with hypertension and/or congestive heart failure, and limitation of milk products in the elderly person with a lactase deficiency. All of the above problems simply emphasize the need for collaboration with colleagues in nutrition and dietetics. Inasmuch as most elderly patients are obese and, indeed, not insulin-deficient, but may have an excess of insulin, proper dietary management is essential for them. In fact, this is perhaps the only aspect of managing the diabetic patient that enjoys an apparent concensus among the specialists in dealing with this disease.

Although rigid adherence to a diabetic diet with the attendant weight loss in the obese patient is all that is necessary to control most elderly diabetics, there are many patients who will need further measures to control their diabetic symptoms. There is controversy regarding drug therapy of the diabetic patient, particularly the elderly. Recommendations from diabetologists range from advising that the diabetic patient be maintained at a blood sugar of less than 150 mg percent at all times, to ignoring the blood sugar entirely and treating only the symptoms in the elderly diabetic patient. Those recommending "tight control" of the diabetic cite studies indicating that the complications of this disease are significantly limited by controlling the hyperglycemia. Advocates of treating only symptoms of the disease, not the level of blood glucose, also cite research data indicating that complications occur in spite of, or without apparent association with, the level of blood glucose. Regardless, the American Diabetic Association has recently renewed its endorsement of efforts by physicians to control the blood sugar level in their diabetic patients in the hope of postponing complications. However, the clinician caring for the elderly patient with diabetes must attempt this "control" with as little interference and discomfort to the patient's life as possible. The following are recommended as additional steps in the treatment of the diabetic patient:

Oral drug therapy. The use of oral medications in the treatment of the diabetic has been the subject of considerable controversy over the past decade. The University Group Diabetes Program study suggested that oral sulfanylurea therapy not only failed to postpone development of complications of diabetes, but also was associated with an increase in cardiovascular deaths. Many investigators have disputed this study, and its implications in the older diabetic are quite unclear in that "long-term complications" are not a major consideration. Endocrinologist William Jubiz has stated in his recently published text, *Endocrinology—A Logical Approach for Clinicians,* that he prefers to use an oral agent rather than insulin in the obese adult onset diabetic patient for the following reasons:

1. The obese diabetic is resistant to insulin and, unless weight reduction is accomplished, it does not make sense to give more insulin to a patient who is already producing too much and does not respond well to it.
2. To take a pill is more pleasant than to receive an injection of insulin everyday.

Nonetheless, he goes on to explain the oral hypoglycemic agent should not be used indiscrimi-

nately and is only to be considered if there is obvious dietary failure. There are several types of sulfanylurea medications, all of which work by stimulating insulin secretion in the pancreas and enhancing tissue glucose uptake. Table 10-6 shows some characteristics of these drugs. The clinician should be aware of the fact that chlorpropemide has the longest duration of action, as well as the most side effects, including hypoglycemia, which can be difficult to appreciate in the elderly patient. It also has the problem of causing hyponatremia due to inappropriate antidiuretic secretion in approximately 5 percent of patients. The drug, phenformin, was used for many years as an effective hypoglycemic agent, but has been recently withdrawn from the market by the U.S. Food and Drug Administration because of its association with lactic acidosis in the elderly patient.

Table 10-6
Some Facts About Oral Hypoglycemic Agents

Compound	Mechanism of Action	Metabolism	Duration			Side Effects
			Half-life, h	of Action, h	Dose, g	
Tolbutamide	Acutely: stimulation of insulin secretion; Chronically: increase in sensitivity of β-cells, increase in tissue glucose uptake, decrease in gluconeogenesis	Hepatic oxidation and urinary excretion	4–5	6–12	0.5–3.0	3%; GI, hematologic, skin, hypoglycemia, cardiovascular, hypothyroidism
Chlorpropamide	Same as above	Urinary excretion unaltered	35	60	0.1–0.5	6%; GI, hematologic, skin, cholestatic jaundice, hypoglycemia, hyponatremia and water retention, hypothyroidism
Acetohexamide	Same as above	Hepatic reduction to active metabolite; active renal tubular secretion	6–8	12–24	0.25–1.25	GI, hematologic, skin, hypoglycemia, hypothyroidism
Tolazamide	Same as above	Hepatic metabolism and urinary excretion	6–8	12–24	0.1–0.75	GI, hematologic, skin, hypoglycemia
Phenformin	Decrease in GI glucose absorption and increased tissue glucose uptake	One-third hydroxylated in liver and two-thirds excreted in urine unchanged	3–5	6–8	0.05–0.15	Mostly GI; lactic acidosis rare in absence of renal disease

Reprinted by permission from The pancreas and alterations in carbohydrate metabolism, in Jubiz W: Endocrinology: A Logical Approach for Clinicians. New York, McGraw-Hill, 1979, p 173.

Insulin therapy. As indicated above, the majority of elderly diabetic patients will be able to be managed with diet alone, or diet with the addition of sulfan-ylurea medication. If, however, the elderly patient is indeed an insulin-deficient type diabetic, insulin replacement is mandatory. Also, insulin therapy should be considered for any older diabetic who is not responding to the above measures. It is essential to individualize insulin therapy and is most easily done in a controlled setting such as the hospital. However, with the assistance of devoted family members, the cooperation of a community nursing service, and frequent visits with the primary care clinician, insulin therapy may be successfully initi-ated without hospitalization. *Optimal* control of blood sugar cannot be obtained unless regular (short acting) insulin is given before each meal, but this is usually unacceptable to the patient. Relatively good control can be maintained in most diabetics who are insulin-dependent with b.i.d. dosage of intermediate-acting insulin, approximately two-thirds of the dose being administered before breakfast and one-third being administered in the evening. Regular insulin may need to be added to the inter-mediate-acting insulin if hyperglycemia persists in the hours immediately following injection. (Refer to Table 10-7 for the duration of action for the various kinds of insulin.) The difficult-to-manage insulin-dependent diabetic may need to be referred to an endocrinologist for consultation to determine the appropriate level of insulin replacement and fre-quency of administration. The primary care clini-cian should be aware of the phenomenon of the Somogyi effect, i.e., periods of hypoglycemia alter-nating with periods of hyperglycemia, induced by insulin excess. Also, the clinician caring for the older patient must be particularly sensitive to the signs of *hypoglycemia* that might be mistaken as lethargy, depression, or simply "old age."

Additional management problems. A primary care clinician might be given a false sense of confidence if he or she is attempting only to control the blood glucose level in the diabetic patient. Other factors that must be attended to include:

1. *Foot care.* This is at least as important in the care of the older diabetic patient as the level of blood glucose. Patients with a peripheral neuropathy may have a painless sore that can progress to a nonhealing ulceration and, eventually, gan-grene of an extremity. Feet, and particularly the toenails, must be checked regularly for any external lesions. Toenails should be properly cut, i.e., straight across and not too near the

Table 10-7
Insulin Preparations

	Peak Action, h	Duration of Action, h
Short-acting		
Regular	4–6	6–8
Semilente	4–6	12–16
Intermediary		
NPH	8–12	18–24
Lente	8–12	18–24
Long-acting		
Protamine zinc	14–20	24–36
Ultralente	16–18	30–36

Reprinted by permission from The pancreas and alterations in carbohydrate metabolism, in Jubiz W: Endocrinology: A Logical Approach for Clinicians. New York, McGraw-Hill, 1979, p 166.

nail base. They should also be trimmed fre-quently enough so they do not curl, thicken, and develop the potential for self-inflicted wounds on the patient's feet. The patient should be advised to wash his or her feet daily, apply a moisturizing lotion, and wear dry, clean socks. Also, because of the diminished sensation in the lower extremities of older people, it is recom-mended that they pay particular attention to properly fitting shoes and avoid using *hot* water for bathing.

2. *Eyes.* Because of the increased incidence of glaucoma and cataracts in the diabetic patient, eyes should be screened periodically for these problems. Also, funduscopic exams should be done regularly to detect diabetic retinopathy and document progression, if it exists. Laser beam therapy for retinitis proliferans and dia-betic hemorrhage can be remarkably effective in limiting one of the most dreadful complica-tions of diabetes.

3. *Genitourinary system.* Renal function should be evaluated periodically in all diabetic patients. Although renal failure from basement mem-brane thickening (Kimmelstiel-Wilson syn-drome) is rare in the adult-onset diabetic, the normal decrease in renal function in the elderly is indeed aggravated in the diabetic patient. Also, "silent" urinary tract infections are more common and can further compromise the renal status. Therefore, complete urinalysis in addi-tion to serum evaluation of renal status is essen-tial.

4. *Cardiovascular system.* There is a remarkable as-sociation of *arteriosclerotic* vascular disease with diabetes mellitus. This affects the heart and the

peripheral vasculature. Cardiac status and peripheral pulses should be checked regularly in the diabetic. The detection of occlusive peripheral vascular disease at an early stage can lead to definitive therapy, for example, by-pass surgery, which can prevent the loss of an extremity.

In summary, it is obvious that management of the elderly diabetic patient involves considerably more than controlling blood glucose levels. Although this is part of care, these patients should be seen regularly (no less than every three months) for evaluation of their general health status, with particular attention to the potential problems listed above. The effects of diabetes mellitus can be demonstrated in virtually every organ system of the body, and the reader is referred to a text in endocrinology for a more definitive discussion. In spite of the serious complications of diabetes, many of which are eventually fatal to the patient, it is emphasized that the majority of older diabetic patients are completely independent and capable of normal activity. This should be the focus of patient management, and patients should be encouraged to pursue as normal a lifestyle as possible. Indeed, exercise is a very helpful adjunct in managing the diabetic patient—it improves well-being, limits the need for drugs (both sulfanylureas and insulin), and can assist the patient in achieving weight loss. As with dietary recommendations, this exercise should be encouraged in the form that the patient most enjoys and is capable of, e.g., walking, dancing, bike riding, swimming, etc. With appropriate and supportive management of diabetic patients, this metabolic defect need not result in dramatic changes in their lives.

Community resources can also be of great assistance in managing elderly patients with metabolic problems, particularly the diabetic. Visiting nurses can be very helpful in ensuring proper administration of insulin, in assisting family members with instruction and teaching them how to give injections, and in periodically evaluating the general health status of the patient. Primary care clinicians are advised to be aware of the resources in their community, whether they be self-help groups, home nursing care, Meals on Wheels, or day care centers. The quality of medical care can be significantly enhanced by employing the appropriate programs and agencies available to elderly patients.

HEALTH MAINTENANCE

It will be apparent from the narrative of this chapter that periodic screening of the elderly is essential for health maintenance. It is particularly true for metabolic diseases as so many of the manifestations might be mistaken for "normal aging." It is recommended as part of routine health maintenance that older patients, when undergoing an annual medical evaluation, have a 12-channel chemistry profile and a thyroid panel to detect metabolic disease. These basic tests would be sufficient screening procedures to detect the common metabolic problems, e.g., diabetes mellitus, thyroid malfunction, and hyperparathyroidism. The primary clinician is however, cautioned not to "over interrupt" these results and is referred to the specific section discussing these entities regarding how the results of such tests might be different than in younger patients.

REFERENCES

General References:

Andres R, Tobin JD: Endocrine systems, in Finch, Hayflick (eds): Handbook of the Biology of Aging. New York, Van Nostrand Reinhold, 1977, p 357

Gergerman RI, Bierman EL: Aging and hormones, in Williams RH (ed): Textbook of Endocrinology, ed 5. Philadelphia, WB Saunders, 1974, p 1059

Jubiz W: Endocrinology: A Logical Approach for Clinicians. New York, McGraw-Hill, 1979

Thorn GW: Hormonal disorders: General considerations and major syndromes, in Harrison's Principles in Internal Medicine, ed 8. New York, McGraw-Hill, 1977, p 468

Common Problems:

Asch RH, Greenblat RB: Geriatric endocrinology, in

Reichel, W (ed): Clinical Aspects of Aging. Baltimore, Williams & Wilkins, 1978, p 315

Davis JP: Endocrines and aging, in Reichel W (ed): The Geriatric Patient. New York, Hospital Practice Publishing Co, 1978, p 82

Williams TF: Diabetes mellitus in older people, in Reichel W (ed): Clinical Aspects of Aging. Baltimore, Williams & Wilkins, 1978, p 327

Uncommon and Rare Problems:

Thorn GW et al: Harrison's Principles of Internal Medicine, ed 8. New York, McGraw Hill, 1977

Williams RH: Textbook on Endocrinology, ed 5. Philadelphia, WB Saunders, 1974

11

Cardiovascular System

William C. Fowkes, Jr., M.D.
Virginia Fowkes, F.N.P., M.H.S.

Heart disease is the most significant cause of morbidity and mortality in the elderly. Older patients may develop any kind of heart disease or even have congenital lesions that escaped detection earlier in life.

Considerable evidence suggests that aging affects cardiac function independently from specific disease entities. The peak tension exerted by the aged myocardium is comparable to that in younger persons. The duration necessary to achieve peak tension is, however, longer with the elderly. Gradual stiffening of the myocardium is accompanied by deposits of lipofusion, a pigment associated with aging. Other histological changes include increased vacuolization and neutral fat deposition. With each decade, decreased cardiac reserve results in stepwise reductions of maximum exercise heart rate and cardiac output. Both aortic and mitral valves gradually stiffen. Calcium may infiltrate the mitral annulus and extend into the valve leaflets. Significant obstruction of the aortic orifice occurs more frequently with advancing age. Fibrosis of the myocardium commonly accompanies aging. This process is of uncertain origin and may extend into the conduction system and impair impulse transmission. Amyloid deposition in the myocardium is a poorly understood process associated with aging. This occurs in 50 percent of patients over the age of 90. Since older patients have compromised cardiac function, it is often difficult to separate the effects of normal aging from disease processes.[1]

The heart is influenced by other changes within the vascular system. With age, decreasing vascular compliance results in an increase in blood pressure that may increase myocardial work and oxygen consumption. Geriatric patients may present with typical cardiac symptoms including anginal pain, dyspnea, palpitation, and weakness. More than likely, however, symptoms are atypical and nonspecific. The chest pain associated with acute myocardial infarction may be obscure. Effort dyspnea and anginal pain may be less prominent due to inactivity. Mental confusion, failure to thrive, or becoming bedridden are common presenting problems.

Frequently, the treatment of patients with cardiovascular disease involves use of potent medications. Drug therapy is tolerated less well by older patients than younger ones. Of greatest import is the fact that the older patient may be taking medication given by a variety of heatlh care providers for more than one condition. It is imperative that all medications taken by the patient be reviewed for potential adverse interactions. Review the other side effects and interactions of drugs affecting the cardiovascular system in Chapter 6.

INCIDENCE OF CARDIOVASCULAR DISEASE IN THE ELDERLY

The perceived prevalence of heart disease in the elderly correlates directly with the thoroughness of examination and evaluations. Examination of un-

The authors gratefully acknowledge the assistance of Douglas P. Zipes, M.D., Professor of Medicine, Krannert Institute of Cardiology, Indiana University Medical Center, Indianapolis, Indiana.

selected patients who lived at home and were between ages 65 and 74 revealed significant heart
disease in 40 percent. In 20 percent of patients, the
cardiac condition was a significant cause of disability.
Heart disease occurred in 50 percent of the group
over the age of 75.[2]

Coronary disease and hypertension are the leading causes of death in the elderly. Changes after the
age of 70 make history of hypercholesterolemia or
smoking less reliable as predictors of disease. This
may be related to attrition of patients with coronary
disease and survival of a healthier group.

Although it is impossible to control for genetic
factors, there are populations in whom the incidence of heart disease in geriatric age groups is
quite low or occurs much later than normally found
in the United States and other industrialized countries. There are significant differences in social
structure, diet, and activity in those populations.
Evidence suggests that the prevalence of certain
types of heart disease (coronary disease and hypertension) is related to acculturation in the northern
European way of life. However, the relationship of
this information to cogent strategies in the health
care of older population groups remains proble-
matical.

Comparison of older patients who die of cardiac
disease with normal patients of similar age reveals
multiple problems. Cardiac failure is generally associated with two or more cardiac diagnoses.
Ranked in order of frequency, common pathological
findings are coronary disease, degenerative disease
of the mitral annulus or aortic valve, hypertension,
and senile amyloidosis.[3]

Regardless of the underlying etiology, the geriatric patient generally presents to the health care
system with one of three major clinical syndromes:
congestive heart failure, chest pain, arrhythmia, or
a combination of these problems. With increasing
emphasis on health maintenance and community-
wide detection programs, the elderly patient who
does not have symptoms may be referred with
significant hypertension or pulse irregularity.

EMERGENCIES

Pulmonary Edema

Symptoms and signs of pulmonary edema are
acute dyspnea, hypotension, and wet pulmonary
rales. Management depends on the underlying etiology. This is a medical emergency, and relief is
critical. If an atrial arrhythmia with rapid ventric-

ular response is the contributing cause, management of the arrhythmia is paramount. This should
include, if necessary, immediate DC electrical cardioversion. Oxygen, antiarrhythmic agents, morphine, diuretics, digitalis, and other inotropic agents
may be used. In the older patient, the use of rotating
tourniquets can be dangerous and, if applied incorrectly, can precipitate acute vascular insufficiency.
The peripheral pulses should be checked before
applying rotating tourniquets to the extremities.

Ruptured Aneurysm

Ruptured aortic aneurysm is a disease that afflicts
older patients, especially those who do not have
routine medical care. The rupture of an abdominal
aortic aneurysm has a very high mortality rate in
excess of 50 percent and approaching 85 percent.
Patients present with an acute abdomen, profound
shock, and a palpable abdominal mass. Consultation
should be obtained rapidly while the patient is being
stabilized.

Acute Myocardial Infarction

Acute myocardial infarction, which will be discussed in detail in subsequent sections, is a medical
emergency and a frequent occurrence in the senior
population. Management includes the rapid transfer of the patient to the monitored environment.

Cardiac Arrest

It is important for all primary care providers to
be certified in cardiopulmonary resuscitation. This
includes recognition of cardiopulmonary arrest and
proficiency at ventilation, as well as closed chest
massage of arrest victims. Major therapeutic goals
include institution of resuscitation and stabilization
while the patient is transported to an appropriate
environment. Ideally, patients with chronic illness
should have input regarding decisions about resus-
citative procedures and what they would like to
happen in an arrest. Living wills, which include
specific instructions to the health care provider,
may be developed with interested patients.

UNCOMMON PROBLEMS

Some older patients have atypical conditions associated with cardiac disability. The typical clinical
pattern may be absent. In most instances, this is an
unusual manifestation of a common problem. More
unusual kinds of heart disease may, however, be

present. Congenital heart disease has been noted in 90-year-old patients. Occasionally pericardial disease is associated with unexplained congestive failure. Thyrotoxic heart disease may be well masked in the older patient. A reasonable evaluation of each geriatric patient presenting with cardiac symptoms is appropriate in attempting to define the underlying etiology. This does not mean that older patients should have cardiac consultation, catheterization, and angiography. Careful history and physical examination should be performed. Noninvasive laboratory tests such as the electrocardiogram and chest x-ray should be utilized in the evaluation. This will allow diagnosis in 75 percent of patients. If further evaluation is needed, cardiac consultation should be obtained.

Constrictive Pericarditis and Tamponade

There are multiple causes of constrictive pericarditis ranging from infection to tumor. In most patients, no specific cause is found with chronic constriction. The pathologic process causes gradual increase in the intrapericardial pressure that impedes cardiac filling and lowers cardiac output. Patients complain of fatigue, weakness, dyspnea, or syncope. There is a gradual onset of symptoms that suggest right heart failure or cirrhosis of the liver. These symptoms include abdominal ascites and edema. In both conditions of constrictive pericarditis and pericardial tamponade, it is critical to recognize the presence of low cardiac output manifested by symptoms of weakness and fatigue. A low blood pressure, tachycardia, elevated venous pressure, and pulsus parodoxus (exaggerated drop in the blood pressure during inspiration) are important signs. Kussmaul's sign, paradoxical elevation of venous pressure during inspiration, may be present.

Symptoms develop rapidly with tamponade. The chest x-ray may reveal a water bottle heart configuration suggesting pericardial effusion. Echocardiography is useful in the diagnosis, and consultation should be obtained early. Pericardiocentesis can be life saving.

Congenital Heart Disease

Occasionally the older patient presents with a long-standing congenital lesion. This is usually an atrial-septal defect. The symptoms and signs are not unique in that patients appear with congestive failure and arrhythmias. Clues to this diagnosis are the presence of significant signs of right heart failure, large dilated pulmonary arteries suggesting a left to right shunt, and an abnormal cardiac x-ray silhouette suggesting multiple chamber enlargement. With older patients, it is unlikely that cardiac surgery will be appropriate. Irreversible pulmonary hypertension or other medical illness may make the risk of surgery too great.

DIAGNOSIS AND TREATMENT OF COMMON PROBLEMS

Hypertension

The prevalence and incidence of hypertension increase with age even in healthy older populations.[4] In a nursing home, the prevalence of blood pressures above assumed population normals (140/90) reaches approximately 50 percent. The "normal" blood pressure for the older population is considered to be at a higher level than 140/90, possibly 160/95. With increasing age, there is a gradual stiffening of the central arterial tree and a corresponding increase in systolic blood pressure. Although this is a normal process, elevated blood pressure increases risk of cardiovascular disease, and at some point intervention is appropriate.

The decision to intervene in elderly patients must remain a matter of individual determination in the context of the patient's value system after discussion of risks and benefits. Although there is good evidence of improvement in life expectancy with reduction of elevated blood pressure, the assumption that such results apply to the older patient is presumptuous since only 10 percent of the patients in the 41 published trials of antihypertensive drugs were over the age of 60.[6]

It is probably not appropriate to treat isolated systolic hypertension. Although a significant risk factor, systolic hypertension is largely a manifestation of decreased aortic compliance and is often resistant to therapy.[7] If treatment is pushed aggressively, the diastolic pressure and blood flow to vital organs may be compromised.[8] There is frequently an exaggerated elevation of the systolic pressure in older patients with diastolic hypertension. In general, it is appropriate to offer treatment to older patients with documented hypertension over 160/100.

In the vast majority of patients, elevated blood pressure has no demonstrable specific cause and is therefore called essential hypertension. Sporadic cases of hypertension due to endocrine and renal causes do occur in older people. There is an occasional patient over the age of 50 who has renovascular hypertension associated with atherosclerotic involvement of the lower abdominal aorta impinging upon the renal orifice. This possibility needs to be considered if hypertension worsens, is difficult to control, and when other evidence of significant atherosclerotic disease exists.

SYMPTOMS, SIGNS, AND EVALUATION

Most patients with hypertension are asymptomatic, and elevated blood pressure is identified at the time of physical examination or community screening programs. When symptoms or signs are present, they relate to complications from the disease that include stroke, congestive heart failure, or coronary heart disease. Patients with hypertension may complain of headaches. However, this occurs probably no more frequently than in the normotensive population. In evaluating the patient with hypertension, it is important to consider secondary causes, although these are rare. A history of renal disease is significant and may be causative. Profound muscle weakness and polyuria may be associated with primary aldosteronism. Usually three measurements taken on different days are necessary before a diagnosis of hypertension is confirmed. The blood pressure should be taken repeatedly. Initially, both arms are checked to see if there is a significant difference. It is more likely for the blood pressure to be lower in the left arm because of atherosclerotic obstruction at the bifurcation of the left subclavian artery. The blood pressure should be taken routinely with the patient lying and standing to determine the effect of posture. Funduscopic examination assists in determining the severity and duration of the patient's hypertension. A narrowing of the arteries and nicking of arteriovenous crossover are related to the duration of hypertension. Exudates, hemorrhages, and papilledema are associated with increasing severity. Bruits may suggest the presence of atherosclerotic lesions. Palpable left ventricular hypertrophy or the presence of an S_4 suggests left ventricular hypertrophy, although this may relate to myocardial disease. Any evidence of end organ involvement in the physical examination—such as eye ground, central nervous system, or myocardial findings—or in laboratory studies doubles the risk of complication.[9]

The appropriate evaluation of hypertensive patients has been the subject of much debate.[10] Certain baseline studies are important. These include measurement of the serum electrolytes, a test of renal function, and an electrocardiogram. Blood glucose and uric acid tests may also be obtained, as therapy can affect glucose metabolism and uric acid clearance. More extensive evaluation is appropriate when the patient's history or physical examination suggests the hypertension may be secondary to endocrine or renal causes. Failure to respond to treatment is also an indication for further evaluation.

MANAGEMENT

There are no simple guidelines for monitoring patients with hypertension since the severity of hypertension, complications of associated diseases, and response to treatment determine the amount of care required. The relatively healthy, asymptomatic patient who is satisfactorily controlled on one medication may be followed every three months. A patient who has multiple problems and is taking several medications needs more frequent attention. Laboratory studies such as serum potassium and BUN or creatinine may be done to check for potassium depletion or deteriorating renal function. A decision should be made with the patient or a family member about monitoring the blood pressure at home. This may be appropriate with some patients and not others. If the patient is not interested in monitoring blood pressure, this should be done by office personnel at regular intervals to assess the adequacy of management.

In managing patients with hypertension, therapeutic goals are directed towards reducing morbidity and mortality by preventing complications such as stroke and heart failure. Diverse opinions exist about management of hypertension in older persons. A basic approach is to lower the blood pressure to a level consistent with normal physiologic functioning and absence of side effects from medication. If postural symptoms or other signs of circulatory insufficiency occur, a higher blood pressure should be accepted. It is common for older patients to be disabled or hospitalized because of overzealous management of asymptomatic hypertension.[11] Furthermore, reduced risk of complication from hypertension has been demonstrated with treatment of patients whose blood pressures have not been successfully reduced to normal levels.[12] Adverse reactions to antihypertensive treatment include severe postural hypotension, cerebral symptoms from poor perfusion of the central nervous system, and severe electrolyte disturbance.

Comprehensive management includes modification of risk factors. These are cumulative. For example, an individual who smokes and has hypertension has approximately double the risk of a person who smokes and is normotensive.[13] Weight loss has been shown to ameliorate hypertension and may be all that is necessary to decrease the blood pressure. A 20 to 30-pound weight loss in an overweight individual may result in an average pressure drop of 10–20 mm Hg and eliminate the necessity for drug management.[14] Salt intake should be restricted. Although it is difficult to demonstrate that salt restriction by itself is effective in lowering blood pressure, there is little question that as an adjunct to drug therapy, it is useful. Since severe salt restriction cannot be accomplished without major constraints on diet, simple instructions assist the patient and family in limiting sodium intake. For example, salt should not be added to the food in cooking or at the table. Prepared meats such as lunch meats, ham, or bacon should not be used. Condiments such as ketchup, canned foods, and pickles are eliminated from the diet. A salt substitute may be used except when the patient is taking a potassium sparing diuretic or has severe renal insufficiency.

Meditation and relaxation exercises may be useful adjuncts to hypertensive therapy. Studies indicate these approaches are effective in lowering the blood pressure temporarily or as long as the practice continues.[15] The effects of these techniques for long-term management are questionable. For patients who show interest, however, these techniques can be taught easily and are without side effects. Older patients may be good candidates for those techniques since they are more likely to have time to practice and use them.

The effects of exercise on hypertension are uncertain. An immediate result of exercise is an increase in blood pressure. However, exercise affects weight reduction, and this in turn lowers the blood pressure. There is little evidence to suggest that exercise causes hypertension directly. There are, however, many other benefits from regular exercise. Patients should be encouraged to walk to their tolerance each day. For the older patient brisk walking is the appropriate exercise, though bicycling or swimming are very effective.

Drug therapy is tailored to the individual patient. (See Fig. 11-1.) Diuretics are the best initial approach for older patients, though judicious use of vasodilators and sympathetic inhibitors may be warranted. Side effects or complications of drug therapy are much more likely to occur in older patients. Therefore, initially cautious use of low doses with

SELECTION OF DRUG REGIMEN

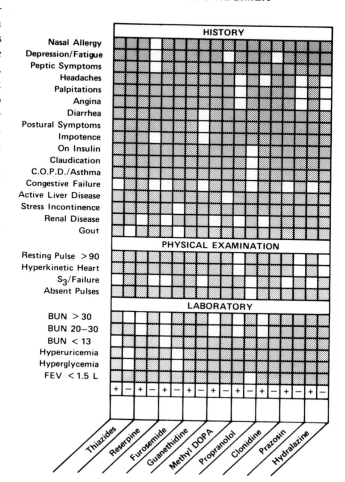

Fig. 11-1. To use the drug selection key, the form should be checked after the patient's history, physical examination, and initial laboratory evaluation are completed. When an item is positive, for example, the patient has nasal allergy or hyperuricemia; the appropriate unshaded square(s) is(are) checked horizontally. When the form is completed, and when all items are reviewed and checked, the vertical columns are totaled and the (−) score subtracted from the (+) score for each drug. The drug with the highest score would be considered useful with the particular patient scored. Drugs that tend to be less expensive and have convenient dosage schedules are placed toward the left side of the evaluation chart and, in general, would be used as first choices. The selection table is not meant to replace the step approach to management; rather, it is to be of assistance especially in selection of a second or third drug.

gradual changes in the regimen is recommended. Frequently, geriatric patients have more than one health problem, and medication must be evaluated for multiple effects. An antihypertensive drug may adversely affect another problem or may have an unexpected therapeutic benefit. For example, hypertension and angina pectoris both may be improved with use of propranolol. A diuretic or vasodilator that decreases pre- and afterload and lowers blood pressure may ameliorate both hypertension and congestive heart failure. If diabetes is present, diuretics may increase hyperglycemia and some adjustment in the regimen may be appropriate. In patients with chronic lung disease, use of beta blockers aggravates airway obstruction and is contraindicated. Table 11-1 summarizes antihypertensive agents which are commonly used.

Congestive Heart Failure

In older people, there is a gradual decline of functional cardiac capacity and consequently a decrease in cardiac reserve.[16] Stress that might be tolerated well by a younger individual may precipitate congestive heart failure in an older person. Stress from infections such as pneumonia or from surgical procedures are common contributing events. Frequently, older patients have more than one cardiac disease. When congestive heart failure occurs, clinicians usually diagnose arteriosclerotic heart disease as the etiology. While this is the most common cause, other conditions should be considered.[17]

The mechanism for congestive failure in the older person is not different from that in younger individuals. The cardiac output cannot be maintained successfully, and end diastolic pressure increases, eventually exceeding the plasma oncotic pressure and resulting in transudation of fluid into the lungs and periphery. The right and left heart may fail independently. The left ventricle, which generates a higher pressure and is intermittently supplied by coronary blood flow, is more susceptible to most disease states. For this reason, the absence of peripheral edema or lack of elevated peripheral venous pressure does not rule out congestive heart failure. The impact of heart rate on cardiac functions is important to consider. Older people with restricted cardiac capacity have relatively fixed systolic ejection times. The ejection period cannot be reduced as effectively with catecholamine stimulation as in younger persons. Therefore, as the ventricular rate doubles from 60–120, the effective diastolic filling period is reduced by approximately one-third. The mean diastolic pressure will increase equivalently. Furthermore, older individuals with poorly compliant ventricles associated with aortic valve disease or hypertension suffer more physiologic impairment from loss of atrial kick. High-end diastolic pressures and adequate filling can be maintained with vigorous atrial contraction into a stiff ventricle while maintaining a relatively low-mean diastolic pressure. With loss of atrial contractions as occurring in atrial fibrillation, congestive heart failure may develop rapidly. Patients with congestive heart failure are susceptible to embolic complications. This is probably the result of a sedentary lifestyle and sluggish circulation, which results in stasis and venous thrombosis. Pulmonary embolism must be considered with anyone whose condition worsens suddenly.

SYMPTOMS, SIGNS, AND EVALUATION

Symptoms of congestive failure may be obscure. Frequently, patients with heart failure present with fatigue, mental confusion, or failure to thrive. Sometimes, the older patient will become bedridden or the family will bring the patient to the office with complaint of weight loss. More obvious symptoms include dyspnea, weakness, fatigue, edema, cough, and occasional paroxysmal nocturnal dyspnea or orthopnea. Some patients complaining of nocturnal dyspnea have Cheyne-Stokes respiration characterized by cyclic hyperpnea alternating with periods of apnea.

Pulse abnormalities may be evident. Atrial fibrillation, premature ventricular or atrial contractions, sinus tachycardia, and pulsus alternans may be found. In the presence of biventricular failure, findings include distended jugular veins, pulmonary rales, hepatomegaly, and peripheral edema. In bedridden patients, sacral edema is likely. Heart murmurs indicating the presence of valvular heart disease may be found with cardiac examination. It is not uncommon for murmurs to be present during acute cardiac decompensation and disappear later. The opposite may also occur whereby the very ill patient has a cardiac output too low to produce murmurs initially; they appear as the patient improves.

Other signs of cardiac dysfunction include a palpable diffuse ventricular impulse with prolonged ejection time. Third and fourth heart sounds are common also.

Table 11-1
Common Antihypertensive Drugs

Drug	Dosage Schedule	Average Dose/Day	Side Effects	Remember	Side Benefits
Diuretics					
Hydrochlorothiazide	bid	50–100	Potassium depletion	Decreases glucose tolerance Hyperuricemia	May improve congestive failure
Chlorthalidone	qd	50–100	Same as above	Same as above	Same as above
Furosemide	bid	40–80	Same as above	Same as above	Same as above
Spironolactone	bid	50–100	Hyperkalemia	Little direct antihypertensive effect	Same as above
Vasodilators					
Hydralazine	qid	40–200	Reflex tachycardia Lupus syndrome	May cause vascular headache	May improve congestive failure
Prazosin	tid	3–15	May cause vascular headache	Tachyphylaxis	Same as above
Sympathetic Inhibitors					
Reserpine	qd	0.25–1	Mental depression, peptic ulcer disease, nasal congestion, impotence	May worsen congestive failure	
Methyldopa	bid	500–2000	Mental depression, impotence, liver toxicity		
Clonidine	bid	0.2–1	Mental depression	Rebound hypertensive crisis	May improve vascular headache
Propranolol	bid	40–160	Bradycardia	May worsen congestive failure, obstructive lung disease, or peripheral arterial insufficiency May block early symptoms of insulin reaction in diabetic patients	May improve vascular headache and angina pectoris

Noninvasive laboratory procedures should be utilized initially to define the underlying etiology. The electrocardiogram may reveal evidence of past myocardial infarction or left ventricular hypertrophy. Echocardiography is useful if there is a question of valvular or congenital heart disease. Further evaluation such as radionuclide imaging or cardiac catheterization may be necessary and should, if contemplated, be discussed with the patient and family.

MANAGEMENT

Management of patients with congestive heart failure depends on the severity of symptoms and may take place in the home or office, or require hospitalization. In the moderately or severely ill person, hospital care and a monitored environment are necessary. This includes patients who are quite uncomfortable, are too ill to be able to care for themselves, have life-threatening problems such as serious premonitory arrhythmias, or have difficulty maintaining normal physiological functions. The ambulatory patient with modest symptoms in whom an etiology has been established can be followed in the outpatient setting. Support systems such as the visiting nurse and home visits may be used to monitor the physical status in marginally ill patients managed at home.

Laboratory evaluation usually includes a CBC, urinalysis, electrocardiogram, chest x-ray, electrolytes, and tests for renal function such as BUN. The BUN is especially useful in monitoring diuretic therapy. Excessive effects from use of diuretics depletes electrolytes and reduces blood volume, as well as cardiac output with resultant prerenal azotemia and elevation of the BUN.

Specific management includes bedrest to reduce metabolic demands and treatment of any precipitating cause such as anemia or infection. In the hospital, oxygen may be useful if hypoxemia is present. Salt restriction is important. This is easily managed in the hospital but more difficult with home care and usually must be supplemented with diuretic therapy. Patient and family education about salt restriction is critical, and a dietician is a helpful consultant. If the patient has atrial fibrillation with rapid ventricular response, digitalis glycosides are used to control the ventricular rate. Persistent atrial fibrillation or flutter may be treated with cardioversion to sinus rhythm. Patients with long-standing atrial fibrillation or flutter usually cannot be maintained in sinus rhythm even if converted successfully. Normally, digitalis is not indicated in patients who have chronic atrial fibrillation with a slow ventricular response. Patients with afterload problems such as hypertension or aortic stenosis usually benefit from this drug.

Diuretics combined with salt restriction remain the mainstay of therapy in older patients. However, they are very likely to become potassium-deficient with diuretic therapy. This is especially so with patients who have additional problems such as hepatic insufficiency, which would further augment aldosterone production and aggravate urinary potassium wastage. The combination of a thiazide with a potassium-sparing diuretic (triamterene, spironolactone) may eliminate the need for potassium supplements. Potassium-sparing diuretics should not be used with salt substitutes, which contain potassium, as hyperkalemia may result. The more potent loop diuretics (furosemide, ethacrynic acid) may be necessary to treat the more severely ill patient or patients with renal insufficiency who do not respond to thiazides. These drugs interfere with the countercurrent exchange mechanism in Henle's loop of the kidney. They are more expensive, have a shorter duration of action, and may be more potent than is necessary. Usually thiazide diuretics are given first before using loop diuretics. Thiazide and loop diuretics are additive in effect and may be used simultaneously for the more seriously ill patient.[18] In patients with severe cardiac disease, afterload

reduction in the form of vasodilators (hydralazine, prazosin) may be used. These medications lower blood pressure, improve cardiac output, and lower diastolic filling pressures in patients with congestive failure.[19]

Arrhythmias

An arrhythmia of any type may be associated with any underlying pathologic condition. Some, such as premature contractions and supraventricular tachycardias, may be present when there is no evidence of heart disease. The impact of an arrhythmia on the older person depends on the degree of cardiac pump dysfunction caused by valvular or myocardial disease, loss of atrial function, and slow or fast ventricular rates. Symptoms are the result of falling cardiac output or congestive failure. Arrhythmias that reduce cardiac output may precipitate or aggravate other problems in older patients. Some examples are chronic brain syndrome, cerebrovascular accident, and postural hypotension. The formation of intracardiac thrombosis and subsequent pulmonary or systemic embolism are other consequences.

Premature Contractions

Premature atrial and ventricular contractions can be observed in a high percentage of older patients and may be unassociated with cardiac disease. Premature contractions may, however, be the first manifestation of cardiac disease or the harbinger of more serious arrhythmias.

Ectopic beats are frequently noticed by the patient and may be picked up with routine pulse examination or an electrocardiogram.

SYMPTOMS, SIGNS, AND EVALUATION

If symptoms are present, there may be a sense of skipping or irregularity. If bigeminy exists and the premature beat is ineffective, symptoms of low cardiac output such as weakness or fatigue may be noted. Although careful physical examination can help in determining the type of ectopic beat, the electrocardiogram is necessary to define the ectopy and to look for other significant problems. Occasionally, in bigeminal rhythm, the ectopic beat produces little or no stroke output resulting in an effective rate in the 30s or 40s. In this instance, the only evidence of the premature beat may be an audible first heart sound and an abnormal jugular venous pulse pattern detected with physical examination.

MANAGEMENT

Asymptomatic ectopic beats rarely need management in the otherwise healthy individual. Tobacco, coffee, or other caffeine-containing beverages may be causative. Potentially toxic drugs in this setting have yet to be proven useful. When the ectopic rhythm is likely to have serious consequence, treatment should be directed towards preventing the serious arrhythmia. Examples are frequent premature ventricular contractions in the presence of acute myocardial infarction or premature atrial contractions in the patient with mitral valve disease and a history of paroxysmal atrial arrhythmias.

A variety of antiarrhythmic agents are available. (See Table 11-2.) Procainamide and disopyramide are frequently effective for premature ventricular contractions. Quinidine and propranolol are more useful in the control of atrial premature beats.

Atrial Fibrillation

Atrial fibrillation is probably the most common significant arrhythmia among older populations. The incidence varies considerably and relates to the characteristics of the population studied.[20] The underlying etiology is usually arteriosclerotic heart disease or cardiomyopathy. Atrial fibrillation may be an asymptomatic and an unexpected finding with routine examination. In this instance, there is usually a slow ventricular response within normal physiologic range. Atrial fibrillation in an older person is a frequent preamble to, or an early manifestation of, congestive heart failure.

SYMPTOMS, SIGNS, AND EVALUATIONS

Symptoms relate to the patient's condition and severity of symptoms is usually related to ventricular rate. They may be absent in healthy persons or severe in patients with a rapid ventricular response. The patient may become bedridden due to weakness or present following a syncopal episode. The patient's pulse is irregular with varied pulse amplitude. Often, there is a pulse deficit when comparing auscultated and palpable pulse rates. (A higher rate is counted by auscultation than at the wrist.) Other physical findings depend on the degree of physiologic impairment. With rapid ventricular response rates, significant congestive heart failure may be present. In this situation, signs will relate to the duration of the problem and include distended neck veins, pulmonary rales, third heart sound, hepatic congestion, and peripheral edema.

The electrocardiogram will reveal fibrillation waves (visualized best in lead V_1) and an irregular

Table 11-2
Common Antiarrhythmic Drugs: Ambulatory Usage (Oral)

Drug	Maintenance/Day	Therapeutic Blood Level	Valuable In	Remember	Benefits
Digitoxin	0.125–0.5 mg	1–2 ng/ml	Atrial arrhythmias	Decrease dose for renal insufficiency	Improves contractility
Quinidine	0.8–1.6 g	2–7 μg/ml	Atrial and ventricular arrhythmias	Hyperkalemia potentiates effect Depresses myocardial contractility	
Disopyramide	400 mg	2–4 μg/ml	Ventricular and atrial arrhythmias	Depresses myocardial contractility	
Procainamide	1–2 g	4–8 μg/ml	Ventricular and atrial arrhythmias	Lupus syndrome common in older patients	
Propranolol	40–160 mg	50–100 ng/ml	Atrial and ventricular arrhythmias	Worsens congestive failure, obstructive lung disease, and peripheral vascular disease	May improve angina

ventricular response. If the rate is fast, aberrant ventricular conduction may stimulate a ventricular arrhythmia. However, the variable R-R interval identifies the arrhythmia. A patient with intermittent symptoms may have a paroxysmal arrhythmia. Holter monitoring is useful in evaluating this possibility. If the interval between symptoms is more than 24 hours, the patient is instructed to turn on the monitor when symptoms occur.

MANAGEMENT

The degree of cardiac impairment determines the patient's management. Treatment may not be necessary when the patient is asymptomatic and has a slow ventricular response with a resting pulse range between 60 and 70. In paroxysmal atrial fibrillation, habits such as coffee or alcohol consumption, which may precipitate the arrhythmia in some patients, should be evaluated and modified accordingly. Immediate DC cardioversion should be considered for treatment of the patient who has an acute myocardial infarction and atrial fibrillation with rapid ventricular rate. With all persons, attempts should be made to define the underlying etiology or precipitating condition causing the arrhythmia.

Because atrial fibrillation is usually accompanied by rapid ventricular response, treatment is directed at slowing the ventricular rate. Digoxin is usually the drug of choice. It is carefully titrated to achieve a resting pulse rate between 60 and 70. With normal renal function, the initial digitalizing dose is 1–2 mg with a maintenance dose of 0.25–0.50 mg daily. With a maintenance dosage, effective blood levels will be achieved in five to seven days. The patient is instructed to withhold the medication if the pulse rate is less than 60 upon awakening in the morning. Some patients with atrial fibrillation have exaggerated increases in heart rate in response to exercise. For this reason, patients who have atrial fibrillation, are being treated with digitalis, and who complain of effort dyspnea should be exercised and checked for such a possibility. A higher dose of digitalis may be necessary if there is an undue increase in heart rate with exercise. Propanolol may also be used to slow the ventricular rate, but, outside the acute situation, it is usually inappropriate because of expense, risk, or side effects. It aggravates chronic obstructive pulmonary disease and must be given two to four times daily.

Elective conversion to sinus rhythm should be considered with the initial diagnosis of atrial fibril-

lation and with the assistance of a cardiologist. Cardioversion is especailly useful in patients with mitral valve disease. In these patients, restoring atrial contraction may afford some protection against embolism. Unfortunately, maintenance of sinus rhythm is difficult in the patient with long-standing mitral valve disease even if successfully converted. Conversion to sinus rhythm is also important for patients with valvular aortic stenosis and who have decreased ventricular compliance. Atrial contraction is critical in ventricular filling and allowing the heart to operate at a lower mean diastolic pressure for a given cardiac output. Following cardioversion, an antiarrhythmic agent—usually quinidine—is given to maintain the sinus rhythm.

Since atrial fibrillation increases the risk of embolism, anticoagulation must be considered. With older people in general, the risk of anticoagulation therapy probably exceeds the benefit of protection from embolism. The exception is the individual with mitral stenosis and chronic atrial fibrillation. These patients have a much greater incidence of systemic embolization and should receive warfarin therapy.

Sick Sinus Syndrome

Sick sinus syndrome is caused by functional or anatomic impairment of the atrial pacemaking mechanism in the region of the sinus node. With intermittent failure of the sinus pacing mechanism, a number of arrhythmias occur. These include bradycardias, either sinus bradycardia or junctional bradycardia, and a variety of escape atrial arrhythmias such as atrial fibrillation, atrial tachycardia, or atrial flutter.[21]

SYMPTOMS, SIGNS AND EVALUATION

Patients with sick sinus syndrome usually have paroxysmal symptoms associated with the bradyarrhythmias or tachyarrhythmias. These are paroxysmal weakness or fatigue, syncope, dyspnea, palpitations, or symptoms associated with congestive heart failure or embolism.

Physical examination may not be helpful since the individual may have sinus rhythm at the time seen. Without a period of evaluation and observation, it is difficult to determine whether or not the sinus bradycardia or atrial fibrillation is the result of sinus node dysfunction. The electrocardiogram may reveal periods of sinus pause, wandering atrial pacemaker, or sinus arrest accompanied by atrial escape rhythms. (See Fig. 11-2.) Holter monitoring is very effective in making this diagnosis.

MANAGEMENT

Management of patients with sick sinus syndrome is sometimes difficult. Antiarrhythmic agents may be ineffective. Early evidence suggested that digitalis glycosides were risky in this condition.[22] More recent studies indicate that digitalis is not harmful and actually may be helpful. It increases atrial automaticity and should be considered in patients with this condition.[23] Treatment of atrial tachyarrhythmias is related to the patient's physiological condition. Cardioversion is avoided since relapse is extremely likely. An atrial arrhythmia, such as atrial fibrillation with slow ventricular response, may be tolerated quite well by the patient and result in cessation of the paroxysmal difficulties. In patients with significant symptoms associated with brady- and tachyarrhythmias, pacemaker implantation is a satisfactory solution. However, pacing frequently must be supplemented by drug therapy to control the condition optimally.

Conduction Disturbance

Usually disturbances with conduction are cuased by fibrosis of the conduction system. Occasionally, patients with coronary heart disease may develop acute and chronic heart block. The development of lesions in the conducting system, including fascicular and bundle branch block, can be observed for a long period of time prior to the onset of complete heart block and associated symptoms. Disturbances of conduction can be physiologic rather than pathologic and due to drug toxicity with digitalis or other substances.

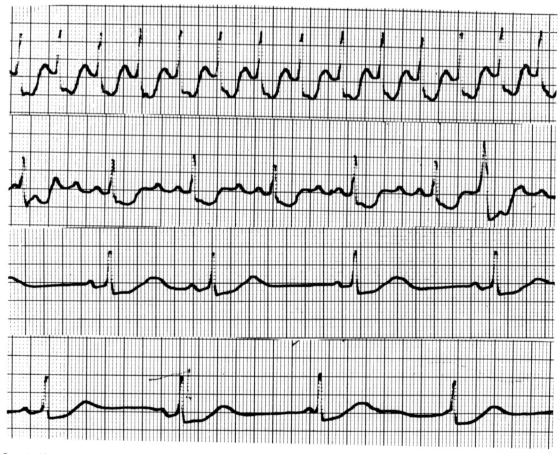

Fig. 11-2. A 67-year-old woman who had aortic valve replacement five years earlier presented with a history of near syncope and palpitations. The top two rhythm strips reveal typical atrial flutter with 2:1 and 4:1 block. The latter two strips reveal sinus bradycardia, sinus pause, and wandering atrial pacemaker consistent with sick sinus syndrome.

SYMPTOMS, SIGNS, AND EVALUATIONS

Symptoms depend on the ventricular rate and status of cardiac output. Syncope or near syncope is common in patients with complete heart block and slow ventricular rates. Other symptoms include postural dizziness or mental confusion. Symptoms associated with congestive heart failure may be present also. With acquired complete heart block, the heart rate is slow in the range of 40/minute. Cannon A waves in the neck, variable first heart sounds, systolic murmur, and systolic hypertension are common findings. Many persons have intermittent symptoms prior to the onset of complete heart block and may present without these typical findings.

The electrocardiograms may reveal varying degrees of heart block. Occasionally, an older patient presents with postural faintness and is discovered to have bifascicular block on the ECG. Other etiologies for the syncope, such as postural hypotension, secondary to hypersensitive carotid sinus, metabolic abnormalities, or central nervous system difficulties, must be considered. Patients who have paroxysmal symptoms suggesting complete heart block or Stokes-Adams attacks should be referred for further evaluation. Evaluation may include Holter monitoring, His bundle studies, and atrial stimulation studies.

MANAGEMENT

In patients with third degree AV block, pacemaker insertion is the treatment of choice. Increased survival of individuals with complete heart block and pacemaker installation, as opposed to controls, has been demonstrated.[24] Individuals with significant conduction abnormalities who have pacemakers implanted live a normal life expectancy.

The transvenous route for pacemaker insertion is the most commonly used method. The endocardial lead is inserted through the jugular vein into the right heart, and the pacemaker electrode is positioned in the apex of the right ventricle. The battery unit is implanted in the subcutaneous tissue beneath the clavicle.

Following insertion of the electrode, several problems may occur, including improper positioning of the electrode, electrode dislodgement, or performation of the right ventricle.

The primary provider should be aware of pacemaker characteristics and problems that may arise with patients who have permanent implanted pacemakers. When these patients develop any new cardiovascular or central nervous system complaint, pacemaker dysfunction should be considered a possibility. This is especially important when the symptoms resemble those occurring with the initial diagnosis of conduction disturbance.

To assess pacemaker function, it is necessary to know the pacemaker's characteristics and to have an ECG of the patient after pacemaker insertion. Patients should be instructed to carry a card that identifies the type of pacemaker and its characteristics, including refractory period and rate. When questions arise, the cardiac surgeon or manufacturer should be contacted.

Pacemaker dysfunction usually has three manifestations. These are failure of impulse generation, failure of demand function, and failure of capture. Failure of impulse generation may result from failure of the power source or fracture of a wire.[25] In this situation, the patient's intrinsic rhythm will resume pacing of the heart and symptoms relate to the effectiveness of this rhythm. The patient's ECG reveals absence of the pacemaker artifact. Absence of the pacemaker spike with a heart rate slower than that set for the pacemaker is also an ominous sign. The patient should be managed with agents such as isoproterenol or temporary pacing until the cardiovascular surgeon can evaluate the situation.

Generally, failure of demand function is not detectable clinically and is noted on the electrocardiogram. Most pacemakers in use are the demand type and function only when needed—that is, when the patient's intrinsic heart rhythm falls below a preestablished rate. This requires a sensing circuit within the mechanism that senses the patient's QRS and prohibits pacemaker discharge. The demand circuits have a refractory period, usually 0.2–0.4 seconds. The patient's QRS may not inhibit pacemaker discharge if the QRS occurs late enough to fall within the pacemaker's refractory period. This possibility should be considered when the patient's spontaneous QRS complex, either of supraventricular or of ventricular origin, fails to inhibit pacemaker discharge. Failure of demand function may be an early sign of battery exaustion. (See Fig. 11-3.)

Failure to capture may result from a variety of problems. With complete failure, the patient's intrinsic rhythm will take over. Intermittent failure of capture can be noted on the ECG with the appearance of a pacemaker artifact without a beat following. This suggests dysfunction and should be evaluated by a consultant. Generally pacemakers are programmed to slow as the batteries become ex-

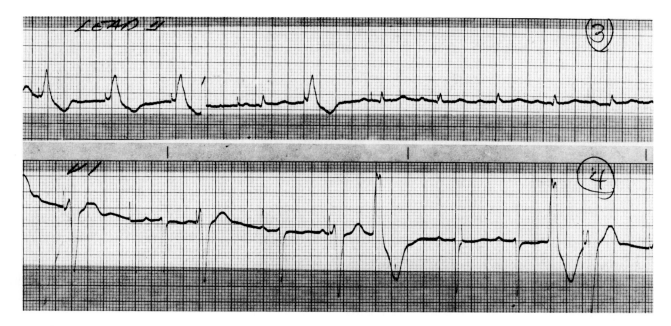

Fig. 11-3. The top strip reveals three normal pacemaker artifacts followed by typical broad pacemaker QRS complexes. The fourth pacemaker artifact fails to produce a QRS. It is followed by a P wave that, after a prolonged PR interval, is conducted to the ventrical producing a QRS. This is followed by a pacemaker-generated beat at a short interval indicating the preceding QRS complex was not sensed by the sensing circuit. Both rhythm strips demonstrate failure of capture and failure of demand function consistent with pacemaker dysfunctions.

hausted. Patients should be instructed to count their pulse and note variations from the intrinsic pacemaker rate (usually 72). A more rapid rate suggests the patient's own rhythm is operative and is not usually a problem. Rates slower than the set rate suggest a problem and should be evaluated. Most modern pacemakers have a life expectancy of more than three years. Frequency of patient evaluation should increase toward the end of expected battery life. There are various technical methods to evaluate pacemaker function. Devices may be purchased to transmit the impulse by telephone to a central site. An inexpensive device using an AM radio tuned to 55 KHZ, a magnet, and a clock with a sweep second hand may be used by the patient to detect and count pacemaker discharge accurately and to report aberrations.[26]

Following the patient with an implanted pacemaker should be a responsibility shared and defined by both the patient and consultant.

In spite of improved shielding, pacemakers remain sensitive to external electromagnetic waves. Appliances such as microwave ovens may interfere with function. The manufacturer's specifications should be observed meticulously.

Angina Pectoris

SYMPTOMS, SIGNS AND EVALUATIONS

Classic angina is characterized by chest pain that is precipitated by effort and relieved by rest. The duration is short, usually less than five minutes, and the syndrome is intermittent. Frequently, the pain is described as an ache or pressure and located in the midchest or substernal region. Some patients have atypical presentations and complain of burning or sharp pain in an unusual location such as the epigastrium or jaw. Exposure to cold, eating a meal, or emotional stress may be contributing factors to an anginal episode. Dyspnea or palpitations may be present. Frequently, patients liken anginal discomfort to indigestion that may be accompanied or relieved by belching.

Most patients will not have any significant physical findings. Some may have signs of conditions such as hypertension or xanthelasama associated with hypercholesterolemia. If the patient is examined during an anginal episode, a fourth heart sound may be present. Rarely, paradoxical splitting of the second heard sound is noted. The ECG may be normal or reveal a variety of abnormalities, including evidence of old myocardial infarction, intraventricular block, or ST and T-wave abnormalities. Changes typical of ischemia are flat, horizontal depressions of the ST segment. These may be present during an acute ischemic episode. Other less specific T-wave changes may be seen. These changes can be confused with nonspecific abnormalities associated with medication such as digitalis and diuretics. Treadmill testing is used to verify the presence of coronary disease where uncertainty exists. Coronary arteriography is warranted if coronary bypass surgery is a consideration. This is rarely appropriate with geriatric patients.

MANAGEMENT

Nitrites are the primary therapeutic modality. Sublingual nitroglycerin is best used prophylactically and prior to an event that the patient recognizes as causing angina. It is also used to treat anginal pain after onset. In this setting, however, it may be more effective simply to stop the activity that precipitated the event. Long-acting nitrites such as isosorbide dinitrite are effective in selected patients. Propranolol, which decreases myocardial oxygen consumption, is quite effective in reducing the frequency of anginal attacks. Conditions such as congestive heart failure and hypertension, which increase myocardial oxygen consumption, should be treated. How vigorous to be in the management of patients with hypertension and coronary heart disease is debatable. Moderately severe hypertension (over 170 systolic and 105 diastolic) should be treated. However, recent evidence suggests that individuals with modest hypertension and coronary heart disease survive longer than individuals who have coronary heart disease and are normotensive.[16] Further studies are needed to make firm recommendations about the vigor of hypertension therapy in the patient with coronary disease.

Coronary artery bypass surgery with a saphenous vein graft is an effective method of managing angina pectoris, which is not controlled by medical means. Surgical mortality has lessened and is approximately 2 percent overall. Morbidity remains significant with a 15–20 percent rate of myocardial infarction associated with surgery and a 15 percent rate of saphenous graft closure.[27] Evidence suggests that there is reduction in mortality and morbidity in individuals with left main coronary artery lesions.[28] This accounts for only 10 percent of all patients with angina pectoris who receive coronary artery surgery. As yet, controlled studies do not

reveal definite prolongation of life in patients who have other than left main stem or triple vessel coronary disease. The procedure itself includes costs, risks, discomfort, and a period of disability. These factors should be weighed carefully. The patient should determine whether or not the disability and discomfort associated with the angina is worth the cost and risk of undertaking bypass surgery.

Myocardial Infarction

SYMPTOMS, SIGNS, AND EVALUATIONS

A diagnosis of myocardial infarction should be considered in any older patient presenting with chest discomfort or symptoms of congestive heart failure. Typical chest pain symptoms may be minimal or absent and the presenting complaint hidden in an array of other problems. In approximately 25 percent of patients with acute myocardial infarction, little or no pain is perceived. If an older individual presents with a sudden ill-defined illness associated with significant disability, a myocardial infarction must be considered. Myocardial infarction occurs in approximately 10 percent of individuals presenting with acute stroke.

Characteristically, patients with acute myocardial infarction have chest pain described as an aching or pressure sensation. Occasionally, it is a sharp or burning pain. The pain may radiate to the neck, jaw, arms, back, or abdomen. Duration and severity differentiate the pain of myocardial infarction from that of angina. With a myocardial infarction, the pain is severe and lasts longer than ten minutes. It is a random event and not necessarily associated with effort as is angina. The onset of pain frequently occurs at rest or awakens an individual from sleep.

Physical findings depend on the severity of the insult and the amount of myocardial damage. With a small myocardial infarction, the physical examination may be relatively normal. Usually a fourth heart sound is present. In a severe case, signs of shock and congestive heart failure may be evident. The classic electrocardiogram changes, including Q waves, elevated ST segments, and inverted T waves, may not be present. Initially, only ST-segment and T-wave abnormalities may be present. These may be the only findings in subendocardial infarction.

Laboratory measurement of enzymes must accompany evaluation of the ECG. The creatinine phosphokinase (CPK), serum glutamic oxaloacetic transaminase (SGOT), and lactic dehydrogenase (LDH) are enzymes most commonly measured. The

CPK is the most sensitive and elevated earliest after acute myocardial infarction. The CPK is also rich in skeletal muscle. Injury to the peripheral muscles, such as that incurred by an injection, may elevate the CPK. Isoenzyme determination is useful to differentiate myocardial from skeletal muscle CPK. Other laboratory findings associated with acute myocardial infarction include an elevated white blood count and sedimentation rate. Low-grade fever commonly occurs on the second or third day. Radionuclide imaging is a new technique that is very accurate in the detection of acute myocardial infarction.

MANAGEMENT

In the United States, standard practice for patient management includes hospitalization in a monitored environment for two to three days with a total period of hospitalization averaging two weeks. The cost effectiveness of hospitalization has yet to be evaluated. In 1971, Mather did a controlled study of myocardial infarction in the United Kingdom. Good risk patients were alternately hospitalized or treated at home. There was no significant difference between the two groups of patients, suggesting that some patients with myocardial infarction could be managed at home safely.[29] The older patient who has a supportive family and does not wish to be hospitalized may be appropriately managed at home. Premonitory rhythms are detected and treated. The hospitalization period should be used both to educate the patient about coronary heart disease and to begin a rehabilitation program. Although most geriatric patients do not return to gainful employment following acute myocardial infarction, it is likely that they can return to their usual lifestyles and should be encouraged to do so. A gradually increasing exercise program in the form of regular walks is planned. Treadmill exercise evaluation may be useful in giving a specific exercise prescription to the patient. Other issues, including diet, medication, and sexual activity, are discussed thoroughly with the patient and family. Dietary advice should be tailored to individual needs. A normal diet is appropriate with modification of fat, if lipoprotein abnormalities exist, and with salt restriction, if congestive heart failure is present. The patient, preferably with spouse in attendance, should be given the opportunity to discuss sexual activity and to ask questions prior to hospital discharge. The patient or couple should be informed that sexual relations may begin whenever desired and that

marital sexual intercourse is no more stressful to the heart than brisk walking. Initially, it is probably wise not to discuss precipitation of angina by intercourse but to question the patient during posthospital office visits and to use prophylactic sublingual nitroglycerin prior to intercourse when indicated. In many metropolitan areas, cardiac rehabilitation programs are available at low cost through agencies such as the YMCA.

Peripheral Vascular Disease: Arteriosclerosis Obliterans

Atherosclerosis may involve the larger peripheral arteries. If the carotid or basilar systems are affected, cerebral ischemic events occur. With involvement of the aorta and vessels to the lower extremities, there may be obstruction of the vessel or weakening of the wall leading to the formation of aneurysms. Acute intestinal infarction, a catastrophic event in the older patient, results from obstruction of the mesenteric arteries. Ischemic colitis may occur. Usually this appears as lower gastrointestinal bleeding. Patients with an abdominal aortic aneurysm may be asymptomatic for many years, although aneurysms invariably progress in size. They are identified as an asymptomatic pulsatile mass in the abdomen or with the catastrophic event of rupture. In the latter situation, the patient has severe abdominal pain and profound shock. Arteriosclerosis obliterans of the lower extremities causes gradual obstruction of peripheral vessels. Symptoms relate to the degree of obstruction and the effectiveness of collateral circulation. Femoral and popliteal disease is present in approximately half the patients. Aortoiliac disease is noted in approximately one-fourth of these patients. Involvment of the tibial and popliteal arteries is much less common. The deep femoral artery is usually spared from the process.

SYMPTOMS, SIGNS, AND EVALUATIONS

Many individuals with peripheral vascular disease are asymptomatic and are detected during routine evaluation. Other patients have symptoms of ischemia. The classic presentation is intermittent claudication. This is characterized by onset of cramping pain in the affected extremity in a specific, consistent manner associated with exercise and relieved by rest. Consistency is important as musculoskeletal problems of the leg or thigh can mimic claudication. In this event, however, the cycle of exercise and pain is not consistent. When the process of atherosclerotic obstruction involves the lower abdominal aorta at the bifurcation of the common iliacs, claudication may involve the thighs and hips with the associated symptom of impotence caused by a decreased blood flow to the genitalia.

Arteriosclerotic vascular insufficiency can cause ulceration. Frequently, this occurs over the lateral malleolus or toes, and if untreated, progresses to gangrene. Occasionally, portions of atherosclerotic plaques ulcerate and embolize to the feet. In this instance, patients have very painful discrete hemorrhagic lesions in the toes.

Physical findings of peripheral vascular disease include the presence of diminished pulses in the affected extremity. With ample collateral circulation, there is a delay in the appearance of the pulse due to the circuitous course of blood flow. Occasionally, patients with lesions in the common iliac system have normal, palpable pulses that disappear with exercise. When arterial insufficiency is severe, signs of chronic ischemia are present. These include loss of hair, thickening of the nails, calluses, dependent rubor, and elevational pallor.

Laboratory procedures allow very good noninvasive evaluation of patients with peripheral vascular disease. They are Doppler evaluation, plethysmography, segmental limb pressures, digital temperature and pressures, and stress testing. These examinations, along with ultrasound and arteriography, assess the severity of the lesions and the degree of anatomical involvement. The vascular surgeon should be involved in the decision to proceed with these studies and their interpretation.

MANAGEMENT

Patients with peripheral vascular disease need to be informed about their condition and contributing factors. Many of these people smoke. Their problems worsen significantly if smoking continues. With cessation of smoking, the condition improves and surgical intervention may be avoided. Lipoprotein abnormalities should be detected and dietary and drug therapy instituted as needed. Drugs such as propranolol, a beta blocker, are contraindicated as they will aggravate the condition. Vasodilators increase skin circulation but have little use in the treatment of peripheral vascular insufficiency. Frequently, bypass grafting is the treatment of choice. Long-term patency is achieved with 75 percent of patients. When surgery is performed for intermittent claudication, initial success is in the range of 80–90 percent with mortality rates of 3–4 percent.[30]

Even in patients over 70 with impending limb loss, salvage is achieved in 70 percent initially and over 50 percent in five years. The surgical mortality rate in this age group is 8.3 percent.[31]

Peripheral Vascular Disease: Varicose Veins

Peripheral veins have one-way valves that facilitate venous flow from the periphery into the central circulation. Varicose veins result from incompetence of these valves. As the valves become incompetent, leg veins remain filled with blood at high pressure. This results in thickening of the venous wall and gradual elongation and tortuosity of the peripheral vein. As the blood remains in the vein for prolonged periods, there is an elevation of the pressure in the venous capillary and chronic stasis. This stasis may cause hemorrhages in the tissues and chronic passive congestion that interferes with normal cellular nutrition. Chronic inflammation and occasionally ulceration of the skin, as well as subcutaneous tissue, are late events. Varicose veins tend to be familial and more prevalent in women since there is an observed increase in severity associated with pregnancy.

SYMPTOMS, SIGNS, AND EVALUATIONS

Varicose veins rarely cause pain but are associated with a sense of heaviness in the extremity. If numerous and severe, swelling and hyperpigmentation are present. Many patients' initial complaint is the cosmetic disfigurement, though this is less common among older patients. Physical examination reveals dilated tortuous veins and hyperpigmentation of the ankles. Frequently, there is edema due to the high venous capillary manifested by a thickening of the skin; a papulosquamous weeping eruption or ulceration may be evident. In general, ulcers are located over the medial side of the lower leg.

Varicosities may involve the greater and lesser saphenous systems. The competence of the deep venous systems should be assessed to locate any incompetent perforators, which are connections between the deep and superficial system. To test deep venous competency, a tourniquet is placed at midthigh and the patient asked to exercise. If the deep femoral system is patent and has competent valves, there is a decrease in the engorgement of the varicosities with exercise. Surgical intervention is not indicated in individuals with an incompetent deep venous system. Trendelenberg's test is used to locate incompetent perforators that may be ligated during surgery. With this procedure, the extremity is elevated and a tourniquet is applied at progressively proximal levels. Following such application, the individual is asked to stand. If, in this position, the perforating system at a given level is competent, the varicosity will fill slowly as with peripheral venous filling. If there is an incompetent perforator, however, immediate engorgement of the varicose veins will occur.

Management of mild cases includes patient education about limb elevation. Tailored elastic stockings may be used. Elastic support should extend from the level of the foot to above the level of the varicosity. Patients with severe venous disease and ulceration may use a paste boot to facilitate healing. A paste boot is a cloth bandage impregnated with medications, zinc oxide, and gelatin. It is applied to the affected extremity like a cast, left in place for two to three weeks, and then removed. Surgical management may be appropriate in the geriatric patient with severe symptoms such as stasis ulcer resistant to treatment. Surgery includes meticulous internal and external venous stripping. Ligation of the vessels may be done. Injection with a sclerosing agent, such as sodium morrhuate, has limited applicability and is ineffective in most instances.

Peripheral Vasular Disease: Thrombophlebitis

Although varicose veins predispose individuals to thrombophlebitis, this problem may occur in entirely normal venous systems. Factors such as recent obstetrical delivery, prolonged bedrest with chronic illness, or the postsurgical recovery period predispose patients to this condition. The stress and stasis from low cardiac output and low flow rates increase coagulability and result in the formation of thromboses. The thrombophlebitis is only a transient local discomfort. However, clots located in the peripheral vein may dislodge and move centrally, causing a pulmonary embolus.

SYMPTOMS, SIGNS, AND EVALUATION

Symptoms may be absent or the patient may have a painful, tender extremity with typical signs of inflammation including erythema, warmth, and tenderness. Careful examination reveals an enlarged calf, a prominent venous pattern, palpable warmth or trace edema over the affected extremity. Studies indicate thrombophlebitis actually exists in less than half the patients with suggestive findings.[32] Noninvasive techniques for evaluation and diagno-

sis include Doppler measures, which reveal change in flow characteristics in the affected limb. Plethysmography or radioactive fibrinogen studies and venograms are more elaborate methods of evaluation.

MANAGEMENT

The patient with thrombophlebitis is at significant risk for developing pulmonary embolism. If the diagnosis is confirmed, a period of anticoagulation for three months is generally necessary. Standard treatment includes administration of heparin, during which the whole blood partial thromboplastin time is maintained at approximately twice normal. Following a week of heparin, anticoagulation therapy is continued with warfarin. Patients and family members should be cautioned not to massage the painful extremity.

Valvular Heart Disease

With older persons, valvular heart disease is the result of a late manifestation of a congenital lesion, a rheumatic condition, or, more commonly, calcification of the aortic and mitral valves. The aortic and mitral valves gradually stiffen with age due to calcium deposition. The prevalence of significant gradients at the aortic valve increases with age. This process also involves the mitral annulus and gradually extends into the substance of the mitral valve, causing mitral stenosis or insufficiency. A common dilemma facing the clinician is the older patient who has nonspecific symptoms such as failure to thrive, weight loss, dyspnea, or fatigue. Examination reveals a murmur that suggests aortic or mitral valvular disease of uncertain significance. The hemodynamic significance of this finding must be evaluated in view of the patient's symptoms. Aortic stenosis is the most commonly missed significant valvular lesion after the age of 50.[33]

SYMPTOMS, SIGNS, AND EVALUATIONS

The patient may have typical cardiac symptoms relating to the underlying valvular lesion. These are dyspnea, palpitations, and those of congestive heart failure. If the underlying lesions involve the aortic valve, the patient may have angina or syncope. If the mitral valve is affected, atrial fibrillation, congestive heart failure, or embolic complications are more common.

The physical examination is helpful in locating the lesion and assessing its severity. With involvement of the aortic valve, the murmurs of aortic stenosis and insufficiency may be evident. The murmur of aortic stenosis is an ejection type and midsystolic. It has a crescendo–decrescendo characteristic and is most prominent at the base of the upper chest, radiating to both carotids. In older patients, the murmur may be heard well at the cardiac apex and confused with mitral insufficiency. Clues that suggest the lesion is severe include a soft or absent aortic second sound, the presence of a third or fourth heart sound, and peripheral pulse abnormalities (a slow-rising sustained pulse). The murmur of aortic insufficiency is a diastolic murmur that is in most cases best heard along the lower left sternal border and has a decrescendo characteristic. In the older patient with increased anteroposterior chest diameter, the murmur may be best heard in the neck or at the apex. The severity of aortic insufficiency is assessed by the extent of the pulse pressure and diastolic blood pressure. Patients with serious aortic lesions have a high pulse pressure which frequently exceeds 100 mg Hg and a low diastolic pressure of less than 50 mg Hg. To a lesser degree, these blood pressure changes also occur as a result of the aging process and decreased compliance of the central aortic vascular tree.

Mitral valve disease usually takes the form of mitral insufficiency. The murmur of mitral insufficiency is holosystolic and heard best at the cardiac apex and radiating toward the axilla. It is more difficult to assess the severity of the valvular damage since murmurs of mitral insufficiency occur as a result of congestive heart failure or cardiac dilation. In the latter situation, the intensity of the murmur decreases significantly as the patient improves. A vigorous apex impulse and hyperkinetic circulation, manifested by a quick rising, brief pulse, suggest the lesion is in the valve rather than due to a failing myocardium. Left ventricular hypertrophy without systemic hypertension or persistent left atrial enlargement on the electrocardiogram suggests a significant valvular lesion. The echocardiogram is of further help in both mitral stenosis and insufficiency. This permits visualization of valve and myocardial movement and chamber size.

MANAGEMENT

If there is a question about the significance of the lesion, cardiology consultation should be obtained. Valve replacement is a procedure of low risk and good results if patient selection is judicious. This decision should be made in the context of the patient's total life situation and considered carefully with the patient and family. Further evaluation may not be appropriate in a person whose limited life expectancy is due to another disease. Furthermore, valvular heart disease, which is hemodynamically significant, improves with standard medical management. Noninvasive studies and cardiac catheterization may be indicated if the patient seems a possible surgical candidate. Additional approaches used to control symptoms include digitalis, diuretics, vasodilators for congestive heart failure, and nitrites for angina. Propranolol is not appropriate in the management of angina associated with aortic valvular lesions. It is not unusual to find an older patient who is a surgical candidate and can tolerate valve replacement with a satisfying, relatively asymptomatic life thereafter.

HEALTH MAINTENANCE

Risk assessment for the development of cardiovascular disease in older patients differs from that in younger people. Cigarette smoking and serum cholesterol, highly correlated with cardiovascular risk in younger patients, lose their reliability after the age of 65. However, hypertension, obesity, diabetes, and hypertriglyceridemia all continue to correlate individually with risk in older patients. The issue of sedentary lifestyle as a risk factor remains uncertain. Evidence in the Framingham study does suggest that more active older patients are at less risk for coronary heart disease.[13] If it were possible to eliminate cardiovascular disease after the age of 65, five years would be added to the lifespan. Rheumatic heart disease, which is established much earlier, and ill-defined "senile" heart disease account for only a small percent of diagnoses in older persons. The most frequent etiology for heart disease in the elderly is *coronary disease*. Preventive techniques may modify this disease process. A considerable question exists about the reversibility of atherosclerotic lesions, especially in geriatric patients. Most studies reveal no regression of atherosclerosis in spite of aggressive treatment.[34] In one study of older patients housed in a veteran's domiciliary, investigators compared effects of a prudent diet high in polyunsaturates with a standard American diet high in saturated fats. Fewer cardiovascular events occurred in the treated group.[35] However, to recommend diets high in polyunsaturated fats for all older patients is probably not warranted. Risk of increased incidence of cancer[36] and a theoretical risk of central nervous system damage[37] from free radicals associated with polyunsaturates have been suggested. General nutrition is commonly a problem in older patients. Some older individuals develop detrimental dietary habits in an effort to avoid foods high in cholesterol and saturated fats. Specific nutritional advice should be given to optimize weight and to address the special dietary needs of patients with lipoprotein abnormalities. Overzealous instruction, however, may have adverse effects by contributing to nutritional inadequacies.

Despite the lack of a demonstrated relationship between smoking and cardiovascular risk in older patients, it is important to recommend cessation of smoking because of associated risk of bronchogenic carcinoma, peripheral vascular disease, and chronic lung disease. Low-cost behavior modification programs with high degrees of success in cessation of smoking are available in many communities through local heart associations, cancer societies, and religious organizations.

Regular exercise is an important part of health maintenance. Most older patients tolerate brisk walking. In the person with degenerative joint disease of the lower extremities, swimming offers a good alternative.

The most effective approach in the prevention of disease is adequate control of hypertension. Finally, working with motivated persons to develop better ways to manage and reduce emotional stress in their lives is an important therapeutic goal in furthering health and well-being.

It cannot be overemphasized that elders need screening for cardiovascular disease. Those at risk and with disease need a closer follow-up with an individualized health maintenance program. Further ideas and guidelines can be found in Chapter 20.

REFERENCES

1. Reichel W (ed): The Geriatric Patient. New York, New York Hospital Practice Publishing Company, Inc, 1978

2. Anderson SF: Practical Management of the Elderly. Blackwell Scientific Publications, Ltd, 1976, p 128

3. Pomerance A: Pathology of the heart with and without cardiac failure in the aged. Bri Heart J 27:697–71, 1965

4. Stamler J, Stamler R, Wallace F, et al: Hypertensive screening of one million Americans, community hypertension evaluation clinic program. JAMA 235:2299–2306, 1977

5. Veterans Administration Group on Antihypertensive Agents: Effects of treatment on morbidity in hypertension: Results in patients with blood pressure averaging 115 through 129 mm Hg. JAMA 202:1028–1034, 1967

6. Koch-Weser J: Treatment of hypertension in the elderly, in Crooks J, Stevenson IH (eds): Drugs and the Elderly. London, Macmillian, 1979, pp 247–262

7. Tarazi RC, Gifford RW Jr: Clinical significance and management of systolic hypertension, in Onesti G, Brest AN (eds): Hypertension Mechanisms, Diagnosis, and Treatment. Philadelphia, FA Davis, 1978, pp 23–30

8. Koch-Weser J: The therapeutic challenge of systolic hypertension. N Engl J Med 289:481–483, 1973

9. Smith W: Hypertension: Who should be treated? Med Times 106:52–55, 1978

10. Gifford R: Evaluation of the hypertensive patient. Chest 64:336–340, 1973

11. Jackson G, Pierscianowski T, Mahon W, et al: Inappropriate antihypertensive therapy in the elderly. Lancet 2:1317–1320, 1976

12. Taguchi J, Freis E: Partial reduction of blood pressure and prevention of complications in hypertension. N Engl J Med 291:329–331, 1974

13. Kannel W, Gordan T: Evaluation of cardiovascular risk in the elderly: The framingham study. Bull NY Acad Med 54:573–01, 1978

14. Reisin E, Abel R, Modan M et al: Effect of weight loss without salt restriction on the reduction of blood pressure in overweight hypertensive patients. N Engl J Med 298:1–6, 1978

15. Benson H: Systemic hypertension and the relaxation response. N Engl J Med 296:1152–1156, 1977

16. Bruce R, Fisher L, Cooper M, et al: Separation of effects of cardiovascular disease and age on ventricular function with maximal exercise. Am J Cardiol 34:757–762, 1974

17. Logue R, Hurst J: Errors in the recognition and treatment of heart Dis Cir 10:920, 1954

18. Olesen K, Sigurd B: The supraadditive effect of the addition of quinethazone or bendroflumethiazide during long-term treatment with furosemide and spironalactone. Acta Med Scand 190:233–239, 1971

19. Mehta J: Vasodilators in the Treatment of Heart Failure. JAMA 288:2534–2536, 1977

20. Vaida P, Rhosley P, Rao D, et al: Tachyarrhythmias in old age. J Am Geriatr Soc 24:412–414, 1976

21. Rubenstein J, Shulman C, Yurchak P, et al: Clinical spectrum of the sick sinus syndrome. Circul 46:5–13, 1972

22. Rasmussen K: Chronic sinoatrial block. Am Heart J 81:38–47, 1971

23. Zakuaddin V, Miller R, McMillin D, et al: Effects of digitalis on sinus modal function in patients with sick sinus syndrome. Am J Cardiol 41:318–323, 1978

24. Furman S, Whitman R: Cardiac pacing and pacemakers, IX: Statistical analysis of pacemaker data. Am Heart J 95:115–125, 1978

25. Vera Z, Mason D, Hilliard G: Complications of cardiac pacemakers: Diagnosis and management. Geriatr 30:38–43, 1975

26. Dorney E: How to evaluate the implanted pacemaker. Med Times 107:36–39, 1979

27. Mundith E, Austen W: Surgical measures for coronary heart disease. N Engl J Med 298:13–19, 75–79, 1975

28. Takaro T, Hultgren H, Lipton M, et al: The VA cooperative randomized study of surgery for coronary arterial occulsive disease, I: Subgroup with significant left main lesions. Circul 54(suppl):111:111, 107–117, 1976

29. Mather HG, Pearson NG, Read KL, et al: Acute myocardial infarction: Home and hospital treatment. Bri Med J 3:334–338, 1971

30. Barker W, Crawford E, Mannick J, et al: The current status of femoropoplitial bypass for arteriosclerotic occlusive disease. Surg 79:30–36, 1976

31. Reickle, F, Rankin K, Tyson R, et al: The elderly patient with severe arterial insufficiency of the lower extremity: Limb salvage by femoral popliffal reconstruction. Circul 61:24–26, 1979

32. Barnes R, Wu K, Hoak J: Fallibility of the clinical diagnosis of venous thrombosis. JAMA 234:605–607, 1975

33. Lewis K: Heart disease in the elderly. Hosp Prac 99:106, 1976

34. Blankenhorn D: Studies on regression/progression of atherosclerosis in man. Adv Exp Med Biol 82:453–458, 1977

35. Dayton S, Pearce M: Prevention of coronary heart disease and other complications of atherosclerosis by modified diet. Am J Med 46:751–762, 1969

36. Mann G: Diet-heart: End of an era. N Engl J Med 297:644–650, 1977

37. Harman D, Hendricks S, Edd D, et al: Free radical theory of Aging: Effect of dietary fat on central nervous system function. J Am Geriat Soc 24:301–307, 1976

RECOMMENDED RESOURCES

Mead WF: The aging heart. Am Fam Physician 18:73–80, 1978

Wallace DE, Watanabe AS: Drug effects in geriatric patients. Drug Intell Clin Pharm 11:597–603, 1977

12

Genitourinary System

Leona Judson, F.N.P., M.H.S.
Thomas Novotny, M.D.
Jack McAninch, M.D.
Joseph C. Scott, Jr., M.D.

The genitourinary system is the site for significant pathology in the elderly. Incontinence especially can greatly hamper the lifestyles of the elderly and their families. Because of the potentially embarrassing nature of genital problems and the time involved in undressing the patient for adequate examination in a crowded and busy office, genitourinary problems are frequently overlooked by both the patient and the health provider.

An appreciation of the normal aging process as it is manifested in the genitourinary tract will help the clinician to deal with some of the common health problems that arise in the elderly.

The Kidneys

There is a gradual loss of functional nephrons. The nephrons become atrophic and are not replaced; the remaining nephrons compensate to a certain degree by becoming enlarged. It is estimated that by the time a person is 85 years of age, there is a 30–40 percent decrease of nephrons. Due to this gradual loss of nephrons, there is a corresponding loss of kidney function. The glomerular filtration rate decreases on the average of 46 percent between the ages of 20 and 90.[1]

The Bladder

Brocklehurst has done much to contribute to present day understanding of the aging bladder.[2] There is an increased incidence of uninhibited bladder contractions, frequently secondary to generalized cerebral changes consistent with arteriosclerosis. Such contractions lead to decreased bladder capacity. Residual urine also increases. In men, bladder diverticuli are fairly common, probably secondary to bladder outlet obstruction, which in turn causes increased intravesical pressure with resultant bladder wall hypertrophy and trabeculation. In women, there is funneling of the bladder neck, probably secondary to relaxation of the pelvic floor. Both subjective and objective findings in bladder function are summarized in Table 12-1.

The Prostate

This gland functions as a supplier of the main seminal fluid vehicle. All men have some hypertrophy occurring beyond the age of 40, 30 percent of which is palpable on rectal exam. This glandular hypertrophy is normally smooth and is the result of stromal hyperplasia and atrophy of the smooth muscle fibers in surrounding adenomatous tissue. These changes occur in a patchy, irregular way with some areas of the gland remaining unaffected. There is also a loss of bacteriocidal secretions from the prostate, a factor which seems to contribute to the increased incidence of bladder infection in men.[3]

INCIDENCE OF GENITOURINARY PROBLEMS IN THE ELDERLY

The primary disability of the genitourinary system in the elderly focuses on incontinence and its associated causes. Urinary incontinence is probably

Table 12-1
A Comparison of the Normal Range of
Cystometrographic Findings in Old Age and Younger
Adults

	Old Age	Younger Adults
Residual urine	0–100 ml	None
Bladder capacity	250 ml+	500–600 ml
Onset of desire to micturate	Late onset— often at limit of capacity	At about half bladder capacity
Presence of uninhibited bladder contractions	Frequently present	Not present

Reprinted from Brocklehurst J: The urinary tract, in Rossman I (ed): Clinical Geriatrics. Philadelphia, JB Lippincott Co, 1971, p 221. By permission.

a major reason for admission of the elderly to nursing homes. It has been estimated that approximately 38 percent of all elderly hospitalized patients are regularly incontinent. Of nonhospitalized individuals, only 3–7 percent are regularly incontinent. The biggest variable in maintaining continence seems to be mental alertness.[4]

Cancer of the urinary tract takes its toll, with cancer of the prostate and bladder being among the most common in men over 50 years.

The incidence of urinary tract infection (UTI) also increases with age. In women, the incidence is fairly stable until the age of 65, when there is an accelerated rate of increase to approximately 23 percent of all women over 65. In men, the incidence of urinary tract infection is less than half that of women, but rapidly increases after the age of 70 to about the same level as for women. The incidence of UTI in both men and women is even higher in the institutionalized setting.[4]

Common Lab Values

The most commonly employed diagnostic tool of the urinary tract, urinalysis, is not markedly different in the elderly as compared with the general population. There is a moderate decrease in the ability to concentrate urine. A representative maximum specific gravity in youth of 1.032 drops to approximately 1.024 by the age of 80.[1] The BUN rises with age. By the age of 80, 65 percent of individuals will have a BUN greater than 20 (normal range is 10–20). Serum creatinine remains stable. It should be noted, however, that there is a reduction

in muscle mass with resultant decrease in creatinine production. Therefore, the serum creatinine may not rise in proportion to the fall in renal function. Creatinine clearance is probably a better indicator of renal function in the elderly.

As noted in Table 12-1, there is an increase in urinary residual and a decrease in bladder capacity. The patient who presents with specific urological complaints may need more definitive workup and/or referral. A brief description of some commonly used diagnostic procedures follows.[5]

THE RESIDUAL URINE

This is a catherterized specimen collected after the patient has urinated completely. Any quantity greater than 50 cc is considered significant.

THE THREE-GLASS URINE

This is most useful in males to localize the site of infection or hematuria. The patient voids up to 15 cc in the first container and a suitably larger quantity in two subsequent containers. The first glass contains urethral washings, the second glass from the area above the bladder neck, and the third glass is obtained after prostatic massage to obtain a culture in suspected cases of prostatitis.

UROFLOWMETRY

This is useful in the workup of obstruction. In this study, a male patient may simply be observed urinating. His maximal urinary flow rate can be obtained by timing a measured quantity of urine production. Ten cc/second is considered borderline for a diminished flow rate. An average flow rate may be obtained by timing a 300 cc specimen; the average flow rate is approximately 16–17 cc/second. (See Fig. 12-1.)

THE CYSTOMETROGRAM

This evaluates bladder detrusor function. It is most helpful in assessing patients with suspected stress incontinence to rule out uninhibited, neurogenic bladder. Cystometrograms are often performed in the urologist's office or in association with voiding cystourethrograms. (See Fig. 12-2.)

RADIOLOGIC STUDIES

These start with the intravenous pyelogram (IVP) and, with the addition of nephrotomography, help to outline renal lesions such as cysts and carcinomas. The urethropelvic angle in females may be observed radiologically by inserting a chain into the urethra

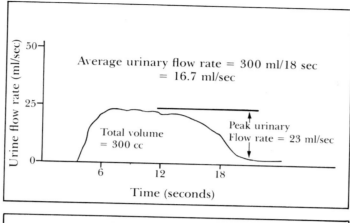

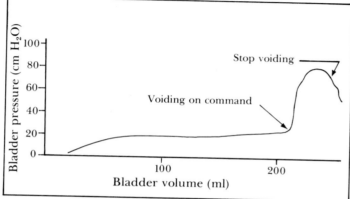

Fig. 12-1. (top) Uroflowmetry, showing total volume and peak urinary flow rate. Average urinary flow rate is determined by dividing the total voided volume by the total duration of micturition.

Fig. 12-2 (bottom). Normal cystometrogram. The primary purpose of cystometry is to determine the presence or absence of the detrusor reflex and whether such reflex is voluntary or uninhibited.

[Both figures reprinted from Pearson RM, Noe HN: Why urodynamic studies are important in urologic problems of the elderly. Geriatrics 34:43–53, 1979. By permission.]

and obtaining a lateral film, both with and without the valsalva maneuver. This study is useful in evaluating women with stress incontinence. The post-void residual film will help to determine the presence of residual urine. One might also consider the use of a retrograde urethrogram to evaluate the male urethra for strictures or prostate enlargement.

ULTRASONOGRAPHY

Diagnostic ultrasound has emerged as a useful tool in assessing abdominal masses as well as renal contours. Mass lesions or cystic lesions may be delineated with considerable accuracy.

SUPRAPUBIC ASPIRATION

When clean catch midstream urines are difficult to obtain, this is a safe procedure that may be performed in the office to obtain urine for analysis and culture in suspected cases of chronic cystitis in the elderly. The abdomen midline above the symphysis pubis is prepped with povidone-iodine, and a 10 cc syringe with a 22 gauge needle is used to obtain urine by inserting the needle 1½ to 2 finger breadths above the symphysis pubis. The depth of the needle's insertion is gauged by the thickness of the subcutaneous tissue. The needle is pointed slightly caudad. The procedure is most productive when there is a full bladder.

Emergencies

Genitourinary emergencies in an elderly population will primarily be related to urinary obstruction and sepsis secondary to urinary infection. When one considers both that indwelling catheters will, if left in place for as short as 72 hours, cause bacteriuria in 100 percent of cases and the fact that there is significant asymptomatic bacteriuria present in the elderly, the frequency of sepsis is understandable.[6,7,8] Because of a rather fragile host response to infection, which has become bloodborn, an elderly patient with a positive urine specimen, a fever, confusion, and possibly even hypotension due to impending endotoxin shock, should be treated vigorously. The initial workup would include blood cultures drawn at three separate time intervals, CBC, catheterized urine culture, the establishment of IV fluids, and the initiation of broad-spectrum antibiotic coverage. Ampicillin or a cephalosporin plus an aminoglycoside such as Gentamicin would be adequate coverage for the usual and unusual gram negative organisms in the urinary tract. This double-drug coverage could be reduced as sensitivities become available.[9]

Urinary obstruction is another common urologic emergency in the elderly, particularly in men. Palpation of the abdomen will reveal a possibly tender, distended bladder that may extend to the umbilicus in severe cases. To prevent hydronephrosis, further bladder decompensation, as well as infection due to stasis, it is essential to drain the bladder utilizing an indwelling catheter. Initially, a soft rubber catheter, with the larger bore being more effective, may be attempted, but often a Coudé catheter, which is more rigid and curved, will be needed to bypass prostatic obstruction. Insertion of this catheter could provoke significant bleeding and should not be performed by untrained personnel. Concomitantly, 15 cc of KY jelly is injected through an irrigating syringe into the meatis, thus serving to lubricate and dilate the urethra. The catheter is inserted through the extended penis and curved around the obstruction. Catheter guides, stylets, or filiforms and followers should never be used due to the possibility of trauma to the urethra. If urethral catheters fail, a suprapubic cystostomy may be performed utilizing commercially available kits such as the Bonano catheter.

One must recognize the entity of postobstructive diuresis in catheterizing the chronically obstructed patient. This may lead to severe water and electrolyte imbalance; with successful catheterization of the bladder, special attention must be given to IV replacement of fluid and electrolytes. There is no benefit to be gained by clamping the catheter after drainage of the bladder is underway.

DIAGNOSIS AND TREATMENT OF COMMON PROBLEMS

Urinary Tract Infection

Urinary tract infection is a common problem in primary care settings, and there is an increased incidence of infection with advancing age. Many reasons have been postulated for the increased incidence of UTI in the elderly. None have been proved. Factors that have been implicated in this increased incidence have to do with changes that occur in the aging bladder. In men, there seems to be a loss of bactericidal secretions from the prostate, with a resultant decrease in natural defenses. Residual urine is frequently present, though its importance in urinary infections has been questioned. Bladder ischemia, in combination with anatomical functional outflow obstruction, has also been suggested as a factor in the development of UTIs by Brocklehurst.[4] Increasing immobilization, poor nutrition, and general frailty also seem to play their roles.

The consequences of urinary tract infections need to be viewed in light of whether the patient has a chronic, stable, or acute UTI. If the patient presents with sudden onset of confusion, rapidly rising BUN, fever, or classical symptoms of UTIs such as dysuria, frequency, incontinence, and urgency, then urinary infection should definitely be worked up and treated appropriately. Many elderly individuals may have chronic asymptomatic bacteriuria. If this is not causing distressing symptoms or contributing to incontinence, it is debatable whether antibiotic treatment is indicated. There is no proven association between chronic bacteriuria and deteriorating renal function.[10]

If a UTI is suspected based on a screening urinalysis, then the patient should be closely questioned regarding symptoms and a repeat clean-catch urinalysis and culture done. If culture results grow out less than 100,000 colonies/cc, or more than one organism, then contamination should be suspected and the patient should be recultured. Simple and economic dip-slide office culture kits are available that will lower the cost of such screening and correlate well with standard methods of culturing. It is often difficult, however, to obtain an adequate clean-catch specimen in the elderly. If infirmity precludes patient cooperation, then an attempt should be made to obtain a clean-catch specimen with the patient in the lithotomy position and with an assistant to cleanse the urethra. This, too, may prove difficult, for many patients and catheterization, either urethral or suprapubic, will need to be performed.

Generally, 100,000 colonies/cc on an office culture of a single organism indicates urinary tract infection, even in the asymptomatic patient. In 30 percent of individuals, less than 100,000 colonies of a single organism may represent a urinary infection if they are very carefully collected specimens such as a suprapubic aspirant. In these situations, a trial of antibiotics is indicated to assess the effects of urinary tract infection on the patient's general health. It is to be emphasized, however, that ambulatory geriatric patients will respond better than bedridden patients to infection control because of, for example, the improve bladder emptying while standing.

A follow-up visit with the treated patient to ascertain the subjective effect of treatment, such as improvement in incontinence, and to reculture the urine is indicated. Any contributing factors to the development of UTI should also be evaluated at this time (such as chronic urinary obstruction), particularly in men. The health provider should look for ways to improve the patient's general well-being, particularly to find ways of increasing fluid intake and general nutrition. Working with other family members to make them aware of the importance of these factors will also be helpful in controlling chronic UTI and related problems.

Incontinence

Urinary incontinence is a distressing symptom for both the elderly and their families. Incontinence contributes to physical and social isolation of the elderly and, uncontrolled, will usually lead to admission to extended care facilities. The health provider has a unique opportunity to assist in maintaining the quality of life of the individual and his or her family and even in preventing expensive hospitalization by investigating and managing this common and bothersome problem of urinary incontinence.

Understanding the physiology of micturition will help the clinician to sort out the factors contributing to incontinence. In normal micturition, there are stretch receptors in the bladder wall that stimulate the bladder center in the posterior sacral segments. This creates a reflex arc and is the sole voiding mechanism in infants and paraplegics. As children develop, afferent pathways from the sacral center to the brain are established, thus bringing awareness into the act of micturition and ultimately, conscious inhibition of the sacral reflex arc.[11] See Fig. 12-3.

The main predisposing factor in the development of incontinence in elderly is the presence of varying degrees of an uninhibited neurogenic bladder. Loss of neurons and deterioration in global cerebral function results in a faulty inhibition of the sacral

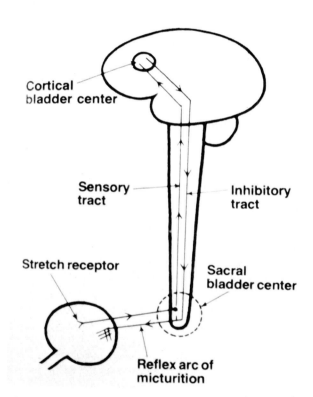

Fig. 12-3. Nervous pathways servicing micturition showing the sacral reflex arc of micturition and the micturition center in the frontal cortex, which exerts an inhibitory effect over the reflex arc. [Reprinted from Brocklehurst JC: Differential diagnosis of urinary incontinence. Geriatrics 33:36–39, 1978. By permission.]

reflex arc. Subjectively, the individual may recognize the need to void but may be too late to inhibit contractions effectively, and thus urinary precipitancy results. This type of bladder is frequently present in people who have had a stroke or have mental confusion, significant cerebral vascular insufficiency, or even frontal lobe tumor.[11]

Another less common type of neurogenic bladder is the atonic bladder. Here, there is loss of afferent fibers at the level of the posterior sacral segment. The individual is totally unaware of bladder filling, resulting in overdistension of the bladder and overflow. Such lesions are present in tabes dorsalis and, to a lesser extent, diabetes mellitus. Cystometry shows a large residual urine, no desire to void during filling, and spontaneous, ineffective bladder contraction.[12]

OTHER FACTORS CONTRIBUTING TO INCONTINENCE

There are other factors that may contribute to incontinence, the main one being alteration of the individual's life situation, such as confinement to bed or a transient confusional state. Such a change will upset a delicate balance the individual has been able to maintain and provoke incontinence in an unstable bladder. Also, such localized changes as atrophic vaginitis, trigonitis, or urethritis may cause some degree of urinary precipitancy. Bladder outlet obstruction leading to retention overflow needs to be considered in the etiology of incontinence. Fecal impaction or prostatic hypertrophy may be likely causes of this entity. Stress incontinence is usually the result of pelvic relaxation in women and may be amenable to surgical repair.

With a basic understanding of the altered physiology of the aging bladder and its relationship to incontinence, a logical approach to investigating and managing the problem of incontinence in the elderly can begin. If a patient complains of intermittent incontinence, or if this is brought to the attention of the health provider through a family member, as is frequently the case, then an appropriate data base is outlined. See Table 12-2.

A stepwise approach to management of incontinence is first the treatment of contributing causes such as UTI, atrophic vaginitis, and underlying obstruction leading to overflow. If there is a significant degree of pelvic relaxation, a trial of Kegel's exercises to strengthen the pelvic floor may be tried. Specifically, the patient should be instructed to con-

tract her perineal and rectal muscles to the point of stopping the urine stream up to 100 times, three or four times a day. In comtemplating surgery to correct stress incontinence, the examiner will place two fingers, one along each side of the urethra, to simulate reestablishment of the anterior vaginal support as would be accomplished by an anterior repair. Have the patient cough and observe for urine leakage. If there is no incontinence with this maneuver, the patient may be a good candidate for surgery.

Drug therapy may also be considered. This is aimed mainly at controlling the uninhibited bladder spasms with the use of anticholinergics. Anticholinergic drugs affect many body systems and are not specifically for bladder wall muscle. Contraindications for the use of such drugs are the prior presence of glaucoma, urinary obstruction, and severe congestive heart failure. Frequent side effects of most drugs in this category include dry mouth, blurred vision, tachycardia, and constipation. Commonly used drugs are: propantheline (Pro-Banthine), flavoxate (Urispas), hyoscyamine sulphate (Cystospaz), or oxybutynin chloride (Ditropan). Generally, it is wise to start out with the lowest dose. Gradually increase the dosage over several days, looking for undesirable side effects and/or therapeutic response. If there is no significant improvement in the incontinence in a three-to-four-week trial, then the drug should be discontinued. If incontinence only occurs at specific times (i.e., only at night) then the drug can be administered at bedtime only.[2]

Transient incontinence, which frequently occurs with enforced bedrest or acute illness, needs no specific treatment other than assisting the patient back to the accustomed living situation as quickly as possible. Altering the environment of the elderly to facilitate safe toileting may be all that is needed to prevent occasional incontinence. Such measures include the use of a bedside commode, night light, administration of a diuretic drug earlier than at bedtime, etc. Here, family members or a home visit by a public health nurse or social worker may be helpful in evaluating what simple alterations might be useful for a given patient and in working with family members to deal with the incontinent individual.

A program of bladder retraining can be instituted if incontinence persists or if the patient has episodes of forgetfulness and confusion.

Table 12-2
Data Base for Evaluation of Incontinence

Subjective	Objective

1. Degree of incontinence, i.e. nocturnal, situational, chronic, stress, etc.
 	
2. Urinary system review—dysuria, stress incontinence, hesitancy, nocturia, etc.
 	
3. Neurologic/mental status system review—are there localizing signs suggesting a stroke, frontal lobe tumor, etc.
 	
4. Presence of related illnesses—diabetes mellitus, cerebrovascular insufficiency, dementia
 	
5. Drug history—drugs contributing to urinary retention/frequency are anticholinergics, antidepressants, hypnotics, etc.
	1. Physical examination to include the following:
	  a. Mental status evaluation
	  b. Neurologic exam
	  c. Rectal exam—R/O fecal impaction, prostatic enlargement
	  d. Pelvic exam in women—R/O atrophic changes, pelvic relaxation
	  e. Clean-catch urinalysis and culture—R/O UTI
	  f. Serum creatinine and BUN or creatinine clearance if renal failure suspected (likely if significant obstruction present)
	  g. Fasting blood sample if diabetes mellitus suspected
	  h. Acid phosphotase in men if urinary obstruction suspected or prostate enlarged
	  i. Special studies: Cystometric studies—if surgery for stress incontinence contemplated or if there is question as to type of neurogenic bladder present

Bladder Retraining

A program of bladder retraining should be preceded by a careful record of the incontinence pattern in a 24-hour period for as many days as it takes to determine a pattern, if any. The patient should be checked every two hours and notation made whether he or she is dry or wet and what prior activity the patient was engaged in (e.g., sleeping, walking, etc.). Next, this record can be reviewed for any obvious patterns. For instance, if the patient is always incontinent at 8:00 a.m. but dry the rest of the time, then simply awakening the patient at 7:00 a.m. and offering the commode may be all that is necessary. Otherwise, regularly scheduled toileting needs to be arranged, corresponding as closely as possible to the times the patient was found to be incontinent. Next, maintaining adequate fluid intake to at least 2,500 cc/day is crucial. It is wise, however, to restrict fluids after the evening hours. Adequate hydration alone may frequently correct incontinence, since fluid intake helps prevent fecal impaction, dehydration, and resulting confusion, and aids in the treatment of underlying urinary infection.

The use of positive reinforcement when the patient succeeds in maintaining continence may also prove useful in bladder retraining. Offering the patient a cigarette, a favorite snack, or a five-minute uninterrupted visit with a favorite nurse will go towards reinforcing the patient's continent behavior. Such reinforcements should quickly follow the desired behavior and be truly seen as "positive" by the patient.[13]

If the patient seems unable to remain dry for less than two hours at a time, the addition of anticholinergic drugs, as described previously, should be tried.

Only after six weeks of a diligent trial program should any conclusions be drawn as to the success or failure of bladder retraining. If such a program is carried out in an extended care facility, as is frequently the case, the success of such a program will rely on the motivation and good communication with the entire nursing staff. While at first this process may actually increase nursing time, a successful bladder retraining program will ultimately save nursing time and cost. See Table 12-3.

Urinary Retention and Obstruction

In virtually all elderly patients, there is some degree of urinary retention. This may be related to actual obstruction or neurological causes. Almost all men over 40 have prostatic hypertrophy but in only 10 percent is there significant obstruction.[14] In addition, the size of the prostate may not correlate with the degree of obstruction and, therefore, further investigation should be carried out to rule out neurological causes of retention. The differential diagnosis of obstruction is as follows:

1. In females, especially with dementia, fecal impaction may be a common source of lower urinary tract obstruction.
2. Prostatic hypertrophy is the most common cause in males.
3. Atonic neurogenic bladder.
4. Urethral stricture.
5. Drugs contributing to urinary retention.
6. Bladder neck contracture may cause obstruction due to hyperplasia of muscle and fibrous tissue in the bladder neck; this is usually found in men in their 40s and 50s.
7. Prostate cancer with or without hypertrophy.

Complications of urinary obstruction are decompensation of bladder muscle with trabeculation and diverticula formation contributing to large residual urines. There may be progressive disruption of the ureterovesical junction with secondary hydronephrosis, infection, and sepsis.

Obstruction may present as a myriad of symptoms such as incontinence due to overflow, urgency, hesitancy, dribbling, nocturia, diminished size of urinary stream, and even inguinal hernia.

Nocturia is present in 64 percent of elderly men but may be associated more with unstable or inhibited neuropathic bladder, as well as obstruction.[15] The differential diagnosis between retention and obstruction should include an appropriate data base for each possibility, but the residual urine that shows more than 50 cc remaining in the bladder after catherization will be one of the more significant findings in clinical obstruction.

Urethral stricture, a chronic entity, is usually associated with a previous history of venereal disease, instrumentation, and indwelling catheters. One should ask the patient about a diminishing stream size, dysuria, and a sense of incomplete urination. A history of balanitis may point to a problem with distal stricture and obstruction in the uncircumcised male. Objectively, a three-glass urinalysis with uroflowmetry will document urethral obstruction. A rectal and genital examination should be performed as well. Treatment would consist of cystoscopy, if not yet performed, and dilation on a repetitive basis as needed.

Prostatic Hypertrophy

As previously stated, all men above the age of 40 have some degree of prostatic hypertrophy; above the age of 60, foci of adenocarcinoma may develop. Both conditions may or may not lead to obstruction, and it is important to ascertain the degree of disability caused by the obstruction before launching into an intensive urological workup. Up to 8 percent of all elderly male deaths may be prostate-related, but these encompass such complications as pulmonary emboli, sepsis, uremia, and operative complications.[3] A potentially reversible cause of hypertrophy is prostatitis, which is statistically present in 16.3 percent of men in the ninth decade of life. Also, one must remember that in a previously prostectomized patient, there may also be prostatic hypertrophy, since 3–5% of these prostates may regrow. There are no medical modalities to slow or arrest hypertrophy once it has occurred.[14]

Indications for surgery for prostatic hypertrophy include: severe subjective symptoms of obstruc-

Table 12-3
Protocol for Bladder Retraining

1. Careful record of the incontinence every two hours over a 24-hour period
2. Determine a toileting schedule based on the pattern of incontinence
3. Record intake and output
4. Encourage fluids to at least 2,500 cc/day
5. Restrict oral intake between 8:00 P.M. and 6:00 A.M.
6. Provide positive reinforcement when successful in maintaining any incontinence
7. Anticholinergic drugs on a trial basis if the patient has difficulty staying dry between toileting
8. Maintain retraining program for at least six weeks before considering the patient intractable

tion—confirmed with findings of bladder decompensation and prostatic enlargement; diminished renal function; large residual urine; abnormal uroflowmetry; atonic bladder; recurrent urinary tract infection; bladder calculi; and recurrent bleeding. See Table 12-4 for a protocol for hypertrophy.

In counseling patients for surgical treatment, it is important to inform the patient both that the prostatectomy in benign prostatic hypertrophy actually refers to the removal of adenomatous tissue surrounding the prostate and that this does not disturb the enervation of the erectile system. The incidence of impotence postoperatively is as low as 5 percent. In radical perineal prostatecomy, however, even as many as 71 percent of males retain potency, according to Finkle and Priam.[16] The myth of total impotency after prostatectomy is simply untrue. In metastatic disease, antiandrogenic therapy is indicated, meaning estrogens, testosterone antagonists, or orchiectomy. Eighty-five percent of prostate cancers are hormone dependent, and these measures (if withheld until metastases do appear) therefore provide great relief of pain and prolong life. Impotence and lack of sexual interest, however, can be expected in most cases with this treatment. There are both permanent and inflatable prostheses available for selected patients.[17,18]

Catheter Care

The indwelling Foley catheter is both a necessary therapeutic modality and a potential death sentence in the elderly. Much has been discussed as to optimum care of the chronic indwelling catheter, but one must recognize two points in particular: (1) adequate drainage of the bladder is a more important indication for indwelling catheters than is the control of simple incontinence; (2) virtually all bladders become infected after 72 hours of catheterization.

It has been shown that carefully maintained closed-catheter drainage systems can alleviate some bacteriuria. A closed system is one in which (1) the catheter, tubing, and collection bag are treated as an inviolable system from the time of insertion through chronic maintenance; (2) the junctions in the system are not broken either by intermittent irrigation or by the collection of urine specimens; (3) the drainage bag is not allowed to spill urine into the collection tubing of the system above the bag.

In general, unless catheter irrigation is performed

Table 12-4

Protocol Useful in Evaluating Prostatic Hypertrophy

Subjective

Presence of:	1.	Dribbling
	2.	Decreased streams
	3.	Greater than 2 times/nocturia.
	4.	Frequency
	5.	Groin pain
	6.	Bloody urine
	7.	Dysuria
	8.	Bone pain

Objective

1. Rectal exam, Nodular or enlarged prostate
2. Three-glass urine to determine source of hematuria and culture of prostatic secretions
3. Serum creatinine or creatinine clearance
4. Acid phosphatase with prostatic fraction
5. Catheterize for residual urine
6. IVP cystogram and post-voiding film

Assessment

1. Significant obstruction is present if greater than 50 cc residual urine, hydronephrosis, trabeculation and large residual evident on IVP
2. Prostatic nodularity may need biopsy and cystoscopy to R/O carcinoma, as well as hematuria

Plan

1. Transurethral or suprapubic
2. Bone scan if biopsy positive to determine type of therapy
3. Counseling as to catheter care and sexuality

in a continuous fashion, it does not seem to help in preventing bacteriuria, mainly because it disrupts the integrity of the system. In a practical sense, however, some irrigation may be necessary to maintain patency. This would utilize a half percent acetic acid solution or antibiotic solution introduced in a sterile fashion by a specially trained team on a biweekly basis.[19] Homebound debilitated patients may need visiting-nurse attention for such procedures and for the periodic changing of the catheter itself. Silastic catheters, though expensive, are in the long run less traumatic than standard rubber catheters. Their biggest advantage, however, is lack of encrustation, thus requiring less frequent catheter changes. A Silastic catheter may function for two or three months without requiring a change. It is important also to encourage the nursing staff to cleanse the catheter and the urethral meatus twice daily to prevent encrustation and to apply an antibiotic ointment, such as povidone-iodine.[7,8]

Catheter stabilization is important in that the normal anatomic position of the penis is in extension (i.e., cephalad) and the catheter should be taped to the abdomen instead of the leg. There are available abdominal catheter belts that anchor the catheter without urethral stress, and these may be preferable. Some men prefer leg bags that can empty from the bottom without breakage of the closed system, thus allowing ambulation or concealment of the catheter apparatus to avoid social embarrassment. In women, the catheter should be fixed to the leg by tape or velcro belt.

Systemic antimicrobrials have been shown to be beneficial only in the first several days of catheter placement. After this, resistance rapidly develops. Many authors feel that the infections, as long as they are not systemic, should be allowed to remain without costly antibiotic treatment, especially in an elderly patient whose life expectancy may not be longer than one year.[19]

Condom catheters, or Texas catheters, are useful in uninhibited incontinence due to neuropathic bladder. They probably should not be used unless the bladder is at least partially emptying without the extreme of overflow incontinence.

Intermittent catherterization may be suitable for some patients if hospital or family resource personnel are available. Small Robinson catheters or thin glass catheters made by Rausch are commonly employed for patients with atonic neurogenic bladder.

After catheters are removed following prostate surgery, there may be some urgency, which is transitory, and this should be pointed out to the patient.

Suprapubic cystostomy is a good alternative to urethral catheterization, especially in nonoperative candidates with lower urinary obstruction secondary to such causes as stricture, postradiation scarring, and prostatic hypertrophy.

Sexual activity in the catheterized patient is certainly a problem; the only legitimate answer would seem to be temporary removal of the catheter or the use of intermittent catheterization as described above.

Hematuria

Complete urological evaluation is mandatory in an elderly patient with hematuria, even if it is microscopic to the degree of 1 or 2 RBCs per highpowered field on urinalysis. Presence of certain drugs, foods, hemoglobinuria, and myoglobinuria may mimic hematuria. A history of trauma, infection, stones, preexisting renal disease such as glomerulonephritis and polycystic kidney, or blood dyscrasia may help differentiate the pathology involved. An algorithm may be useful in diagnosing urinary causes of hematuria. See Fig. 12-4 (algorithm).

In general, if hematuria is present on repeated samples with negative culture, negative IVP, and possibly even negative exfoliative cytology, the patient should be referred to a urologist for definitive workup. All hematuria, especially painless hematuria, should be considered carcinoma until proven otherwise.

Testicular Masses

Testicular masses in the elderly are less common than in younger males. The most serious ailment presenting as a mass would be lymphoma. Varicoceles are however, a common testicular mass and are usually found on the right. If they are found on the left, one is alerted to the possibility of a left renal carcinoma because of an obstruction producing a lesion on the left side of the scrotum.[20] Hernias and hydroceles may be present and transillumination is helpful in differentiating solid versus cystic lesions. Hydroceles may be aspirated but are definitively treated with surgery; they may be commonly associated with hernia and are repaired through the same incision.

HEALTH MAINTENANCE

Many elderly people, for reasons of inadequate transportation, disability, finances, and embarrassment, do not seek routine health maintenance care and may wait until the symptoms become extreme before seeking medical advice. The 75-year-old man who has noted gross hematuria does ultimately seek help but possibly too late. A routine urinalysis done on a yearly basis might have spotted microscopic hematuria and prompted a workup with subsequent treatment and cure at a much earlier stage of his disease.

Therefore, because of the special problems of the elderly in seeking health care, we would like to advocate the use of a simple health maintenance protocol to aid in the orderly screening of problems. Such a protocol can even be utilized during visits

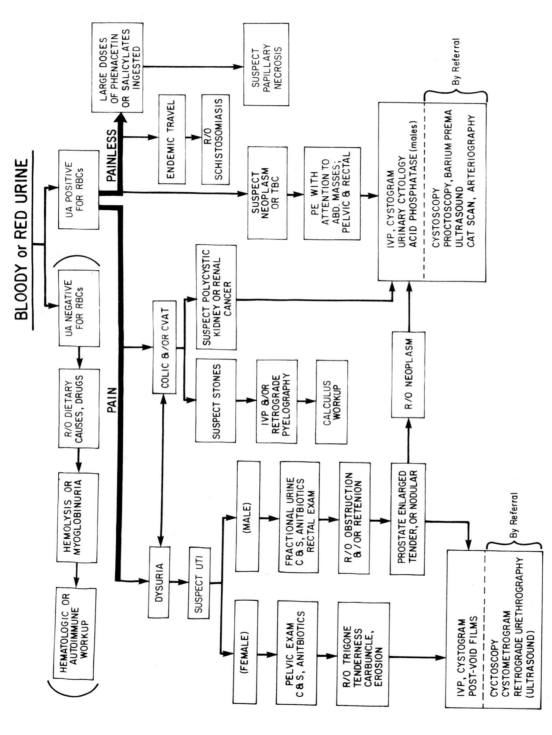

Fig. 12-4. Urinary causes of hematuria (algorithm).

179

unrelated to the genitourinary system. Table 12-5 is a health maintenance guideline that relates to the genitourinary tract.

WOMEN'S HEALTH PROBLEMS

Women beyond child-bearing years will still seek medical attention for a variety of gynecological problems. Many women, because of timidity over the possibly embarrassing nature of their problem or concern over the inevitable pelvic exam, will frequently be reluctant to seek early consultation, let alone preventive health services. The attitude and gentleness of the health provider will have a significant impact on the older patient's decision to return for necessary follow up visits. Specific questioning as outlined in Table 12-5 will aid the clinician in uncovering problems at an earlier stage.

A review of the normal physiological changes occurring in the postmenopausal woman will also help the health practitioner to diagnose and treat common gynecological problems in the older woman.

Most postmenopausal changes have to do with the greatly decreased circulating estrogen produced by the ovaries. As a result, there is an increase in pituitary gonadotrophins. It is theorized that this increased level of gonadotrophins may result in conversion of androgens to estrogens. Peripheral conversion of androstendione to estrogens does occur in the postmenopausal woman. The amount of androgens converted to estrone seems to vary among women. All postmenopausal women, however, seem to experience some degree of estrogen lack, as evidenced by atrophic changes in their reproductive system.[21]

Specifically, in the vagina, one will find decreased rugation, a pink, washed-out looking vaginal mucosa that is dry and even somewhat friable. No longer stimulated by estrogen, glycogen—a major component of the vaginal epithelial cells—is absent. As a result, the pH of the vagina is somewhat higher than in a younger woman, that is, somewhere between 6.5 and 7.5, creating an environment capable of supporting a host of bacteria. These atrophic changes may lead to dyspareunia, and this may be one of the presenting symptoms for the practitioner. The cervix will be markedly involuted in the postmenopausal woman but should be able to be visualized on speculum examination.

The uterus in the postmenopausal woman will be smaller in size than in the premenopausal woman,

and any enlargements may be considered abnormal. As for other pelvic masses, any palpable mass will be considered abnormal because the ovaries involute such that they should not be palpable at all in the geriatric patient.

In the postmenopausal woman, the breasts involute due to the lack of cyclic stimulation of estrogen and progesterone. The alveoli, which are progesterone dependent, disappear and the mammary ducts, which are estrogen dependent, decrease in number. The ducts are filled with connective tissue, and preexisting fibrocystic changes regress almost entirely. In women who are on exogenous estrogen therapy, there may be hypertrophy of the breasts, making examination somewhat difficult.

INCIDENCE OF GYNECOLOGICAL PROBLEMS IN THE ELDERLY

Cancer of the female genital tract increases with age especially after the fourth decade, with cancer of the breast, uterus, and ovary being among the most common.[20]

There are some important age considerations in breast disease, both in the menopausal and postmenopausal woman. In general, benign lesions occur in the premenopausal woman most commonly, and with increasing age there is an increase in malignancy, such that 20 percent of all female cancers in the age group of 75–99 years are breast carcinoma. One out of 13 women can expect to develop breast cancer.[22]

Table 12-6 summarizes the incidence of breast disease found according to age group. Breast cancer is not, however, a random disease, because, as summarized in Table 12-7, there are certain identifiable risk factors to which the physician should direct particular attention.

The perimenopausal woman with hypermenorrhea is at high risk for endometrial carcinoma. This incidence, however, is decreased after the seventh decade. Additional factors, such as delayed menopause past the age of 50, will provide a twofold increase in the incidence of carcinoma of the endometrium. Certainly, prolonged unopposed estrogen stimulation has been well documented to cause changes in the endometrium, which may also lead to carcinoma.[23]

Ovarian and, more rarely, tubal pathology concerns carcinoma, which is the fourth most common

Table 12-5
Health Maintenance Protocol

Subjective	Objective
Men	
1. Have you ever noticed any change in the force of your urine stream?	1. Rectal exam with stool guiac—done yearly
2. Do you have trouble starting and stopping your urine stream?	2. Urinalysis–done yearly
3. Do you have trouble obtaining or maintaining an erection?	3. Acid phosphatase—done yearly if history suggests urinary obstruction or if prostatic enlargement is palpable on exam
	4. Breast exam–done yearly
Women	
1. Do you experience any leakage of urine with coughing or straining?	1. Pelvic exam—done yearly
2. Have you noticed *any* vaginal bleeding since menopause (change of life)?	2. Rectal exam—done yearly, preferably with a stool guiac test
3. Have you experienced pain with sexual intercourse?	3. Urinalysis—done yearly
4. Are you bothered with any vaginal discharge or itching?	4. Pap smear—done every 2–3 years
5. How many times have you been pregnant all together?	5. Breast exam–done yearly
6. How old were you when you completed menopause (change of life)?	
7. Have you ever had a pap smear that is abnormal?	
Men and Women	
1. When you have the urge to urinate, do you have trouble controlling leakage?	
2. Do you experience burning with urination?	
3. How many times do you get up at night to urinate?	
4. Have you ever noticed any dark or bloody urine?	
5. Has decreased urinary control caused you any significant inconvenience?	

cancer death in women in the 65–75-year-old age group. However, 60 percent of these tumors occur in the 40–60 age group, and the remaining 40 percent are equally distributed below and above 60 years of age.[20]

Common Problems

The more common concerns that bring postmenopausal women to seek medical attention are similar to that of younger women. Among these concerns are vulvitis and vaginitis, with problems associated with atrophic changes being especially frequent. Symptoms associated with such common entities are itching, dyspareunia, urinary urgency, stress incontinence, and even vaginal bleeding. Vaginal bleeding is another frequent concern of women, a presentation with many important etiologies needing a careful workup. Practitioners should question the older woman on the occurrence of even minimal vaginal bleeding, for many women may tend to

Table 12-6
Age Periods and Median Age for 5,604 Breast Operations*

Type of Breast Lesion	Age Period (Median Age)
Fibrocystic disease	20–49 years (30)
Fibroadenoma	15–39 years (20)
Intraductal papilloma and duct ectasia	35–55 years (40)
Gynecomastia	Puberty (14) or 50–65 years (55)
Cancer	40–71 years (54, female; 60, male)

*Performed at New York Medical College, Flower and Fifth Avenue Hospitals from 1960–1975.
From Leis HP: Cancer in old age. Ca-A Cancer J Clin 27:209–231, 1977. By permission.

ignore slight bleeding as being insignificant. Breast lumps, which are commonly malignant, are encountered both by the patient as well as by the health provider on routine screening exams.

Less common problems are the vulvar dystrophies and other vulvar lesions. Such conditions cause a great deal of patient discomfort, and although rare, carcinoma of the vulva must be ruled out. Ovarian cancer is unusual but not a rare occurrence. This cancer frequently presents initially as an abdominal

Table 12-7
Patients at High Risk of Breast Cancer

- Women
- Those over 40 years of age
- Patients with a familial history of breast cancer
- Nulliparous women or those with first parity after age 34
- Patients with a previous cancer in one breast
- Those with a precancerous mastopathy type of fibrocystic disease
- Women with an adverse hormonal milieu
- Patients with lowered immunological competence
- Those with excess exposure of the breast to ionizing radiation
- Patients exposed to carcinogens
- Those with other organ cancers, especially the endometrium
- Patients with a high dietary intake of fat
- Patients with chronic psychological stress
- Those living in the western hemisphere or a cold climate, belonging to the upper socioeconomic group and of the white race

From Leis HP: Cancer in old age. Ca-A Cancer J Clin 27: 209–231, 1977. By permission.

mass or with the patient complaint of abdominal enlargement.

DIAGNOSIS AND TREATMENT OF COMMON PROBLEMS

Vulvitis

A common complaint that brings older women to seek medical consultation is pruritis of the vulva, which has many causes. A careful examination of the vulvar area may reveal a monilial infection that can be effectively treated with topical creams such as nystatin. Intertrigo may be present and is a common problem with obese women or those with a significant degree of chronic moisture between skin folds. This can frequently coexist with monilia or tinea cruris. Treatment should be aimed at promoting dryness. Using an astringent compress, such as Burrows solution, and the use of cotton underwear and talcum powder may be helpful. Any externally applied deodorants, ointments, perfumes, or sprays should be avoided. If chronic moisture is caused by incontinence, examining ways to control this would be a logical approach to treatment.

Vulvar Dystrophies

These are characteristic skin changes that involve the vulva and can cause severe pruritis. Most of these lesions have a whitish appearance and may be associated with premalignancy, though this has not been proved. There are basically three different categories of dystrophies, which are outlined in Table 12-8. All three types of vulvar dystrophies can occur in the postmenopausal woman, though lichen sclerosis is probably slightly more common. Figures 12-5 and 6 illustrate the common appearance of these lesions. Biopsy is generally needed to rule out carcinoma in situ as well as to define the type of dystrophy present. Treatment varies with the diagnosis. Lichen sclerosis seems to respond well to the use of topical applications of testosterone cream, usually on a maintenance basis. In resistant cases, alcohol blocks may be used to control the pruritis. In hyperplastic dystrophy, topical corticosteroids are the mainstay in treatment. Frequently, once these lesions clear they may not recur.[24]

Cancer of the vulva cannot be differentiated from the dystrophies. Therefore, it cannot be overem-

Table 12-8

Classification of Vulvar Dystrophies Adopted by the International
Society for the Study of Vulvar Disease

	Clinical	Histologic
Lichen sclerosis	Pruritic, thin, parchment, "atrophic," introital stenosis	Thin, loss of rete, homogenization inflammatory infiltrate
Hyperplastic*	Pruritic, thick, gray or white plaques, skin or mucosa	Acanthosis, hyperkaratosis, inflammatory infiltrate
Mixed*	Areas compatible with both forms may be present at the same time	

*Atypia may accompany hyperplastic dystrophy and is graded mild, moderate, or severe.

Reprinted from Friedrich E: Vulvar Disease. Philadelphia, WB Saunders, 1976, Vol 9. By permission.

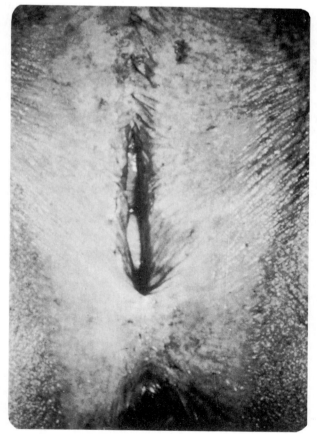

Fig. 12-5. Lichen sclerosis of the vulva. [Reprinted from Woodruff JD: The Vulva, in Famous Teachings in Modern Medicine, New York, Medcom Inc, 1972. By permission.]

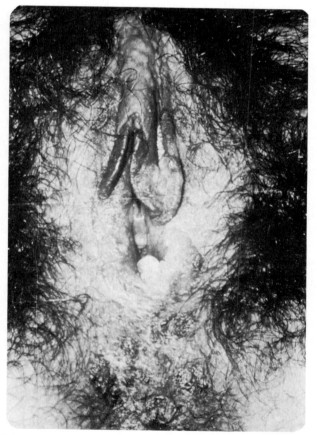

Fig. 12-6. Carcinoma in situ of the vulva. [Reprinted from Woodruff JD: The Vulva, in Famous Teachings in Modern Medicine. New York, Medcom Inc, 1972. By permission.]

phasized that a simple biopsy is critical in making accurate and timely diagnoses. Any suspicious lesion that does not respond to treatment within two to three weeks should be considered for biopsy, a procedure that can easily be performed in the office using a punch biopsy. The 4 or 5 mm size is most useful in vulvar lesions.[24]

Vaginitis

Atrophic vaginitis is the most common complaint associated with the vagina; itching, possibly a pinkish discharge, and dyspareunia are the most common symptoms. The vagina should be inspected for suspicious lesions or ulcerations that may be biopsied under local anesthesia. A KOH prep can be performed to rule out monilial vaginitis that may be present in such illnesses as diabetes mellitus. Trichomonas may be diagnosed with a saline slide examination. Screening culture of the cervix to exclude gonorrhea is also advised. A maturation index may be obtained by using vaginal cytology to assess the state of the estrogen dependent epithelial cells. Treatment of atrophic vaginitis is generally aimed at reestablishing the estrogen-primed environment with the use of vaginal estrogen creams, initially on a nightly basis and then maintained on approximately twice-weekly basis. In addition, a sulfa preparation may be added initially to correct any intercurrent bacterial infection. Vaginal rugation will generally take place in approximately 4–6 weeks following the regular use of topical estrogens. The use of oral estrogens is somewhat controversial but probably is not needed for atrophic vaginitis. It has been shown, however, that there is an absorbed level of estrogen even with the topical preparations.

If dyspareunia is the only presenting symptom, water soluble lubricants during sexual intercourse may be recommended without the use of estrogen creams. Table 12-9 outlines the typical findings and treatment of common types of vaginitis. Other etiologies of vaginitis can also be present in the elderly female.

Abnormal Vaginal Bleeding

Vaginal bleeding is an alarming symptom that has many etiologies, endometrial carcinoma being among the most significant. Other sources of bleeding include leiomyomata, cervicitis, vaginitis, endocervical polyps, ovarian cancer, use of drugs such as digoxin, Coumadin, and, most importantly, estrogen. Even with conjugated equine estrogens, the incidence of cancer of the endometrium is 5–14 times the risk compared to the general population.[23]

In general, a thorough approach must be taken with a woman exhibiting postmenopausal bleeding and should include a fractional D and C; this is the only means of ruling out endometrial carcinoma as the source of bleeding. If bleeding continues, subsequent outpatient endometrial biopsy samples may be obtained on a serial basis.[23]

If a woman is experiencing severe vasomotor menopausal symptoms requiring estrogen therapy, she should be treated for a one-to-two-year period with subsequent gradual withdrawal. Such women should be advised of the increased risk of cancer and monitored with regular office endometrial biopsies.

There have been some recent alterations in the recommendations concerning how estrogen should be administered to the perimenopausal and postmenopausal woman. The changes suggest that the use of progesterone in more physiologic fashion given towards the end of the cycle of estrogen stimulation would provide some benefit both in preventing endometrial cancer by the elimination of "unopposed estrogen" effects, and possibly even in suppressing the tendency towards breast cancer, which is thought to be at least partially hormone-dependent.

Some clinicians currently prefer to give a suitable dose of estrogenic therapy for a 21-day period while starting medroxyprogesterone 10 mg (Provera) bid on day 14, continuing at least through day 21. With this addition of progesterone, a previously proliferative endometrium stimulated by the estrogen is changed into secretory endometrium. Certainly, in the woman who has no uterus or ovaries and is receiving estrogen replacement, one should use the smallest dose that will control the vasomotor problems associated with an estrogen lack. With progesteron therapy, one may inhibit the carcinogenic potential of estrogens even further.[25,26,27]

Ovary

Ovarian tumors often become manifest at a late stage unless a pelvic mass is determined earlier on bimanual exam. Frequently, ascites heralds a widespread lesion that may be diagnosed on paracentesis or culdocentesis by cytologic examination. Any palpable pelvic mass should be referred for evaluation.

Table 12-9
Common Types of Vaginitis

Vaginitis	Character and Discharge	Odor	Vulva Itching Erythema	Vaginial pH	Wet Preparation	KOH	Treatment
Candida albicans	Scant to moderate, curdy white	0	++++	<5	Hyphae, spores, many lacto bacilli	Hyphae, spores	Nystatin supp., clutrimazole
Trichomonas	Watery, yellow-green, frothy	+++	++	5–7	Trichomonads, WBC	Neg	Flagyl-oral
Hemophilus vaginalis	Minimal to moderate, grey, creamy	++++	0–+	5–6	Clue cells, small rods	Neg	Sulfa vaginal cream, ampicillin
Atrophic vaginitis	Scant, thin, yellow, blood tinged	0–+	0–+++	6.5–7.5	RBC, ±WBC, round parabasal epithelium	Neg	Estrogen vaginal cream

One should be suspicious of carcinoma if nodularity is palpated in the cul de sac. A sonogram will help confirm physical findings, and the patient should have a barium enema, IVP, and possibly an upper GI series. With ovarian tumors, irregular or postmenopausal bleeding is occasionally noted and should be worked up with respect to both endometrial and ovarian sources.

Breast

Benign breast disease more frequently occurs in the premenopausal woman. In the postmenopausal woman, the clinician can make a tentative assessment of a breast lump through palpation and review of risk factors. See Table 12-6 for an age-related review of common causes of breast pathology.

Common clinical presentations of fibrocystic disease include bilateral multiple lumps, characterized by some vague pain and a sense of fullness that increases premenstrually. These are usually found in young women, and they may well be cystic, though they do clinically mimic breast cancer. Fibroadenomas are rubbery, well-delineated, nontender lumps found, again, in young women usually in a multiple and bilateral presentation. Intraductual papilloma presents usually with a yellow, pink, or bloody discharge that is unilateral and without associated discreet lumps. Duct ectasia presents also with a discharge that is more sticky in nature, and there may be an associated itching or burning pain in the affected breast. Breast cancer usually presents as a solitary-unilateral–solid-irregular, and a poorly delineated mass that is nonmobile, painless in its early stages, and nontender to palpation. The most common anatomical area affected is the upper outer quadrant. In advanced stages, there may be axillary or superclavicular nodes, retraction of the nipple, bloody discharge, or dimpling.

Subjectively, in breast cancer, women most commonly complain of a lump or mass, and 11 percent of these will be associated with pain. The second most common presentation will be associated with nipple symptoms, that is, discharge, retraction, elevation, etc. The third most common reaction will be skin changes; dimpling, erythema, edema, ulceration, lymphadenopathy. Symptoms of metastasis are signs of advanced disease.

The physical exam should consist of a complete history, physical, and an orderly evaluation of breasts. This should start with inspection, both sitting and supine, both with arms elevated and at the sides. Palpation should begin with the supraclavicular node area, and, while in the sitting position, a bimanual exam of each breast is performed with the patient resting her hands against the clinician's shoulders. The axillary nodes are then palpated for masses with palpation extending into the axilla. A similar procedure is performed on the other side, and, if any lumps are felt, transillumination may be carried out, with cystic masses allowing transillumination but with cancer always presenting as opacity. The nipples are squeezed to produce any discharge, and this discharge may be sent for cytologic examination.

Evaluation of a breast lump in an elderly patient is directed primarily at carcinoma. Even though there have been great advances in the use of xeromammography, most breast masses still need excisional biopsy for definitive diagnosis. In an elderly, otherwise debilitated patient, a needle biopsy may suffice, or a local incision may be all that is required for definitive diagnosis. In a patient reluctant to undergo biopsy, mammography may be performed. In a patient who has had multiple biopsies or who has no lump but does have symptoms of pain and discharge, mammography may be performed to outline preclinical lesions that then should be biopsied. Mammography is not without hazard in terms of x-ray exposure and therefore is not used as a routine screening device. However, in patients over 50 who have multiple risk factors, one may consider mammography a more useful tool in that the benefits will outweigh the risks of radiation exposure.

Therapeutically, breast biopsy may be performed in the office unless there is a strong suspicion of widespread disease. When pathologic diagnosis is made, mastectomy should be considered within the next few days. Currently, there is controversy over what is the best operation for breast cancer. Some physicians will elect for a modified radical mastectomy allowing the pectoral muscle to remain in place; others will opt for a simple mastectomy that has better cosmetic results. The radical mastectomy is more rarely performed today because of the disfiguring consequences of muscle removal. In an elderly patient, a local excision with follow-up radiation may be preferable to a much larger operation. In addition, simple mastectomy and, perhaps even modified radical mastectomies with node dissection, could be performed under local anesthesia if the patient is otherwise a medical risk for major surgery.

Because the fear of disfigurement can be overwhelming, many women may neglect to report breast masses to their health practitioner. It needs to be emphasized, however, that in the early stages of the disease (that is, stage 0 through 2), there may be anywhere from a 38–79 percent 10-year survival if the disease is caught early.[22] Therefore, patients should be encouraged to report any abnormal masses, discharge, or tenderness to their physician as soon as possible.

In the postoperative management of a mastectomy patient, the woman should be made aware of community resources that may include referral for breast constructive surgery, use of external breast prosthesis, or counseling services to assist the wom-

an and her family in dealing with this disfiguring surgery.

In summary, one should remember that breast cancer rises in incidence with increasing age, peaking out at the age of 85.[22] It is a treatable disease with definitive diagnosis usually made on direct tissue sampling, but that diagnosis is often missed because the patient may rely on the physician's yearly examination rather than the monthly self-breast examination. In the elderly, it should not be ignored as a common source of disease since one out of every 13 women will develop breast cancer sometime in her life.

HEALTH MAINTENANCE

Pelvic Exam—Modifications

The pelvic examination should be performed as a routine screening procedure once a year as before, but the pap smear may be deferred to an every two-to-three-year time interval because the incidence of cervical cancer becomes less significant in this age group. Because of the atrophic changes of the vagina with resultant discomfort of a speculum exam, the narrow-bladed Pedersen speculum could be used instead of the wider Graves speculum. If there are arthritic changes in the hips, the patient may be more comfortably examined in the left lateral Sims position. On bimanual examination, one may use a finger in the vagina and a finger in the rectum to assess the pelvic organs adequately, especially if the patient experiences tenderness on a standard two-fingered exam. A gentle examination will be more important in encouraging the patient to return on a regular basis than a vigorous bimanual examination.

A breast examination should be a routine part of the yearly examination as well. The technique for this is outlined in the section about breast disease. In the postmenopausal woman, a regular day should be set up for breast examination by the patient, perhaps on the first of the month or on a numerical day of the patient's birthday. The American Cancer Society publishes numerous pamphlets concerning correct self-examination of the breasts, but the health provider should also emphasize the need to perform the exam properly by a one-to-one instructional effort.

REFERENCES

1. Goldman R: Decline in organ function, ed 1, in Rossman I (ed): Clinical Geriatrics. Philadelphia, Lippincott, 1971

2. Brocklehurst JC: The urinary tract, ed 1, in Rossman I (ed): Clinical Geriatrics. Philadelphia, Lippincott, 1971

3. Basso A: The postate in the elderly male. Hospital Practice 12:117–123, 1977

4. Lye M: Defining and treating urinary infections. Geriatrics 33:71–77, 1978

5. Bennett AH: Current methods for diagnosing urological disease. Geriatrics 29:56–63, 1974

6. Marshall S: Urology in the office. Emer Med 11:143–172, 1979

7. Garibaldi RA, Burke JP, Dickman ML, et al: Factors predisposing to bacteria during indwelling urethral catheterization. N Engl J Med 291:215–219, 1974

8. Edwards L: Troutt PA: Catheter-induced urethral inflammation. J Urol 110:678–681, 1973

9. Kunin CM: Detection, Prevention and Management of Urinary Tract Infection, ed 3. Philadelphia, Lea & Febiger, 1979

10. Brocklehurst JC: Urinary infection: Not all patients need treatment. Mod Geriatr 7:33–36, 1977

11. Cope R: Aging: Its complex management. Hagerstown, Maryland, Harper & Row, 1978

12. Pearson RM, Noe HN: Why urodynamic studies are important in urologic problems of the elderly. Geriatrics 34:43–53, 1979

13. Maney TY: A behavioral therapy approach to bladder retraining. Nurs Clin 11:179–188. 1976

14. Brossman SA: Benign postatic hypertrophy: When should you consider postatectomy for your patient. Geriatrics 34:25–34, 1979

15. Brocklehurst JC: Differential diagnosis of urinary incontinence. Geriatrics 33:36–39, 1978

16. Finkle AL, Priam DV: Sexual potency in elderly men before and after postatectomy. JAMA 198:139–143, 1966

17. Scott FB: Management of erectile impotence using implantable and inflatable prostheses. Urol 2:80–82, 1973

18. Small MP: The small-casion penile prosthesis. Urol 5:479–486, 1975

19. Warren JW, Pratt R, Thomas RJ, et al: Antibiotic irrigation and catheter-associated urinary tract infection. N Engl J Med 229:570–573, 1978

20. Lew EA: Cancer in old age. CA-A Cancer J Clin 28:2–6, 1978

21. Goldfarb AF: Geriatric gynecology, in Rossman I (ed): Clinical Geriatrics. Philadelphia, Lippincott, 1971

22. Leis HP: The diagnosis of breast cancer. CA-A Cancer J Clin 27:209–231, 1977

23. Gusberg SB, Fick HC: Carcinoma of the endometrium: Diagnosis and histogenesis and classification and treatment. Corscaden's Gynecologic Cancer Robert Kreiger, Huntington 4:265–336, 1978

24. Friedrich E: Vulvar Disease. Philadelphia, WB Saunders, 1976, Vol 9

25. Campbell S, McQueen J, Minard J, et al: The modifying effects of progesten on the response of the posmenopausal endometrium to exogenoun estrogen. Postgrad Med J 54(Suppl):58–84, 1978

26. Aylward M, Maddock J, Parker A, et al: Endometrial factors under treatment with estrogen and estrogen/progestogen combination. Postgrad Med J 54:74–81, 1978

27. Maddison J: The practical application of estrogen-progestogen regimens for pre and post menopausal women. Posgrad Med J 54(Suppl):91, 1978 (abstr)

RECOMMENDED RESOURCES

American Cancer Society Series: Facts on Bladder Cancer, Facts on Colorectal Cancer, Facts on Uterine Cancer, Facts on Postate Cancer, Facts on Breast Cancer, Facts on Testicular Cancer, 1978

Dolan T: The vulva in clinical oncology: A multidisciplinary approach. The University of Rochester School of Medicine and Dentistry. American Cancer Society 5:126–129, 1978

Frease AS: Protecting Yourself from Prostate Problems. #381 Public Affairs Committee Inc, New York, 1976

Kirk E: Dealing with the Problem of Incontinence. Unpublished work, Ohio Department of Health, 1971

The menopausal years. Patient Information Library, Physician's Art Service Inc, Daly City, California, 1980

Willson JR: Aging in women. Clin Obstet Gynecol 20:193–222, 1977

13

Respiratory

Gibbe H. Parsons, M.D.
Lynda White, P.A., M.H.S.
Glen A. Lillington, M.D., F.R.C.P.(C), F.A.C.P.

The primary function of the respiratory system is to allow gas exchange, oxygen uptake, and carbon dioxide removal, across alveolar walls. A thin sheet of moving capillary blood adjacent to alveoli forms a surface area roughly the size of a tennis court for this process to occur. Normally, the lung is not the organ limiting exercise ability, since even at maximal exercise only one-half of the normal ventilatory capability is being used. Pulmonary diseases that reduce gas exchange surface area (e.g., emphysema) or impair air movement (e.g., asthma, COPD) eventually will limit exercise capability. Aging alone reduces surface area and air movement but not sufficiently to limit exercise in the absence of disease.

During a single day about 8000 liters of air are moved in and out of the lung. Local defense mechanisms must operate efficiently to warm and humidify the gas, trap inspired particles—pollens, dusts, bacteria, and viruses—and move airway-deposited particles mouthward on a mucus blanket propelled by the moving cilia of respiratory epithelium. Effective coughing aids this process. A properly functioning swallowing mechanism is needed to prevent aspiration of ingested material and saliva. Aging results in impairment of normal defense mechanisms in several ways. Coughing is often impaired due to changes in respiratory muscles and loss of elastic recoil. Ciliary action may be impaired, especially if there is a smoking history. Secretory immunoglobulin IgA, a local defense for nasal and respiratory mucosa, decrease with advancing age. Finally, other diseases that occur in the elderly (e.g., stroke) can impair swallowing resulting in aspiration. These impaired defenses result in increased frequency of pneumonias, often fatal, in the elderly.

Lung carcinoma, usually seen in persons with a cigarette-smoking history, almost certainly is related to long-term inhalation of carcinogens. Elderly smokers, because of duration of exposure, suffer a higher incidence of this disease than younger adults.

The pulmonary circulation, a low-pressure system in comparison to the systemic circulation, carries the entire cardiac output through pulmonary capillaries. Alveolar hypoxia, most commonly the result of chronic obstructive pulmonary disease, results in precapillary arteriolar constriction, pulmonary hypertension, and eventually right heart failure. Peripheral venous thrombophlebitis with clot formation, a disease seen with immobility, venous stasis, and many other predisposing factors common in the elderly can result in pulmonary embolism.

Thus, the elderly experience changes in respiratory structure and function that in the absence of disease go unnoticed; however, diseases of the lung are not uncommon in the elderly and contribute significantly to overall morbidity and mortality.

INCIDENCE OF RESPIRATORY DISEASE IN THE ELDERLY

Excluding acute upper respiratory tract infections, the most common and certainly the most debilitating respiratory disorder in the elderly is chronic obstructive pulmonary disease. A survey in two towns in the United States demonstrated that the frequency of chronic bronchitis was about 10–15 percent of the adult population—twice as common in patients over 40 as in patients in the third decade.[1] The frequency of chronic bronchitis is higher in men than women, reflecting smoking habits. Chronic obstructive pulmonary disease as a listed cause of death has tripled over the past 20 years from about 7/100,000 population in 1956 to about 20/100,000 population in 1976.

The incidence of lung cancer has shown a parallel increase over time. Recent figures[2] show that in 1976 lung cancer accounted for 86,000 deaths—more than any other type. Lung cancer was the most common fatal tumor in men over 55 and nearly equal in incidence to colon and rectum cancer (second only to breast) in women of the same age.[2]

The exact incidence of pulmonary embolism is unknown, but one estimate is that 500,000 cases of pulmonary embolism occur annually. Although not a disease limited to the elderly, pulmonary embolism occurs in conditions seen frequently in the aged—hip fracture, postoperative states, immobility, etc.

Common Lab Values

Although the effects of aging on the lung are not entirely understood, it is clear that most of the parameters normally measured in pulmonary function testing deteriorate with age.[3] Therefore, tests of lung volumes, flow rates, and blood gases must be assessed using normal tables that take patient age into account.

The forced expiratory volume in one second ($FEV_{1.0}$) decreases about 30 ml/year after age 25;[4] the $FEV_{1.0}$ as a percentage of forced vital capacity ($FEV_{1.0}/FVC$) falls from 77 percent at age 45–49 to 71 percent at age 65.[5] Cigarette smoking accelerates these normal changes.[6] Maximum voluntary ventilation and diffusion capacity, a measure of surface area available for gas exchange, also decrease with age.

Arterial oxygen tension (PaO_2) is highest around age 20 (92–108 mm Hg) then declines about 0.4 mm Hg/year so that at age 80 the low normal PaO_2 is 66 mm Hg. One formula for predicting normal PaO_2 is 109–0.43 (age) with a standard deviation of 4.1 mm Hg.[7] Arterial PCO_2 is, by contrast, unchanged with advancing age.

These age-related reductions in pulmonary function do not usually result in symptoms that the elderly individual perceives as abnormal. Complaints of dyspnea usually reflect pulmonary disease rather than the aging process.

In a general practice of medicine dealing primarily with the elderly, chronic obstructive pulmonary disease is the most common *chronic* pulmonary problem. Upper and the more serious lower respiratory infections represent the most common *acute* problems. Pulmonary emoblism almost certainly occurs much more frequently than is recognized. Because pulmonary embolism is a life-threatening event and may masquerade as pneumonia (infarction), dyspnea, pleurisy, and myocardial infarction, the key to diagnosis is a high index of suspicion. Lung carcinoma is the most common tumor in men over 55 and very nearly the second most common malignancy in women of the same age. These common problems, which constitute the majority of chest problems encountered in the elderly, are reviewed in greater detail in a subsequent section.

Uncommon Problems

PULMONARY TUBERCULOSIS

Pulmonary tuberculosis presents special diagnostic and therapeutic problems in the aged. The clinical presentation and radiological findings are often atypcial; in some instances the tuberculin skin test is negative despite the presence of active infection. To reduce diagnostic error, sputum smears and cultures for tubercle should be obtained in all elderly patients with lung disease and a productive cough. Active pulmonary tuberculosis is now more common in the elderly than in the young, and particularly in debilitated or chronic alcoholic patients.

Isoniazid hepatotoxicity is a much more common problem in elderly patients, and the ototoxicity of streptomycin is magnified in old age. Careful monitoring will ensure compliance and allow early detection of toxic effects of the drugs.

CHRONIC ASPIRATION PNEUMONITIS

Recurrent, chronic, or migratory pneumonias may result from repeated aspiration of ingested foods or retained esophageal contents. The occurrence of aspiration is often undetected and unsuspected. Underlying predisposing factors include obtundation, neuromuscular disorders affecting swallowing, pharyngoesophageal diverticulum, achalasia, and regurgitant esophagitis.[8]

A special problem is the lipoid pneumonitis (paraffinoma) due to recurrent aspiration of mineral oil used to treat constipation. The radiological appearance simulates bronchogenic carcinoma. The detection of lipophages in the sputum strongly suggest the diagnosis, which can be confirmed by transbronchoscopic lung biopsy.

DIAGNOSIS AND TREATMENT OF COMMON PROBLEMS

Assessment of Lung Function

Office spirometry is a simple and inexpensive method of assessing and following patients with pulmonary problems. This technique allows one to measure or calculate expiratory flow rates, the forced vital capacity (FVC), forced expiratory volume in one second ($FEV_{1.0}$) and the ratio $FEV_{1.0}$/FVC. The potential reversibility can be assessed by performing the test before and after the administration of aerosolized bronchodilator.

Obstructive airways disease is suspected if $FEV_{1.0}$ is reduced and is confirmed if the $FEV_{1.0}$/FVC ratio is reduced. In such cases, the diagnosis of asthma can be established if there is significant improvement in flow rates following bronchodilators. In most asthmatics, bronchodilators cause improvement in flow rates but not normalization.

A low FVC and $FEV_{1.0}$, associated with relatively normal flow rates and a $FEV_{1.0}$/FVC ratio higher than normal, indicates *restrictive* lung disease.

ACQUIRING THE DATA BASE

Certain aspects of the medical history are important in defining the type of pulmonary problem. A checklist of relevant historical facts is provided in Table 13-1. The symptom pattern provides valuable clues to the diagnosis and aids in the selection of appropriate diagnostic tests.

The physical examination should be comprehensive and not limited to the thorax. In most cases, the presence of obstructive airway disease is readily apparent.

Chest roentgenography is an essential diagnostic modality. It helps elucidate the cause of the patient's symptoms and often reveals the presence of unsuspected or asymtomatic cardiopulmonary disease.

Although the aged lung is subject to most of the pulmonary diseases that occur in younger adults, several conditions are sufficiently common to warrant special mention. These include pulmonary embolism, COPD, bronchogenic carcinoma, and pulmonary infections.

Table 13-1
Important Aspects of the History

I. Symptoms
   Dyspnea—related to what degree of activity?
   Wheezing
   Orthopnea—Positional dyspnea?
   Fatigue
   Cough—dry? Productive? Time of day?
   Sputum—frequency, quantity, color
   Chest pain—pleuritic, anginal, musculoskeletal
   Ankle swelling
   Weight change/appetite loss
II. Past history
   Current and past therapy—nature and
      effectiveness
   Previous pulmonary problems
   Previous chest films or pulmonary function tests
   Occupational exposure—type and duration of
      occupation, hobbies, etc.
   Smoking history—pack years
III. Family history
   Cancer, heart disease, asthma, atopic dermatitis,
      allergic rhinitis, emphysema, chronic bronchitis,
      causes of death.

Pulmonary Embolism

The classical predisposing factors for venous thromboembolic disease (immobility, congestive failure, fractures, surgical operations, venous insufficiency, and carcinomas) are particularly common in the aged. If the patient is not already in the hospital at the time the embolism occurs, the severity of the clinical picture usually results in hospital admission.

Symptoms occurring in the ambulatory or house-confined patient, which should suggest the possibility of embolism, include one or more of the following: unexplained dyspnea, shock, cyanosis, acute congestive failure, chest pain, and hemoptysis. Further consideration of the appropriate diagnostic investigations[9] is beyond the scope of this presentation.

The importance of establishing a definitive diagnosis in the patient suspected to have suffered pulmonary embolism is magnified by the increased morbidity and mortality of anticoagulant therapy in the aged.

Family members should bring to the attention of the physician signs of thrombophlebitis or symptoms suggesting pulmonary embolism.

Chronic Obstructive Pulmonary Disease (COPD)

This encompassing term refers to a group of conditions characterized by reduced expiratory flow rates and is due to increased airway resistance or loss of elastic recoil. Included among these conditions are chronic asthmatic bronchitis, chronic bronchitis, emphysema, bronchiectasis, and cystic fibrosis. Bronchiectasis is now uncommon, and patients with cystic fibrosis rarely survive to late adulthood.

Some very simple pulmonary function tests can help determine if severe obstructive disease is present:

1. A forced expiration with the mouth wide open will fail to extinguish a lighted match at a distance of 6 inches.
2. Prolonged expiratory time: a forced expiration timed by auscultation over the trachea will exceed six seconds.

Emphysema

Emphysema is characterized by increase beyond the normal in the size of air spaces distal to the terminal bronchiole with destruction of their walls. The breakdown of alveolar walls produces "holes" in the lung. Bronchial walls that are poorly supported by alveolar tissue collapse prematurely on expiration, slowing expiratory flow and resulting in incomplete emptying of the lung. The volume of air trapping may be as much as 50 percent of the total lung capacity. In the earlier stages of the disease, there is a compensatory increase in the volume of ventilation per minute. This contributes to the patient's sensation of dyspnea.

Distribution of ventilation and perfusion is often relatively well matched since the capillary network is destroyed along with alveolar walls. This, coupled with the increased volume of ventilation per minute, may account for the relatively normal levels of blood gases in the compensated state. Hypoxemia and CO_2 retention may not be prominent until the disease is far advanced, unless there is a concurrent illness. These noncyanotic individuals who complain bitterly of dyspnea have been termed "pink puffers."[10]

Clinically, the emphysema patient is a thin, cachetic person with a relatively large, hyperinflated chest, who is struggling to breathe. Nonproductive coughing, prolonged expiratory phase of breathing, often with audible wheezes and the absence of cyanosis or cardiomegaly in the earlier stages, are the clinical hallmarks. The chest x-ray is a relatively unreliable diagnostic tool in emphysema, with many false positives and false negatives.

The presence of emphysema may be simulated by the increased anteroposterior diameter of the chest, which commonly occurs in the elderly. In such cases, the auscultatory findings and spirometric values are normal.

Chronic Bronchitis

Chronic bronchitis is defined as a chronic or recurrent increase in the volume of mucoid bronchial secretions sufficient to cause expectoration on most days for at least three months per year in two successive years. Chronic bronchial irritation, usually due to smoking, results in hypertrophy of the bronchial mucous glands, edema of the bronchial mucosa, and increased sputum production. Sputum tends to obstruct the small airways, and loss of support for their walls contributes to obstruction.

The physiological consequences in severe cases may include alveolar hypoventilation, ventilation/perfusion imbalance, hypoxia, and carbon dioxide retention. Hypoxia results in pulmonary hypertension, polycythemia, right ventricular hypertrophy, and eventually right heart failure and peripheral edema. These cyanotic, often edematous, individuals have been referred to as "blue bloaters."[10] Comparison of these two types of patients are noted in Table 13-2.

It must be emphasized that chronic bronchitis and emphysema usually have the same etiology (smoking) and frequently coexist in the individual patient. In many cases, a bronchospastic (asthmatic) factor is also present.

MANAGEMENT OF EMPHYSEMA AND CHRONIC BRONCHITIS

Although there is no therapy that can reverse the lung destruction of emphysema, symptomatic improvement may result from treatment directed towards the bronchitic and asthmatic components of the COPD syndrome. It is possible that such therapy may decrease the rate of progression of the emphysematous process. The therapeutic program is outlined in Table 13-3.

Table 13-2
The "Blue Bloater" and The "Pink Puffer"

	Chronic Bronchitis (Blue Bloater)	Emphysema (Pink Puffer)
Definition	Clinical: sputum production	Anatomic: destruction of alveolar walls
Airway irritants	Almost always a smoking history	Usually a smoking history
Presenting symptom	Persistent cough and sputum	Progressive dyspnea
Dyspnea	Variable in degree	Persistent, effort-related
Respiratory infections	Frequent episodes of wheezing, dyspnea, and purulent sputum	Infrequent respiratory infections
Physical exam	Overweight, often edematous, cyanotic and wheezing	Thin, not edematous or cyantoic. Decreased breath sounds. Barrel chest
Chest film	May be normal, but often increased bronchial markings	Hyperinflation with low flat diaphragms and narrow vertical heart
Pulmonary function tests	Reduced $FEV_{1.0}$/FVC Normal diffusion capacity	Reduced $FEV_{1.0}$/FVC Reduced diffusion capacity
Arterial blood gases	Hypoxia and CO_2 retention	± Hypoxia and no CO_2 retention

Bronchodilators. Bronchodilators are ineffective for emphysema, sometimes helpful in chronic bronchitis, and often markedly beneficial in asthmatic bronchitis. Aminophylline derivatives are well tolerated by the elderly if dosage is adjusted properly and serum levels are monitored. If severe bronchospasm and dyspnea continue, even with optimum oral theophylline therapy, consider adding aerosolized bronchodilators (isoproterenol, isoetharine, metaproterenol), or oral beta adrenergic agents (metaproterenol, terbutaline). Even in patients who appear to have "pure" emphysema, beta adrenergics may achieve mild bronchodilation for which the elderly patient may be very grateful.

Mobilize Secretions. Adequate hydration is the single most effective method of thinning secretions. If the adequately hydrated patient continues to have difficulty handling secretions, add postural drainage and chest percussion. A family member can easily be taught to position and "cup" the patient 2–4 times a day. Such chest physical therapy treatments should be timed to follow inhaled bronchodilator administration. Expectorants, which are probably of little value in most cases, include glyceryl guaicolate and potassium iodide.

Reduce Inhaled Irritants. The practical benefits obtained by stopping smoking include decreased volume of sputum and decreased susceptibility to respiratory infection. In some patients, dyspnea is improved. It is widely believed that cessation of smoking helps slow the progression of COPD, but this has never been clearly demonstrated.

There is no doubt that atmospheric pollutants can exacerbate respiratory symptoms, particularly high atmospheric levels of sulphur dioxide. Epidemological studies indicate, however, that cigarette smoking is a far more important factor than other forms of pollution.[11] Patients with COPD should stay indoors and avoid exercise on days when ambient air is highly polluted.

Infection. Treat respiratory infection (whether "colds" or other infections) promptly with tetracycline or ampicillin. Patients should be given polyvalent influenza vaccine (on an annual basis), as well as pneumococcal vaccine, and should avoid contact with friends and relatives with upper respiratory infections.

Cardiac Failure. In bronchitic patients, recurrent episodes of cardiac failure occur; frequently these are precipitated by respiratory infections. Although right ventricular failure (cor pulmonale) is the classic cardiac manifestation, left ventricular dysfunc-

Table 13-3
Therapy for Chronic Bronchitis and Emphysema

Goal	Modality
Relieve bronchospasm	Bronchodilators
	Theophyllines
	Beta adrenergic agonists
Mobilize secretions	Adequate hydration
	Avoid cough suppressants
	Use percussion and postural drainage
	Avoid drying agents, e.g., antihistamines
Reduce airway irritation	Stop smoking
Control respiratory infections	Flu immunization, pneumococcal vaccination
	Antibiotics for purulent sputum
Reverse congestive heart failure	Duiretics
	Digitalis
Maintain muscular fitness	Regular exercise
Treat hypoxemia if present ($PaO_2 < 50$)	Low flow oxygen
	1–2 liter/min to avoid CO_2 retention

tion may occur in some instances.[12] A good response to diuretic therapy is often seen in the earlier stages. A low sodium diet may be helpful. Eventually a state of chronic cardiac failure may supervene. As noted below, administration of supplemental oxygen is often the most effective therapy for cor pulmonale.

Exercise. The dyspneic person tends to avoid exercise. The resulting loss of fitness may itself contribute to exertional dyspnea. A vigorous training program can improve the exercise tolerance of COPD patients.[13] Lung function is not altered, indicating that improved muscle efficiency is the explanation. Although exercise does not alter the long-term prognosis, it does improve morale and maximizes self-sufficiency. This regular exercise training may include walking and simple calisthenics. A dose of bronchodilator before the exercise may help improve exercise tolerance.

Many patients live for several years with such poor lung function that even slight exertion causes severe breathlessness. These people may benefit from dyspnea control exercises. Pursed lip breathing and relaxation exercises may help the patient to

control his or her respiratory rate and flow rates consciously and may allow a reduction in the work of breathing.

Supplemental Oxygen. Chronic oxygen supplementation may allow the patient with exertional hypoxemia to increase his or her physical activity, and the clinical manifestations of cor pulmonale are often improved, presumably by reduction in pulmonary vascular resistance. Before beginning chronic O_2 supplementation, the patient's condition should be carefully evaluated by a pulmonary disease specialist.

The causes of acute worsening of the patient with emphysema or chronic bronchitis are often obscure, but the development of acute viral or bacterial infection is the most common factor, closely followed by injudicious use of sedatives (Table 13-4).

Home Care and Family Responsibilities. The goal of treatment in these severely affected patients is to keep the patient comfortable, active, and out of the hospital or nursing home. Pulmonary rehabilitation programs, if available, should be considered. Education of patients and families about the disease process, medications, diet, and exercise are vitally important for continued self-sufficiency. Family members should be taught techniques of percussion and postural drainage if sputum production is a prominent symptom of the illness. If home oxygen

Table 13-4
Causes of Acute Clinical Deterioration in Emphysema and Chronic Bronchitis

Pulmonary—chest wall
  Infections—viral or bacterial
    Pneumothorax
    Cough fracture of rib with pain and splinting
    Pulmonary embolism
    Bronchospasm
Cardiac
  Left heart failure
    Cor pulmonale—right heart failure
    Arrhythmias
    Polycythemia
Drugs
  Depression of respiratory center—valium, codeine, phenobarbital
    Induction of bronchospasm—propranolol

or IPPB machines are needed, training in the proper techniques of cleaning, assembly, and use of equipment is necessary.

Asthma and Chronic Asthmatic Bronchitis

Asthma is a condition of hyperreactivity of the bronchi, manifested by increased airway resistance that changes in degree, either spontaneously or in response to medications. Asthma occurs in about 1 percent of the population, may appear at any age, and is characterized by episodic paroxysms of dyspnea, coughing and wheezing. Coughing may be the sole manifestation of asthma. In the elderly, however, asthma is usually chronic and associated with persistent sputum production (chronic asthmatic bronchitis). It rarely shows complete reversibility on bronchodilator therapy and therefore fits in the category of COPD. Many patients with chronic asthmatic bronchitis also have emphysema, particularly if there is a smoking history. Eosinophilia is usually present, and the presence of increased numbers of eosinophiles in peripheral blood and sputum, as well as significant improvement after bronchodilators, are the critical diagnostic tests.

Table 13-5 outlines factors that can precipitate an asthmatic attack or aggravate bronchospasm in the patient with chronic asthmatic bronchitis.[13]

TREATMENT Of ASTHMA

Four classes of drugs are available to treat asthma: theophyllines, beta adrenergic agonists, cromolyn, and steroids.

Aminophylline, the ethylenediamine salt of theophylline, is the most commonly used theophylline preparation. Therapeutic blood levels (10–20 mg/ml) can be achieved in most adults with 5.6 mg/kg orally q6h.[14] However, patients with liver disease, heart failure, or the elderly may require only 2 mg/kg q6h. Toxicity from overdose results in the symptoms noted in Table 13-6, easily remembered because they parallel symptoms of a structurally similar common drug, caffeine.

If theophylline alone is not adequate therapy a beta adrenergic agent should be added (Table 13-7). These are administered orally or by aerosol inhalation. Untoward reactions to beta-adrenergic agents are more common and more troublesome in the elderly, particularly if administered orally.[15]

Disodium cromoglycate (cromolyn) is an inhaled

Table 13-5
Precipitating Causes of Asthmatic Exacerbation

Allergen exposure—pollens, etc.
Infection—sinusitis, URI
Aspirin intolerance
Isoproterenol abuse
Exercise—induced
Irritant inhalation—smoke, cold air, dusts, pollutants
Emotional upset

powder that prevents allergic bronchospasm in perhaps 50 percent of cases of extrinsic asthma. It is prophylactic only and must be used for 6–8 weeks before its full effect can be assessed. It has little value in the management of chronic asthmatic bronchitis in most instances.

Oral prednisone may be added to the regimen when other drugs fail to control the disease. In alternate-day AM doses of 5–20 mg, prednisone is often effective without excessive side effects. Beclomethasone, a topically active inhaled steroid, causes less adrenal suppression than daily prednisone and may allow reduction in prednisone dosage or even discontinuation of the drug. In maximal recommended doses, however, beclomethasone is only equivalent to 5–10 mg of daily prednisone. It can cause hoarseness and oral candidiasis. It is not suitable for treatment of the acute asthmatic attack.

Although it is well known that emotional upset may trigger an asthmatic attack, the much more common sequence is anxiety appropriately associated with the dyspnea of wheezing. The treatment of the anxiety is not tranquilizers but, rather, bronchodilators and, if necessary, low flow oxygen.

Bronchogenic Carcinoma

Bronchogenic carcinoma is a major problem in smokers over the age of 40. It has long been the most common cancer in males and is now approaching the second most common cancer in females, reflecting increased smoking by women.

Table 13-6
Side Effects of Theophylline

GI:	Nausea, vomiting
CNS:	Insomnia, irritability, tremor, *seizures*
Cardiac:	Tachycardia, arrhythmias
GU:	Diuresis

Table 13-7
Beta Adrenergic Agents

Epinephrine
  Inhaled or subcutaneous—short acting
    α and β effects occur
Ephedrine
  Oral administration only
    CNS and cardiac stimulation limit usefulness
    Often combined with Theophylline (Tedral, etc.)
Isoproterenol
  The most potent β agent
    Has β_1 (cardiac) as well as β_2 (bronchodilator)
      activity
    Aerosol route
    Short duration of action
Isoetharine
  Greater β_2 specifity than isoproterenol
  Aerosol only
Metaproterenol and Terbutaline
  Nearly identical in actions and side effects
  The best oral agents for β_2 specificity
  More β_2 specific as aerosols than tablets
  Commonly cause tremor
  More prolonged bronchodilator effect than
    isoproterenol

The overall five-year survival of only 5–15 percent indicates that most cases are already inoperable or incurable at the time of diagnosis. Although this would suggest that prompt diagnostic intervention by the primary care physician has little value, it must be emphasized that certain clinical presentations are often a manifestation of relatively early disease and are associated with a much higher cure rate. Recognition of these presentations (Table 13-8) by the primary care physician is an indication for prompt referral of the patient for definitive studies.

Even if the disease is obviously inoperable (Table 13-9) recent advances in radiation therapy and

Table 13-8
Clinical Presentations of Lung Cancer Suggesting Early
or Curable Disease

1. "Occult" lung cancer—negative chest x-ray with positive sputum cytology
2. Solitary pulmonary nodule
3. Recurrent pneumonia in the same lobe or segment
4. Hemoptysis with peripheral lung lesion or negative chest x-ray
5. Lobar or segmental atelectasis

chemotherapy may achieve significant palliation and prolongation of survival.

It is important that both the patient and family participate in the choice of therapies available. For bronchogenic carcinoma not curable by surgery, the prognosis is poor, but the physician still has important care to render. Assurance that the patient will not be deserted and that pain can be controlled are important. When life expectancy is short, use of potent narcotic analgesics should not be withheld for fear of addiction. The hospice movement, aimed at humanized home care of the terminally ill, is available in some areas. The local cancer society may be a source of information for other supportive community services.

Pneumonia

Incidence. Although upper respiratory infections are not more common, lower respiratory infections occur in the elderly with increasing frequency and with advancing age, claiming a high mortality. For patients over 70 years of age the pneumonia-related mortality is 25 percent.[16]

Pathophysiology. Elderly or debilitated patients are more susceptible to pneumonia due to impaired defense mechanisms (e.g., ineffective cough, decreased respiratory IgA), and frequent coexisting disease (heart disease, renal insufficiency, COPD). Aspiration pneumonias also occur more commonly in the elderly, due to obtundation, esophageal disorders, and deglutitional difficulties.[8]

Signs and Symptoms. Usual signs of pneumonia such as fever, cough, purulent sputum, chest pain, and leukocytosis may be masked in the elderly. Tachypnea, tachycardia, confusion or shock may be the presenting clinical manifestations.

Management. In all cases of suspected pneumonia, a chest x-ray and sputum studies should be obtained. Interpretation of the roentgenographic

Table 13-9
Lung Cancer—Indicators of Inoperability

1. Malignant pleural effusion
2. Chest wall involvement
3. Mediastinal involvement
4. Tumor within 2 cm of carina
5. Extrathoracic spread

findings is complicated by the frequent presence of pre-existent abnormalities and by the disparity between roentgenographic changes and the clinical severity of the illness that commonly occurs in the elderly.

Interpretation of sputum smears and cultures is complicated by the difficulty in obtaining an adequate specimen from elderly patients and by the frequency with which the specimen is grossly contaminated. The preliminary microscopic examination of the sputum smear will indicate whether the sputum is suitable for cultures. If sputum is unobtainable or inadequate in quality, an ideal specimen for culture can be obtained by transtracheal aspiration.

Blood cultures are sometimes positive in cases of pneumonia, particularly those of pneumococcal origin. If pleural fluid is present, a sample of this material should be taken for culture.

Bacterial pneumonia in the nonhospitalized patient who has not been previously on antibiotic therapy is usually due to the pneumococcus, although Klebsiella infections are not uncommon. Pneumonias that develop in hospitals are frequently due to staphylococcus, klebsiella, or the gram negative enteric bacilli.[17] If the patient is obtunded or has swallowing difficulties, anaerobic infection is likely. Acute pneumonia with negative cultures suggests viral infection, mycoplasma pneumonia, ornithosis or Legionnaire's disease. Chronic consolidations suggest fungal or mycobacterial infection.

Microscopic study of gram-stained sputum helps guide the initial selection of therapy while awaiting the results of cultures, and it aids in the interpretation of the significance of the sputum culture.[18]

Untoward effects from antibiotic therapy occur more commonly in the aged. Careful patient monitoring is essential.

Family members can help by encouraging appropriate immunizations and discouraging exposure to crowds or individuals with respiratory infections.

SUMMARY

Aging alone results in changes in pulmonary function and arterial blood gases that are not apparent to the patient in the absence of disease. Chronic obstructive pulmonary disease and pulmonary infections are common in the elderly, and bronchogenic carcinoma is the most common fatal malignancy over the age of 55. Pulmonary embolism probably occurs much more frequently than is recognized.

Routine office spirometry, annual chest films, appropriate immunizations, and prompt attention to symptoms and signs of respiratory disease are aids to detection and prevention of pulmonary illness.

The primary care physician, by involving patient and family in eldercare, by utilizing community resources, and by recognizing the special needs of the elderly, can provide humanistic and meaningful medical care for the older population.

HEALTH MAINTENANCE

Office spirometry has not become as commonplace as electrocardiography, yet there is a definite need to detect early obstructive airways disease. Elderly smokers with advanced symptomatic COPD usually have stopped smoking on their own. Less symptomatic smokers may view abnormal spirometry as a motivation to quit and can find help in smoking-cessation clinics or at local health agencies (e.g., the American Lung Association). Although an elderly smoker may not prolong life or improve pulmonary function by quitting, reduction in sputum production, bronchospasm, and frequency of infections usually occurs. Ninety percent of smokers want to quit, and the physician should be able to offer encouragement and help.

An annual chest roentgenogram is of most value in detecting asymptomatic peripheral lung tumors at a stage when curative resection is possible. Indolent pneumonias or tuberculosis may be detected in a relatively asymptomatic patient.

Annual flu immunizations are recommended for the elderly or patients with significant cardiorespiratory disease. The pneumococcal vaccine should be given once to high risk elderly patients. The exact duration of immunity is as yet unclear but probably exceeds five years.

Screening for tuberculosis exposure with the PPD skin test is appropriate for contacts of an active case or patients suspected of having the disease. A PPD should not be given, however, if a previous PPD was positive, as another positive reaction adds no helpful information and may result in an intense local reaction.

Avoidance of crowds or individuals with viral illnesses can prevent what in the elderly may be a very debilitating illness.

REFERENCES

1. Thurlbeck WM: Chronic Airflow Obstruction in Lung Disease. Philadelphia, WB Sanders Co, 1976, pp 235–287
2. Cancer statistics, 1979: CA-A Cancer J Clin 29:6–21, 1979
3. Bates DV, Macklem PT, Christie RV: Respiratory Function in Disease. Philadelphia WB Saunders Co, 1971, pp 96–100
4. Morris JF, Koski A, Johnson LC: Spirometric standards for healthy non-smoking adults. Am Rev Resp Dis 103:57, 1971
5. Schlesinger Z, Goldbourt U, Medalie J, Oron D, Neufeld HN, et al: Pulmonary ventilatory function values for healthy men aged 45 years and over. Chest 63:520, 1973
6. Ashley F, Kannel WB, Sorlie PD, Masson R: Pulmonary function: Relation to age, cigarette habit and mortality, the Framingham study. Ann Intern Med 82:739, 1975
7. Sorbini CA, Grassi V, Solinas E, Muisean G: Arterial oxygen tension in relation to age in healthy subjects. Respir 25:3, 1968
8. Lillington GA, Parsons GH: Tips on the management of aspiration. Consult 19:98, 1979
9. Lillington GA, Parsons GH: Acute pulmonary embolism. Hosp Med 11–20 July, 1980
10. Marks A: Chronic bronchitis and emphysema: Clinical evaluation and diagnosis. Med Clin North Am 57:707, 1973
11. Anderson DO, Ferris BG: Air pollution levels and chronic respiratory disease. Arch Environ Health 10:307, 1965
12. Baum GL, Schwartz A, Llamas R, Castillo C: Left ventricular function in chronic obstructive lung disease. N Engl J Med 285:361, 1971
13. Woolf CR, Suero JT: Alteration in lung mechanics and gas exchange following training in chronic obstructive lung disease. Dis Chest 55:37, 1969
14. Mathison DA, Stevenson DD, Tan EM, Vaughan JH: Clinical profiles of bronchial asthma. JAMA 224:1134, 1973
15. Piafsky KM, Ogilvie RI: Dosage of theophylline in bronchial asthma. N Engl J Med 292:1218, 1975
16. Mufson MA, Chang V, Gill V, Wood SC, Romansky MJ, et al: The role of viruses, mycoplasmas and bacteria in acute pneumonia in civilian adults. Am J Epidem 86:526, 1967
17. Garb JL, Brown RB, Garb JR, et al: Differences in etiology of pneumonias in nursing home and community patients. JAMA 240:2169, 1978
18. Elder HA, Sauer RL: Infectious disease aspects of respiratory therapy, in Burton GG, Gee GN, Hodgkin JE (eds): Respiratory Care: A Guide to Clinical Practice. Philadelphia, JB Lippincott Co, 1977

RECOMMENDED RESOURCES

Ayers LN, Whipp BJ, Ziment I: A Guide to the Interpretation of Pulmonary Function Tests. New York; Roerig-Pfizer; 1975

Burton GG, Gee GN, Hodgkin JE (eds): Respiratory Care: A Guide to Clinical Practice. Philadelphia, JB Lippincott Co, 1977

Patient Education Materials:

"Helping smokers quit" kit. (Obtained free from: Office of Cancer Communications, National Cancer Institute Bethesda, MD 20014)

Modrak M, Moser KM, Archibald C, Hansen P, Ellis B, et al: Better Living and Breathing: A Manual for Patients. St Louis, CV Mosby Co, 1975

Petty TL, Tyler ML: If you have emphysema or chronic bronchitis, this booklet is written for you. Breon Laboratories #8266, 1979

The do's and don'ts of walking. Breon Laboratories #8996, 1974

What you need to know about cancer of the lung. DHEW Pub No (NIH) 78-1533 (Obtained from Office of Cancer Communications, National Cancer Institute, Bethesda MD 20014)

14

Gastrointestinal System

Walter Morgan, M.D.
Corinne Thomas, F.N.P.
Marvin Schuster, M.D.

Gastrointestinal complaints are very common in elders. Perhaps no other system expresses stress as frequently as the gut. The many stresses and losses with aging in America result in a myriad of digestive complaints. Overnutrition in adult years and undernutrition in elder years takes their toll. Multidrug use (both prescription and over-the-counter) is common, with adverse effects.

Gastrointestinal symptoms are of great concern to elders. Dyspepsia, flatulence, and diarrhea are emotionally burdensome to them and others around them. Fear of colon cancer may bring elders to seek care for minor symptoms, or conversely may scare them away, afraid "to find out." Many functional complaints mimic serious organic diseases. The clinician is particularly challenged as elders frequently present with atypical history and physical findings. Pain is often atypical in location, character, and intensity.

Aging has both general and specific effects. The loss of teeth and grinding ability, coupled with diminished taste and smell, often result in a decreased interest in food. There is diminished motility and secretions. Secretion of hydrochloric acid and the digestive enzymes of the stomach, intestines, liver, and pancreas diminish. There is a decrease of mucous secretion and muscle atrophy of both the small and large intestine.[1] (See Table 14-1).

Normal aging is not responsible for all changes, but rather a lifetime of assault by stress, certain habits, foods, food processing, chemicals, and drugs. Geographic and subgroup epidemiology studies are beginning to implicate life-style rather than race) as contributory. This is most notably true of diverticulosis.

INCIDENCE OF GASTROINTESTINAL PROBLEMS IN THE ELDERLY

Acute gastrointestinal problems occur in over 7 percent of people over 45 years of age per year.[2] The National Health Survey[3] reports 9 percent of people aged 65 and older had limited activity because of gastrointestinal problems; 2.8 percent were because of hernia symptoms; 1.6 percent due to peptic ulcer; probably 0.7 percent due to gastrointestinal cancer; 0.4 percent due to hemorrhoids; and 3.6 percent due to other gastrointestinal problems. According to other studies, some 32 percent of the elders report a constipation problem, and 10 percent will have a peptic ulcer at some time. Diverticulosis will afflict 40 percent of 70-year-olds and 70 percent of 80-year-olds; gall stones appear in 38 percent of people by the seventh or eighth decade.[4] Hiatus hernias become increasingly frequent after 50 and have been reported in 67 percent of elders over 60.

One gastroenterology clinic[5] found 56 percent of elders with GI symptoms had functional gastrointestinal complaints; 10 percent had gastrointestinal malignancy, 8 percent gall bladder disease, 7 percent duodenal ulcer, 3 percent gastric ulcer, 3 percent diverticulosis symptoms, and 13 percent had other gastrointestinal problems.

Depression and weight loss are common psychosomatic problems that present with gastrointestinal signs and symptoms. Anorexia, constipation, and somatic pains are cardinal signs of depression and mimic primary gastrointestinal disease. Decreased

Table 14-1
Gastrointestinal Changes of Aging[1]

Change	Complication or Association
Loss of teeth	Poor intake, large bolus
Loss of tongue papilla, taste and smell	Poor appetite, weight loss
Reduced salivary ptyalin	Slightly reduced carbohydrate digestion
Reduced esophageal peristalis	
Irregular nonperistalitic esophageal waves	Delayed emptying, presbyesophagus
Poor relaxation of esophageal sphincter	
Hiatal hernia	Esophagitis, bleeding
Thinned gastric mucosa and muscularis	Atrophic gastritis, iron deficiency anemia, pernicious anemia, ulcer, carcinoma
Decreased gastrin, gastric acid, pepsin, intrinsic factor	
Decreased colonic muscle tone	Constipation
Decreased colonic motor function	
Diverticulosis	Diverticulitis
Reduced liver weight and blood flow	None
Decreased liver inducible enzymes	Altered drug metabolism
Reduced serum albumin	Weakness, weight loss
Increased globulin	None
Cholelithiasis	Cholecystitis

food intake is usually responsible for weight loss rather than malabsorption or cancer.

Simple constipation is the most common gastrointestinal complaint of the elderly. Gaseousness, flatulence, and vague feelings of fullness and ill-defined indigestion are frequent. "Heartburn," substernal and epigastric burning pain, may be a result of air-gulping, esophagitis, gastritis, ulcer, or gall bladder disease. Chronic or episodic lower abdominal pain, especially in the left lower quadrant, is most likely due to irritable bowel syndrome or diverticular disease. Finally, hemorrhoids are very common problems in elders.

Death is often caused by gastrointestinal problems, most commonly malignancy. Approximately 60 percent[6] of cancer deaths originate from gastrointestinal primary sites. Other causes are cirrhosis, peptic ulcer (usually hemorrhage), hernia and other intestinal obstruction, and cholecystitis. Table 14-2 illustrates the specific death rates for the most fatal gastrointestinal problems. Rates for most conditions increases with age. One exception is cirrhosis, which drops after a peak in the fifth or sixth decade.

Uncommon Problems

Dysphagia, jaundice, and malabsorption are less common problems of elders but are important to recognize and pursue. Causes of dysphagia could be badly chewed food due to poor teeth; lying supine; stomatitis and pharyngeal ulceration; neurological deficit, e.g., basilar artery insufficiency; acholasia; decreased esophageal motility; obstructive bands; esophageal diverticula; esophagitis; or carcinoma of the esophagus. All patients with dysphagia should be investigated with barium swallow and esophagoscopy.

Transient jaundice occurs with infection, shock, or congestive heart failure. Jaundice in elders, however, is much more commonly due to obstruction, either from common duct stones or carcinoma of the head of the pancreas.[7] The former may not

Table 14-2
Death Rates for Selected Gastrointestinal System Causes by Age Group,
United States, 1974 (Per 1000 Population)[26]

	65–74 Years	75–84 Years	85 Years and Over
Neoplasms, GI	224.2	405.0	519.2
Cirrhosis	46.4	29.3	18.5
Peptic ulcer	13.6	29.1	50.1
Hernia and intestinal obstruction	10.1	31.0	70.4
Cholecystitis, cholangitis	5.7	16.9	38.5
Enteritis and diarrheal disease	2.1	6.9	18.2
Appendicitis	1.4	3.0	4.9
Bacillary dysentery	0.1	0.1	0.2

produce the classic colic pain. Cholangitis may complicate stone obstruction and resemble hepatitis. In cholangitis, rapidly falling enzymes (after the stones pass), leukocytosis, and fever help in the differential diagnosis. Jaundice can result from viral hepatitis, which is almost always secondary to blood transfusions. It is serious and usually progresses from insidious onset to acute hepatic failure and death in a high percentage of cases. Drug-induced jaundice may result from methyldopa and isoniazid. Intrahepatic cholestasis also may be caused by oral hypoglycemia drugs, phenothiazines, and anabolic steroids.

Malabsorption affects elders more than younger adults. Steatorrhea is a common symptom in generalized malabsorption. The manifestations of selected malabsorption syndromes and some of their causes are listed in Table 14-3.

Table 14-3
Malabsorption Syndromes

Manifestation	Malabsorbed Nutrient	Some of the Causes
Steatorrhea	Fat	Pancreatic insufficiency, celiac disease, gastrectomy, neomycin
Diarrhea	Fatty acids, bile salts, lactose	Liver disease, gastrectomy, cholestyramine, PAS, lactose deficiency
Weight loss, fatigue	Fat, carbohydrate, protein	Pancreatic insufficiency, liver disease, gastroenteritis, celiac disease
Iron deficiency anemia	Iron	Alcohol, esophageal, web, atropic gastritis
Megaloblastic anemia	Folic acid, B_{12}	Decreased intrinsic factor, decreased gastrin, antibiotics
Bone pain, fractures	Calcium, protein	Decreased gastrin
Bleeding	Vitamin K	Celiac disease, liver disease, mineral oil laxatives
Edema	Protein	Celiac disease
Abdominal cramps, bloating	Lactose	Lactose deficiency, celiac disease, pancreatic insufficiency

Emergencies

Gastrointestinal emergencies are more life-threatening to the older patient, because elders generally are less able to tolerate either the particular crisis or the treatment.[8] Diagnosis of these problems is often more difficult because the history and physical findings may be atypical, particularly pain. In elders, abdominal pathology will often present as pain radiating to the chest, shoulder, or back. Conversely, nonabdominal problems may present as abdominal pain, such as cardiac, pulmonary, or urinary crises.

Gall Bladder Disease is the most common cause of severe acute abdominal pain in elders. Vomiting, fever, right upper quadrant pain, and tenderness, occasionally a palpable mass, and leukocytosis are the classic complex. Jaundice may be present. The general management of cholecystitis is similar to treatment in young patients. Prepare for surgery, however, if the patient does not improve within 24 hours if sonogram or if cholangiogram demonstrates cystic duct obstruction. The elderly patient may tolerate infection poorly and be subject to septicemia. Earlier intervention may be warranted compared to younger patients.

Gastrointestinal Obstruction, usually small bowel, is the second most common cause of serious pain.[7] Half are caused by hernias. The next most common causes are adhesions from previous surgery. Symptoms may be steady pain rather than colic. Bowel sounds, initially hyperactive, soon become silent.

Obstruction of the large bowel is most commonly due to rectosigmoid cancer followed in frequency by sigmoid volvulus. The latter is marked by constipation and distention; men are affected more than women. Decompression sigmoidoscopy may correct the problem in half the cases. Cecal volvulus affects women more than men, with acute onset of pain, vomiting, and distention.

Gallstone ileus is a less common cause of obstruction, but should be considered especially in women with known gall bladder disease.

The general management of intestinal obstruction is similar to that in younger adult patients, except that earlier intervention is frequently indicated because peritonitis develops more rapidly.

Appendicitis is common in the elderly, ranking just below intestinal obstruction as a cause of severe acute abdomen. The symptoms may be initially vague. Vomiting is less common in older patients.[9] Bowel sounds are commonly absent, and there is often a localized ileus. Abdominal and rectal masses, as well as leukopenia, are commonly present. Since many elders delay in seeking care, perforation and death rates are higher. Elders' health status may rapidly deteriorate even to the point of masking the site of origin of their problems.

Acute Pancreatitis increases in incidence with age; the clinician may be misled by the commonly associated lower chest pain, ECG changes, cardiac decompensation, and confusion. Amylase results are usually valid, though often transient. Pancreatic cancer or hyperparathyroidism should be considered in patients with recurrent or nonalcoholic pancreatitis.

Management of acute pancreatitis differs little in the elderly compared to the younger patient; however, the incidence of complicating recurrences, abscesses, and cysts increases with age.[10]

Mesenteric Thrombosis and Infarction classically present with pain, abdominal distention, bloody diarrhea, and rebound tenderness, especially around the umbilicus. The clinical presentation picture may mimic upper intestinal obstruction, although the plain X-ray picture is often relatively airless. Paracentesis may reveal bloody fluid, but only after gangrene begins. Hematocrits and complete blood counts should be performed every six hours on suspect cases. Shift of white cell differential to the left and rising hematocrit (due to hemoconcentration) warrants angiography and rapid surgical intervention.[7]

Hemorrhage. Gastrointestinal bleeding in elders is most often due to hemorrhagic gastritis, duodenal or gastric ulcer. Aspirin ingestion, even small quantities, may precipitate the problem. History of aspirin ingestion should be vigorously pursued, naming many of the hundreds of aspirin-containing preparations on the market. Steroid and nonsteroidal anti-inflammatory medication also leads to hemorrhage. Alcohol abuse is another common precipitating factor. Other causes of gastrointestinal hemorrhage are less common but equally serious.

Profuse bleeding after intense vomiting due to biliary tract of other disease may lead to an esophageal tear.[7] There is a history of bloodless vomiting preceding the hematemesis.

Esophageal varices may bleed profusely in the

elderly. Massive bleeding can also occur from diverticula or carcinoma of the colon, often with no history or preceding symptoms suggestive of these problems.

Rarely, a diffuse intravascular coagulopathy due to gram negative sepsis may first present as gastrointestinal bleeding.

The presentation of gastrointestinal bleeding may be by hematemesis, rectal passage, or both. Bright red vomitus indicates a recent bleed of considerable quantity. "Coffee ground" emesis may be due to bleeding that is equally as massive.

Rectal bleeding will vary from guaiac-positive normal appearing stool, (usually a 25–50 ml blood loss), to a few drops of red blood in the toilet bowl, to red, maroon, or black stools, which usually mean a loss of 200–1000 ml anywhere in the tract. The color is dependent on transit time and digestive factors. Stool can be red from gastric bleeding if passage is within four hours; it will be tarry if it is in the gut for 8–20 hours.[11] A black or red stool is an emergency. Diverticula is a very common cause. General management of massive hemorrhage is similar to that of younger adult patients, except that it is often more extensive. Bleeding is difficult to control in the elderly, partly because of hardened blood vessels. Also, elders develop shock more rapidly because of their less responsive neurovascular systems.

Common Laboratory Values Chart

Unless otherwise noted in Table 14-4, laboratory values are the same for the elderly as for younger adults.[24]

DIAGNOSIS AND TREATMENT OF GASTROINTESTINAL PROBLEMS

Hiatal Hernias

The incidence of hiatal hernias is more frequent after age 50 and has been reported in 67 percent of elders over 60.[1] The diagnosis is made by x-ray, generally as an incidental finding in the evaluation of heartburn or epigastric distress. These symptoms are usually due to esophagitis or ulcer disease, however, and are too often attributed to the hiatal hernia. Management should be directed accordingly.

Table 14-4
Common GI Lab Values[24]

Ammonia	30–70 μg/100 ml		
Amylase	60–180 somogyi units/100 ml		
Bilirubin			
Direct	0.1–0.4 mg/100 ml		
Total	0.2–0.9 mg/100 ml		
Cholesterol, total[8,9]			
Age 60	165–258 mg/100 ml		
Age 70	129–246 mg/100 ml		
Gamma-glutamyl transpeptidase at 25°C	4–18 mU/ml (females) 6–28 mU/ml (males)		
Triglyceride			
Ages 50–59	10–190mg/100 ml		
Transaminase			
SGOT	5–40 units/ml (Sigma-Frankel)		
5–35 units/ml			
Protein[9,10]			
Selected ages	Albumin	Globulin	A/G
21–30	61.65	38.35	1.61
41–50	56.80	43.20	1.32
61–70	52.85	47.15	1.12
Over 70	51.87	48.17	1.08

Esophagitis

The lower esophageal sphincter becomes weakened with aging, allowing reflux of gastric acid into the esophagus.[1,12]

DATA BASE

The patient complains of "heartburn," which is a substernal or epigastric burning sensation. It gradually progresses and often is intermittent. It is usually worse at night and after reclining after a big meal. Regurgitation may be present. The pain can be retrosternal. Dysphagia may develop as scarring occludes the esophagus.

Substernal pain due to esophagitis is easily confused with angina. The former is more often associated with a horizontal position and an empty stomach. Angina is related to exertion, but this distinction is not always true. Also, sublingual nitroglycerin may relieve pain from both conditions.

Esophageal problems may first be discovered when they present as lung complaints; bronchietasis or lung abscess may be due to acute or chronic gastric reflux.

The physical examination is usually normal. A barium swallow may show a damaged esophageal lining and, as the problem persists, a narrowing at the distal end. A barium swallow should be done to rule out cancer. Swallowing acid barium may trigger spasm of the sphincter, which will be visible on fluroscopy. Perfusion of 0.1 NCl through tubes into the esophagus causes increase in manometric pressure. Esophogascopy reveals inflammation.

MANAGEMENT

Body position and antacids are the cornerstones of treatment. Both the head *and* shoulders must be elevated 30 degrees. This can be done by propping up the whole bed or the head-end half of the mattress. The use of more pillows elevates only the head, increasing the reflux. Smoking and alcohol should be restricted, as well as coffee, chocolate, carbonated beverages, pepper and spices.[1,12] Weight reduction is helpful in obese patients.

Antacid therapy is aimed at keeping something in the stomach at all times to neutralize acid. A tablespoonful of antacid can be taken between meals (or two hours after a meal). Elders who don't eat regularly or eat scanty meals can be instructed to "take antacid or eat food every two hours when you're awake." A dose at bedtime is most important.

Alginic acid with antacids (Gaviscon), after meals and at bedtime, makes an effective foam barrier to reflux.

Urecholine (25 mg tid), a cholinergic drug, may help some patients by increasing the tone of the gastroesophageal sphincter. Anticholinergics, on the other hand, tend more to decrease gastric emptying than suppress secretion and are not recommended.

Gastritis and Peptic Ulcer

Stomach motility decreases due to muscular thinning in elders. Acid and pepsin decrease, contributing to decreasing iron and B_{12} absorption. This may cause reduced natural protection against gastric polyps and cancer. Mucosa thinning leads to atrophic gastritis, which increases the risk of gastric cancer 20 times.[13] Atrophic gastritis is probably the most common gastrointestinal condition in elders and is usually asymptomatic. If symptomatic, there usually are vague epigastric discomfort, nausea, and flatulence.[1] If discovered in an elder, they should be watched closely for occult blood.

Peptic ulcer affects 10 percent of the elderly, the same percent as younger adults. However, the ratio of duodenal to gastric shifts from 10:1 to 2:1,

possibly due to reduced gastric mucin protection. Men are affected more than women, but the ratio narrows from 11:1 in middle age to 5:1 in elders.[13]

DATA BASE

Symptoms and signs in the elderly vary from the young in that, though epigastric burning predominates, the classic empty-stomach timing may not be so strong. Fever, leukocytosis, and other typical signs may be absent even when there is perforation. Drug-induced ulcers are common. (See Chapter 6.) The differential diagnosis between gastric ulcers and cancer is especially important. Initial symptoms may be similar but weight loss, anemia, and occult blood suggest cancer.

MANAGEMENT

Management of stomach problems differs from the young in two important respects.[14] First, as gastric cancer is far more prevalent, gastric ulcers deserve follow-up fluoroscopy or endoscopy to make sure they are healed. Most gastric ulcers heal in four to six weeks with adequate therapy. Delayed healing warrants repeat gastroscopy with cytology and biopsy. Benign polyps can be removed with a fiberoptic gastroscope.

Secondly, bleeding, though not more common, is far more severe, possibly due to the thinned mucosa of the arteriosclerotic vessels. When bleeding occurs, mortality rises to 65 percent in the elderly. Therefore, careful surveillance for bleeding is important. Regular stool guaiacs are indicated during the management phase. Anticoagulant therapy for cardiovascular problems is particularly risky. Melena and hematemesis deserve hospital care, surgical consultation, and early intervention.

Therapy involves frequent small, bland meals and antacids for both gastric and duodenal problems. Antacids are given one hour after each meal and at bedtime. Tablets are less effective than liquids. Choice of antacid may need more thought for the elderly than for the young. They may be more sensitive to the constipating effects of aluminum hydroxide or the diarrhea-causing effects of magnesium hydroxide. The clinician can accordingly choose an antacid with different composition. (See Table 14-5.)

Also, sodium content of the antacids may be a problem in some patients with cardiovascular or renal problems. Calcium-containing antacids cause rebound hyperacidity and also hypercalcemia in

Table 14-5
Selected Antacids[25]

Product	Neutralizing Capacity mEq/ml	Aluminum Hydroxide	Magnesium Hydroxide (H) or Trisilicate (T)	Sodium
			(mg/5 ml tablet)	
Alka Seltzer*				276
Aludrox susp	2.81	307	103 H	1.5
tab		233	84 H	1.6
Amphogel susp	1.93	320		6.9
tab		300,600		1.4,1.8
AMT susp	1.79	305	625 T	7.2
tab		104	250 T	3.5
Cremalin tab†	2.57	248	75 H	41
Di-Gel susp, tab	2.45	282†	87 H	8.5,10.6
Gelusil susp, tab	1.33	250	500 T	8
Maalox susp	2.58	225	200 H	2.5
Mylanta susp	2.38	200	200 H	3.9
Riopan‡				0.7
Rolaids§				53
Tums‖				2.7
WinGel susp, tab	2.25	180	160	2.5

*Sodium and potassium bicarbonate, citric acid.
†Codried with magnesium carbonate.
‡Magaldrate.
§Dihydroxyaluminum sodium aminoacetate.
‖Calcium carbonate 500 mg.

many patients. Most antacids interfere with the absorption of tetracycline, digoxin, and enteric-coated tablets.

Antacids can be used prophylactically for patients on high regular aspirin or steroid and nonsteroid antiflammation medication to prevent ulceration associated with these drugs.

Anticholinergics should work physiologically, but double-blind studies produced conflicting results. The side effects of increased glaucoma, urinary retention, hypo- or hypertension, gastric retention, arrhythmias, and confusion are very common and obviously much more significant in the elderly.

Cimetidine, the histamine (H_2) antagonist, effectively reduces acid production and hastens healing of duodenal and gastric ulcers.[13] If unsuccessful after a six-week trial, further investigation is warranted. Cimetidine may cause confusion in patients with reduced renal or hepatic clearance.

Patient education should be to inform patients that their condition is best managed by the practice of dealing with stress in constructive ways, avoiding stresses that they cannot deal with comfortably.

They should eat frequent small meals of bland foods, take antacids and other medications as directed, avoid alcohol, caffeine, tobacco, aspirin and other irritants, and immediately report increase in pain or black stools or vomiting.

Constipation and Diarrhea

Bowel habit changes often include both constipation and diarrhea in the same patient, alternatively and intermittently. Usually, one symptom predominates over the other. It is difficult by history and physical exam alone to determine if the cause of the symptoms is serious pathology or a functional problem. Therefore, any change in bowel habits, especially when steadily persistent or progressive over several weeks, or when accompanied by weight loss, fever, or pain, should be thoroughly investigated with proctosigmoidoscopy, barium enema, and other appropriate studies. (See Table 14-6.)

The gastrointestinal tract experiences a steady progressive loss of neurological response and motility with aging. This does not, however, cause

Table 14-6
Common Causes of Bowel Movement Change

Constipation	Both	Diarrhea
Inactivity	Functional	Infection
Low fiber diet	Cancer	Ulcerative colitis
Dehydration	Diverticulosis	Crohn's disease
Debilitation	Antacids	malabsorption
Rectal fissure, pain	Fecal impaction	Hyperthyroidism
Hypothyroidism	Diabetes	Drugs:
Hypercalcemia	Ischemia	
Hyperparathyroidism		Clindamycin
Barium for x-ray		Colchicine
Drugs:		Laxatives, stimulant
		Lincomycin
Alum, calc. antacids		Lithium carbonate
Codeine		Magnesium antacids
Flagyl		Mefenamic acid
Quinacrine		(Ponstel)
Belladonna		Tetracycline
Lomotil		Vitamin D
Diuretics		Guanethidine
Sedatives		

serious bowel problems in most elderly people. Many that do have problems also have contributory decreased physical activity, decreased fiber bulk and water in their diet, and too many bowel-effecting medicines. A diet change may be due to many situational problems such as improper dentures, inability to prepare accustomed foods, or recent dependency on someone else's food preparation. Prevention of constipation and diarrhea can be accomplished through exercise and stress reduction (see Health Maintenance section in this chapter).

A thorough history and examination of the abdomen are warranted. A thorough diet and drug history often provides important clues to other diagnosis. Some subjective and objective characteristics of different causes of bowel habit change are listed below.

Laxative Abuse is a common cause of both constipation and diarrhea. History of the type and duration will be helpful, and gradual withdrawal of all except bulk-formers is usually indicated.

A majority of *drugs* have some effect on bowel habits, and a careful history of both the patient's prescription and nonprescription drugs is necessary. (See Table 14-6.)

Fecal Impaction may present with watery "overflow" stools or incontinence rather than the expected constipation. Antidiarrheal drugs would certainly be contraindicated. Abdominal and rectal exams are usually diagnostic, and removal of the impaction both confirms and cures the immediate problem. The practitioner must seek the cause of the impaction and give attention both to diet and medications to prevent recurrence.

Infectious Diarrhea is usually of sudden onset, often with fever. Close relatives or associates may be similarly affected. Giardiasis may be the cause, which may lead to colonic ulceration seen on sigmoidoscopy.

Lactase Deficiency, manifested by diarrhea and cramping on eating dairy products, develops in many people as they age. The deficiency may be asymptomatic until stressed by an unusually high dairy meal or by other gastrointestinal problems. A lactose tolerance test may be performed but a three-week therapeutic trial of dairy product avoidance is usually better.[15]

Irritable Bowel Syndrome, with its classical abdominal pain associated with diarrhea alternating with constipation, rarely begins after the age of 60, but symptoms may increase in later life. Mucus often floats in the toilet or in the stool. There may be nausea, belching, and flatulence. Diet and stress reduction are the basic treatment.

Diverticular Disease affects up to 70 percent of the over 80-year-old population and is usually asymptomatic. When symptoms do occur, constipation is more common than diarrhea. Pain may develop, but this is due more to spasm than to diverticulitis. Active diverticulitis usually presents with an increase in localized pain, usually over the left lower quadrant, and is often cramplike. There may be a palpable left lower quadrant mass, muscospasm, and rebound tenderness. Leukocytosis and fever are common. A barium enema is usually indicated. Diverticulitis may cause strictures that are radiographically indistinguishable from cancer, which must always be considered. Medical management for acute disease includes bedrest, nothing by mouth, parenteral fluids, antibiotics, analgesics, and sedatives. Chronic and preventive management includes better diet, exercise, and bowel habits.

Cancer is a major cause both of constipation and diarrhea. See the section on Cancer below.

Ischemic Bowel Disease affects the splenic flexure and the rectosigmoid areas most commonly. Abdominal distention and severe pain with constipation often occurs 15–30 minutes after eating. This rapidly progressive disease results in ischemia and infarction of the colon. Early surgery may be life saving but the prognosis is poor.

Inflammatory Bowel Disease rarely begins during advanced age, although it may persist into that period. Exacerbation of ulcerative colitis may be associated with emotional distress.

Appendicitis, Volvulus, and Intussusception may present initially with bowel habit change alone, most commonly diarrhea. Physical examination hopefully will be diagnostic, but radiographs, blood counts, and frequent reevaluations are often necessary to make a diagnosis in atypical cases. (See Emergency section of this chapter.)

Systemic Disease may cause bowel habit change. Diabetes causes both constipation and diarrhea. Diabetic diarrhea may be nocturnal and associated with steatorrhea. Hyperthyroidism may cause diarrhea, and hypothyroidism, as well as hypercalcemia, may cause constipation. All of these should have other signs and symptoms as well, but bowel symptoms may be the patient's chief complaint.

MANAGEMENT OF CONSTIPATION

Once obstruction and metabolic disorders have been ruled out, the following measures can be instituted[16]:

- Progressively decrease stimulant laxatives if the patient is habituated to them.
- Consider alternatives if medication of other conditions is a possible contributor.
- Increase physical activity of the unnecessarily sedentary patient.
- Increase fluids to 3 quarts a day until improved, then 1–1½ quarts a day maintenance.
- Increase diet fiber (fruit, vegetables, whole wheat). (See Health Maintenance section in this chapter.)
- Institute bowel training. Reestablishing the gastroileocolic response is very important. The patient should spend five to ten minutes a day trying to defecate after a breakfast or dinner, which includes hot fluids (a stimulant).
- Prescribe bulk laxatives.
- Establish a reasonable goal, i.e., three movements a week. Encourage patient concurrence.

Suppositories include glycerin, which is a lubricant and a mild stimulant, and Dulcolax, a stimulant. These are effective on most patients and safe if used infrequently.

Bulk or Stool Laxatives, such as hydrophilic mucilloid (Metamucil) may be necessary; one or more tablespoonsful a day. Dioctyl sodium sulfosuccinate (Colace) may be taken orally with or immediately following meals so it mixes with the food. The dose should be reduced as soon as possible. Chronic use of other types of drugs, including Senna and Cascara, should be avoided as they may cause permanent damage to the gastrointestinal neural system.

Enemas are given every other day to patients on regular diets after attempts to defecate have failed. Enemas can be given less often (once a week) to patients with neurogenic colons and low-residue diet. Enemas should be given with the following considerations[17]:

Types:

- Soap suds, though still commonly used, are not safe and should be considered obsolete.[16]
- Tap water enemas are effective but, because they are hypotonic, may cause volume and electrolyte problems in patients with renal or

heart disease. Isotonic saline is safer for patients except those who retain sodium. Isotonic saline is easily made by adding 2 teaspoons salt to 1 liter of water.

- Commercially prepared enemas such as Fleet and Tucks are hypertonic and made with sodium phosphates. They draw water into the colon. Sodium absorption may be a problem in some patients with cardiac or renal failure.

Administration[17]:

1. Volume should be 500–1000 ml, not more than 3 in succession. More may cause shock or perforation of diverticula.
2. Temperature should be approximately 105° F (lukewarm) for comfort.
3. Patient should be informed of what to expect, relaxed, and in a place of privacy.
4. Position of the patient is not critical; most common is to be positioned on the left side, then repositioned to encourage proximal flow.
5. Well-lubricated tip is inserted gently with a slight twisting motion.
6. Container should be no higher than 24 inches above the patient. Higher elevation causes dangerous pressure levels.
7. Administration rate is based on patient comfort.

Fecal Impaction.   Mass of stool in rectum, too large and hard to pass through anus, requires mechanical fragmentation or softening by local medications or both, followed by a large cleansing enema.

The following sequence may be used until impaction is relieved[17]:

1. Digital fracture or indentation of mass, with attempted partial removal, stopping short of causing pain.
2. Instillation of 4–16 oz of mineral oil to be retained one to two hours.
3. Trial of 1000 ml tap water enema or further manual removal.
4. Instillation of 4 oz of osmotic enema (e.g., Fleets) retaining as long as possible.
5. Meanwhile, 2–4 oz mineral oil by mouth q6–8h.
6. Repeat trial of 1000 ml tap water enema.
7. Repeat digital enema and extract stool.

MANAGEMENT OF DIARRHEA

Tests should be performed to rule out obstructive lesions, infections, ulcerative colitis, hyperthyroidism, diabetes, and drug side effects. Parasite studies,

cultures, sigmoidoscopy, and barium enemas are appropriate. Management of functional diarrhea or irritable colon may consist of reassurance and emotional support alone. Brief but repeated primary care psychotherapy sessions can be aimed at helping patients better deal with life stresses.

When lactase deficiency is expected, a simple therapeutic trial of excluding dairy products is usually adequate. If found to cause diarrhea, dairy products need not be totally eliminated, but reduced or least bothersome ones selected.

Kaopectate, not very helpful in acute explosive diarrhea, does help moderate chronic diarrhea. Antispasmodics, such as the anticholingergics belladonna and atropine, may be helpful but have considerable side effects in especially the elderly, including increased glaucoma, arrhythmias, and urinary retention. They should be used very infrequently. Bulk formers such as psyllium (Metamucil), methylcellulose, and bran are effective. Therefore, these products are good both for diarrhea and constipation, and by the same mechanism, namely, binding water. Diphenoxylate HCl (Lomotil) is not addictive and is safe for chronic diarrheas. Opiates are indicated only in severe chronic diarrheas and when other modalities are unsuccessful.

Minor Functional Complaints

Belching.   Most patients who have excessive belching swallow the air just before belching, apparently an unconscious act that is a nervous habit or is used to adjust abdominal pressures to modify some vague discomfort. The swallowing and belching becomes a vicious cycle and is accompanied by increasing worry. Assurance of normalcy may help, as may behavior modification techniques. Swallowing air while eating is not often a cause of excessive belching, except with hurried meals.[18]

Bloating and Abdominal Discomfort.   This syndrome is often attributed to increased abdominal gas, but usually results from a motility problem with no real increase of intestinal gas. Such patients are more sensitive to normal gas content, so reduction of air intake to a minimum seems logical. Patients should stay in an upright position over one and one-half hours after eating. Anticholinergics may help. Lactose intolerance and organic pathology should be ruled out.[18]

Excessive Flatus.   Excessive flatus is composed

most commonly of carbon dioxide and hydrogen derived from colonic bacterial action. Rarely does it consist of nitrogen from aerophagia. Increased CO_2 production may be due to a generalized malabsorptive disorder or a specific one, such as lactose deficiency. A diet high in fermentable polysaccharides also increases CO_2 production. Since this ingredient is a natural part of most high fiber foods advocated to increase stool bulk to improve colon function, it may not be advisable to restrict them if they seem implicated. Reassurance may be all that is necessary, as flatus and cramps due to this type of fiber usually subside in two to three weeks.

Cholelithiasis

Approximately 30 percent of elderly people have gallstones. The incidence increases with age and is more common in diabetes and in women more than men, especially multiparous women or women taking estrogens. The discovery of gallstones usually is the result of an oral cholecystogram ordered to investigate bouts of abdominal discomfort. Pain is the most important symptom of gall bladder diseases. When the radiologist reports cholelithiasis, the question is what to do about it. The gall bladder may or may not have contributed to the symptoms that led to the study, and it may or may not cause problems to the patient in the future. Obviously, 30 percent of the population should not undergo cholecystectomy. The question of which patients should be operated on remains difficult and controversial. Probably only patients with disturbing and recurrent problems warrant surgery. In helping the patient make the decision, the following points are helpful to keep in mind[11,19]:

- Approximately 30 percent of elders with gallstones will develop serious complications.
- The mortality rate of the elective operation is low in the best hands—probably around 1 percent in the elderly. This rate is considerably higher for surgeons who don't perform the operation very regularly.
- The mortality rate for an emergency cholecystectomy during acute cholecystitis is much higher—2.5 to 3.0 percent—and has been up to 12.5 percent for those whose general condition was so poor that a cholecystostomy had to be performed.
- It is generally recommended that any patient who in the past has had bonafide acute cholecystitis also have an elective cholecystectomy if

possible. The future attack rate and complication rate of this group is very high.
- Whether or not the health of the individual patient will likely tolerate the procedure is obviously a major determinant. The expected longevity is also important, although usually difficult to estimate.
- The dissolving of gallstones medically with chenodeoxycholic acid seems to have excellent results. Studies are not yet complete, however, and the drug is not yet on the market.

Hernias

Most new hernias arising in the elderly are direct inguinal or incisional and are due to progressive weakening of muscle and fascial tissue. Recurrent inguinal hernias, even if the original repair was for indirect hernia, tend to be direct. Fortunately, these new hernias are of the diffuse type and are less likely to incarcerate and strangulate than are funicular types, such as indirect inguinal, femoral or umbilical hernias, which pass through tight rings. Nevertheless, many patients reach old age still carrying uncorrected funicular hernias and may be increasingly subject to incarceration as the ring tissues weaken and more abdominal content protrudes. These funicular hernias should be repaired if the patient can tolerate the procedure. Whether the diffuse-type hernia needs repair is more an issue of patient discomfort than risk of strangulation. A new hernia may, however, be a sign of colon cancer.

The symptom of a hernia is usually only a low-grade ache. When hernias incarcerate, the patient may experience more pain or may simply report that the hernia "won't go back inside." Strangulation, or infarction of herniated viscus, causes increasing pain, fever, leukocytosis—signs of obstruction and peritonitis. These symptoms and signs may develop slowly; it is difficult to tell an incarceration from an early strangulation. Certainly, a strangulated hernia is a surgical emergency. Incarcerated hernias, which can strangulate at any time, should be surgically corrected as soon as possible.

Anal Problems

Various anal problems affect especially those patients who suffer constipation and incontinence, and those patients who cannot maintain good hygiene. Patients will often need careful assistance from family members or the nursing staff.

Anal fissures present as acute severe pain, beginning with the passage of a large or hard stool or a more moderate burning or cutting pain. The pain lasts minutes to hours and may be accompanied by a little bleeding. A V-shaped split is seen on the anal mucosa, usually posterior. Management includes stool softener, sitz baths and a steroid ointment or cream treatment. Sitz baths are taken for 15–20 minutes, four times a day, in 6 inches of comfortably warm water. Recurrent and chronic cases require surgical treatment. Pruritis ani is associated with fissures in many people, particularly the elderly.

Cryptitis causes pain on defecation. The pain is not as severe as with fissures, and anoscopy reveals inflamed, dilated crypts. Treatment is the same as for fissures.

Hemorrhoids are usually asymptomatic. When one becomes thrombosed, the patient experiences acute pain. The mass may be visible outside the anus. The vein can be incised to release the clot with or without local anesthesia, often resulting in immediate relief of pain. Pressure is applied for hemostasis, with cautery or catgut sutures, if necessary. Ice bags for 24 hours help, followed by sitz baths.

Sometimes edematous mass of internal hemorrhoids prolapses outside the anus, often not reducible with a finger. Pain may be initially mild, but progresses as the mass becomes more engorged. Management is bed rest in the prone position, preferably 15 degrees head down, with iced witch hazel compresses on the anus. Ultimately, hemorrhoidectomy is indicated.

Internal hemorrhoids produce intermittent symptoms. Discomfort or bleeding with bowel movements, protrusion on straining associated with soiling of undergarments, and pruritis ani are common. Particularly for the elderly, management is directed toward reduction of constipation and production of soft stools. (See Constipation section.) Specific symptomatic hemorrhoids can be ligated with rubber bands and injected with sclerosing 1 percent phenol in the office. Larger, more difficult hemorrhoids require surgery.

Pruritis Ani is merely the complaint of itching around the anus (also see Chapter 19). It may be caused by nervous tension, irritation from stool, associated fissure, cryptitis, hemorrhoids, intestinal parasites, monilia, or other skin conditions. Careful history and examination to disclose the underlying cause is important. The skin may appear irritated or lichenified, in addition to showing possible signs of specific dermatological diagnosis. Epidermal carcinoma should be considered for suspicious lesions. General measures include:

- Avoid toilet paper.
- Wash anal area with soft cloth or cotton after each bowel movement using plain white soap, or use soft facial tissue if washing is inconvenient.
- Dry with soft cloth or cotton.
- Apply zinc sterate talcum powder, corn starch, or other bland powder.
- Change underpants daily.
- Avoid scratching or abraiding the area.
- Triamcinolone 0.1 percent ointment b.i.d. for ten days.

Cancer

Unfortunately, cancer is a common disease of the elderly. Approximately 10 percent of all deaths among the elderly are due to gastrointestinal cancer. Colon cancer makes up 30 percent of cancer deaths; gastric, 10 percent; pancreas, 10 percent; liver, 8 percent; and esophagus, 2 percent.[6] Cancer of the colon is more common in women and cancer of the rectum more common in men.[1] Patients with anorexia, weakness, and chronic constipation should be thoroughly evaluated for cancer. Other nonspecific symptoms and signs may include weight loss, anemia, and development of a new abdominal hernia. Occult blood loss may be the most reliable sign, although obviously there may be a cause other than cancer. Tarry black or red-streaked stools may also occur.

Colon cancer increases steadily in incidence with age. Patients may present with bowel habit changes, narrowing of stool diameter, weight change, vague discomfort, black or red stools, a mass, or an elevated sedimentation rate. Early detection of ascending colon cancer is more difficult than the more common descending colon tumors, as bowel habit change is less common. Serial stool guaiacs should be done on a patient with any new bowel complaints.

The villous adenoma is not a common type of polyp, but may be malignant in 10–15 percent of cases and be associated with colon cancer in up to one-third of cases. Mucus stools are common with tumor. Low rectal polyps may be missed on rectal exams because they are soft.

Situations that raise the index of suspicion of cancer of specific sites are as follows[7]:

- Dysphagia may indicate cancer of the esophagus.
- A nonhealing or recurrent gastric "ulcer" may be a gastric carcinoma.
- Jaundice, together with a palpable gall bladder, is very likely due to cancer of the pancreas.
- Sudden onset of diabetes may indicate cancer of the pancreas.
- Thrombophlebitis may indicate cancer of the pancreas.
- Acute pancreatitis, especially recurrent, may indicate cancer of the pancreas.
- An enlarging liver in an alcoholic may be due to a primary hepatoma.
- Benign rectal polyps or history of familial polyposis increases the risk of cancer anywhere in the colon.

Management of any suspicious problem should include thorough history and physical examination, CBC, stool guaiac, endoscopy, upper gastrointestinal series, proctoscopy, and barium enema. The rectal exam may find 15 percent of colon cancers, and the proctoscope may visualize another 30 percent. The flexible fiberoptic scopes can visualize most of the colon. Stool guaiacs should be repeated at least three consecutive times during one week. If positive, the patient should be placed on a meat-free diet for four days and then the series of three guaiac tests begun. Vigorous investigation of gastrointestinal complaints by the primary care clinician will result in early detection and better prognosis. Most of the tests indicated are safe and not too expensive.

When cancer of the pancreas is suspected, ultrasonography, computed tomography, endoscopic retrograde cholangiography, angiography, and pancreatic function tests have all been somewhat helpful. The choice of which to pursue is based best on local experience with these modalities.[20]

Carcinoembryonic antigen (CEA) tests have not proven to be helpful because of high rates of both false positives and false negatives.

Treatment of alimentary tract cancer is surgical excision. Mortality from the surgery itself may be 5–12 percent in the elderly, 50 percent higher than in younger patients. Survival rates from the cancer are poor and vary with the site and, of course, with the extent of growth and metastasis. Carcinoma of the distal colon, however, has an 80 percent five-year survival when resected early.[21] (Many clinicians consider adding an alternative therapy such as vis-ualization to the approach. Some research indicates their effectiveness. Refer to Chapter 21.)

The management for the incurable cancer patient is centered on carefully preparing the patient and the family for death, with strong support from the entire primary health care team, hospice groups, and other community resources such as the Cancer Society.

Ostomy Care

Many patients face a life with a colostomy or ileostomy with understandable fear, disgust, or depression. Badly damaged body image, fear of accident from soilage, and fear of rejection, especially in the area of sexual intimacy, join the problems of coping with the disease that led to the "ostomy." Impotence is common, the rate depending on the operation. The spouse and other family members share the negative reactions. Averting these problems is best begun long before the ostomy. Preparation should include careful explanation of the physiology involved, maintenance and control procedures, and with ample opportunity to dispel myths and to ventilate feelings. Much written material and some films are available to patients. There is a very active United Ostomy Association with many local chapters, and enterostomal therapists function in many areas. The primary health care team can help locate and coordinate supportive efforts. The spouse should be involved in as much of this preparation as possible.

Excretion from the ostomy depends greatly on its location. Except for left-sided colostomies, drainage is more or less continous and uncontrollable, with collection bags always needed. (For proximal colostomies and ileostomies, fluid and electrolyte loss may need monitoring.) Left-sided colostomies, the most common in the elderly, generally empty only when irrigated and can be covered with a gauze pad or small pouch. Irrigation is with lukewarm tap water, held at shoulder height above the colostomy, run in air-free through aa catheter attached to one of various manufactured cone-shaped devices, and inserted as far as it will comfortably go. Up to one quart fluid is accepted over ten minutes, followed by 30 minutes emptying time. This is done every day or two. Diet should be high in bulk,[11] but coarse fiber, such as corn, may irritate the stoma.

Skin irritation around the colostomy site comes mostly from tape and adhesive mechanical problems; secondly, from fecal contaminant; and thirdly, from allergy to tapes and adhesives. Irritation can be greatly avoided by[22]:

- Fitting ileostomy appliances carefully with shape and size appropriate to the patient. Refitting several weeks after surgery is usually necessary.
- Cleansing of the skin carefully with plain water or very mild soap, allowing air-drying time as long as possible. Avoid rubbing and perfumed soaps.
- Use of Stomahesive as a water-absorbing seal, a barrier to fecal movement onto the skin.
- Applying adhesive backing carefully, in the body position the patient is likely to be in most of the day, gently smoothing out adhesive from stoma outwards.
- Removal of appliance as seldom as possible, generally once every five to seven days.
- Peeling off adhesives gently, as a banana skin.
- Protecting excoriated skin with Hollister Medical Adhesive or Stomahesive.

HEALTH MAINTENANCE

The foundation of health maintenance and prevention of disease in the gastrointestinal tract is good nutrition and stress reduction. Although life long habits have affected the gastrointestinal system, it is not too late to implement a more healthy regimen. Stress reduction and development of better coping methods will reduce the incidence and the severity of peptic ulcer, dyspepsia, and functional bowel syndrome. The elderly have long-established coping patterns that may need to change to help them with the new stresses of aging. The primary health care team can help identify and alleviate many of these. (See Chapter 21.)

The usual American diet is not the most healthful for the gastrointestinal system. Overconsumption can be prevented by development of the attitude—as early in life as possible—that the purpose of eating is to meet nutritional needs. Food can and should be enjoyed, and the enjoyment should focus on the self-satisfying knowledge of good nutrition and taste, not quantity.

Most American diets are low in fiber content. Diet high in fiber content is important to colonic health. Overrefined diet reduces the bulk necessary for effective colon motility. Chronic constipation and diverticulosis result. Assisting elders to include enough fiber in their diet is important. (See Table

14-7.) Colon cancer is more common in Western nations, and the incidence is increasing. Ingested carcinogens are possible reasons. Avoidance of unnecessary chemicals, including food additives and drugs, is a reasonable precaution. Our overly refined, constipating diet has also been suggested as a contributor to colon cancer, possibly by keeping carcinogens longer in the colon.[23]

Regular, frequent, small, and unhurried meals promote better digestion and help to avoid the bloating and inappropriate gastric acid action associated with large, infrequent or rushed meals. Adequate fluid intake—1½ to 2 quarts a day—may enable easier swallowing and may lessen constipation, particularly in elders.

Avoidance of excessive alcohol will prevent alcoholic liver disease and reduce incidence of gastritis, pancreatitis, folic acid malabsorption, and diarrhea.

Good teeth, natural or dentures, avoid the problem of swallowing poorly masticated food and prevent the boredom and subsequent malnutrition that "edentulous diets" often incur. The elderly need particular attention to gum and periodontal hygiene to preserve remaining teeth. (See Chapter 8.)

Cigarettes will aggravate peptic ulcers and other stomach problems. There are many medicines that irritate the gastrointestinal tract and cause considerable distress. Over-the-counter aspirin and laxatives are bad offenders. Many prescription drugs have irritating effects on the gastrointestinal system or cause an allergenic response. When aspirin, anti-inflammatory drugs, or oral steroids must be taken regularly, the atrophic gastric mucosa can be better protected by the concomitant antacids.

Table 14-7
Total Dietary Fiber of Selected Fruits, Vegetables, and Wheat Products in Grams/100 g Fresh Base

Cabbage, cooked	2.83
Carrots, cooked	3.70
Peas, raw	7.75
Tomato, raw	1.40
Banana	1.75
Apple, flesh only	1.42
Pear, flesh only	2.44
Plum, raw, flesh and skin	1.52
Strawberry, raw	2.12
White flour (75%)	3.45
Brown flour (90–95%)	8.70
Whole wheat	11.00
Bran	48.00

The role of exercise in promoting a healthy gastrointestinal tract cannot be overemphasized. Exercise helps colonic motility and facilitates regular bowel movements. Encouragement of elders to walk daily, do isometric exercises or stretching is particularly important. Many elders become increasingly sedentary for nonmedical reasons, and their more naturally sluggish colons need additional stimulation. (See Chapter 21.)

Maintaining regular bowel habits prevents the discomfort of constipation, the strain of irregular movement on weak colon walls and on diverticula, and the stress on hemorrhoids and fissures. "Regular" for the elderly may be less often than when they were young because they are eating less. Establishment of a regular time for movements and encouragement to respond to urges are important. With good nutrition that includes high fiber, fluids, and exercise, they should be able to have regular movements and avoid laxatives. (See Table 14-8.)

There are several practices relevant to early detection and prevention of gastrointestinal problems. Approximately 15 percent of colon cancers are within the reach of the examining finger. The annual rectal examination is also a good time to review the patient's gastrointestinal symptomatology and risk factors, both of which may have subtly changed since the previous examination.

Proctosigmoidoscopy reveals almost 40 percent of colon carcinomas. However, because of poor patient acceptance, time, cost and some risk, the procedure is not appropriate as part of the annual examination of asymptomatic patients with normal risk factors. It has been recommended that everyone have the procedure once over the age of 55 to rule out polyposis. Annual sigmoidoscopy is indicated if the patient has had a polyp, a family history of colon cancer, continued abnormal bowel habits, or continued positive guaiac stools for which no cause is found on more extensive investigation.

An annual stool guaiac test reveals occult bleeding from carcinoma, peptic ulcer, or (rarely) diverticula, which may be otherwise asymptomatic. False positives due to the trauma of the exam or due to recent ingestion of rare meat are common. The patient should perform three serial tests at home on regularly passed stool. Home guaiac tests are also appropriate for patients who refuse a rectal examination.

Table 14-8
Ways to Add Fiber or Bulk to the Foods You Eat*

- The best way—eat bran cereal such as All Bran or Bran Buds. Start with a bowlfull each day for several weeks, then cut the amount down to 2 or 3 tablespoons a day, or whatever is needed for regularity.

- Add bran to things you make—like quick breads, muffins, pancakes, homemade granola (1/2 oats and 1/2 bran). You can also use Raisin Bran or 40% Bran Flakes as a cereal substitute after several weeks on the 100% bran.

- Eat 100% whole wheat bread instead of white bread. Look at the label on the bread you buy—the first ingredient listed should be "whole wheat flour"; if it just says "enriched flour" or "wheat flour," it means white flour.

- Use whole grain cereals such as oatmeal, Zoom, Roman Meal, or Ralston instead of low fiber cereals like cream of rice or cream of wheat. These cereals also are good in meatloaf or meatballs, etc., instead of bread crumbs.

- Cooked dried beans are a good source of fiber, too—try pinto beans, split peas, red beans, other beans, and dried peas in casseroles, soups, dips, fillings for tacos, etc.

- Eat whole fruits, including peels where practical, instead of drinking juice.

- Use salads often. Nibble on raw vegetables like carrots and celery instead of sweet, sugary snacks.

- Also important—use less foods with sugar. Sugar replaces the fiber and other important nutrients in foods. Instead of sweet desserts, try fresh fruit for dessert. Eat a good breakfast so you won't be tempted to grab a donut snack or other sweet food.

*Occasionally, the use of lots of fiber all at once can cause gas in some people. But stick with it—all problems will be gone in one or two weeks.

The instructions to the patient on the Hemocult package are helpful.

Prevention of complications of some gallstones may be achieved by giving chenodeoxycholic acid, which slowly dissolves cholesterol (radiolucent) gall stones. Currently only in some research centers, this drug may soon be generally available.

A Final Word

Several issues of importance to keep in mind when treating elders with gastrointestinal problems:

- Gastrointestinal problems are very common in the elderly.
- These problems often present differently in the elderly than in younger patients.

- Problems are often functional rather than organic.
- It is often difficult to tell the difference.
- Many of the organic problems are critical to the patient's life—especially cancer, ulcer, and cholecystitis.
- Thorough investigation of complaints is therefore warranted.
- Functional complaints often respond well to simple measures.
- Most of the problems are preventable.
- The whole primary health care team, community resources, the family, and, most importantly, the patient can be effective in promoting a healthier individual.

REFERENCES

1. Schuster MM: Disorders of the aging GI system. Hosp pract 11(9):95–101, 1976
2. US National Health Survey: Acute Conditions. DHEW Pub No. (PHS) 79-1560, Sept 1979, p 14
3. Wilder CS: Limitation of activity due to chronic conditions, United States, 1974. Vital and Health Statistics: Series 10, Data from the National Health Survey; No. 111, DHEW Pub No. HRA 76-1537. June 1977, p 18
4. Bhamthumnavin K, Schuster MM: Aging and gastrointestinal function, in Finch CE, Hayflick L (eds): The Biology of Aging. New York, Van Nostrand Reinhold, 1977, pp 709–723
5. Sklar M: Gastrointestinal diseases in the aged, in Reichel W (ed): Clinical Aspects of Aging. Baltimore, Williams & Wilkins, 1978, pp 173–182
6. Morton JH: Alimentary tract cancer, in Rubin, P (ed): Clinical Oncology. American Cancer Society, 1974
7. Steinheber FU: Interpretation of g.i. symptoms in the elderly. Med Clin NA 60:1141–1157, 1976
8. Ferris P: Surgical management of the elderly. Hosp Prac 11:65–71, 1976
9. Yusuf MF, Dunn E: Appendicitis in the elderly: Learn to discern the untypical picture. Geriatr 34(9):73–79, 1979
10. Gardner B: Acute intra-abdominal inflammatory disease, in Shaftor GW, Gardner B (eds): Quick Reference to Surgical Emergencies. Philadelphia, Lippincott, 1974, pp 211–228
11. Spiro HM: Clinical gastroenterology, ed 2. New York, Macmillan, 1977, pp 308, 916–928, 872
12. Fisher RS, Cohen S: Gastroesophageal reflux. Med Clin NA 62:3–20, 1978
13. Chapman ML: Peptic ulcer. Med Clin NA 62:39–51, 1978
14. Narayanan M, Steinheber FU: The changing face of peptic ulcer in the elderly. Med Clin NA 60:1159–1172, 1976
15. Kohli D: Lactose intolerance, add milk to your g.i. suspect list. Pat Care 10(2):116–126, 1976
16. Brocklehurst JC: How to define and treat constipation. Geriatr 32:85–87, 1977
17. Hogstel M: How to give a safe and successful cleansing enema. AJ Nurs 77:816–817, 1977
18. Bond JH, Levitt MD: Gaseousness and intestinal gas. Med Clin NA 62:155–171, 1978
19. Pearlman BJ, Schoenfield LJ: Gallstones. Med Clin NA 62:87–105, 1978
20. Go VLW, Sheedy PF: Ultrasonography, computed tomography, endoscopic retrograde cholangiography and angiography in the diagnosis of pancreatic cancer. Med Clin NA, 62:129–140, Jan 1978
21. Peterson BA, Kennedy BJ: Aging and cancer management, I: Clinical observations, cancer. Cancer J Clin 29:322–332, 1979
22. Lazar P et al: Recognizing, Treating and Preventing Ostomy-related Skin Problems. Chicago, Hollister, 1977
23. Southgate DAT, Bailey B, et al: A guide to calculating intakes of dietary fiber. J Human Nutr 30:303–313, 1976
24. Wallach J: Interpretation of Diagnostic Tests, ed 2. Boston, Little Brown & Co, 1974, pp 8–9
25. American Pharmaceutical Association: Handbook of Non-prescription Drugs, ed 5, 1977, pp 6, 13–17
26. National Center for Health Statistics: Vital Statistics. DHEW (PHS), 1974

RECOMMENDED RESOURCES

Finch CE, Hayflick L (eds): The Biology of Aging. New York, Van Nostrand Reinhold, 1977

An excellent review of changes and relationship to symptoms and disease processes. See especially Chapter 27, Aging and the gastrointestinal function, by K. Bhanthumnavin and M. Schuster.

Shafton GW, Gardner B (eds): Quick Reference to Surg-ical Emergencies. Philadelphia, JB Lippincott, 1974
Clear, precise guide to diagnosis and management.

Spiro HM: Clinical Gastroenterology, ed 2. New York, Macmillan, 1977
Exceptionally pleasant writing and well organized.

Steinhaber FU: Interpretation of g.i. symptoms in the elderly. Med Clin NA 60:1147–57, 1976
Excellent differential diagnosis.

15

Musculoskeletal System

JoAnn Trolinger, F.N.P., M.H.S.
David Daehler, M.D.
Andre Calin, M.D., M.A., M.R.C.P.

The cornerstone of the care of elders with musculoskeletal conditions is aimed at keeping patients mobile and independent in their home environment. The most gratifying and important physical sign to see in the older person is ambulation. The patient should enter into planning appropriate therapeutic regimes to encourage his or her cooperation and effort to attain that goal. It is equally important to involve family and friends in these plans so they may help the patient to maintain his or her independence through encouragement in treatment programs.

Normal aging brings degenerative changes in joints, tendons, and muscles. Most joints lose range of motion, although some may increase mobility due to stretched ligaments. The spine may lose up to half its range. The decrease in muscle mass results in less skill and strength as worn tendons can easily rupture. Bone atrophies with loss of mineral content.

INCIDENCE OF MUSCULOSKELETAL PROBLEMS

The normal changes in locomotion result in many aches and pains; muscle strains and joint pains are the most common problems encountered, and manifest themselves in a variety of complaints.

Progressive kyphosis adds abnormal stress on posture and gait, requiring extension of the cervical spine and aggravating painful shoulders. Degenerative changes in joint structure frequently result in stiffness and pain. These syndromes will result in decreased use, which leads to further immobility and atrophy.

Elders have many muscle strains and fractures. The progressive sensory losses of hearing and visual acuity, coupled with some unsteadiness, dizziness, and loss of muscle coordination, make the elderly much more vulnerable to these problems.

Fracture of the neck of the femur is a very common occurrence. Prior to the age of 50, such fractures are negligible in numbers, but double with each five-year period above the age of 60. They occur 2.4 times more frequently in females than males. The complications of fractured hips remain among the common precipitating events leading to death. Other common fractures are of the wrist and vertebrae.[1]

Osteoarthritis affects 50 percent of persons in their 50s and 85 percent in their 70s. Rheumatoid disease has been reported in 15 percent of women and 5 percent of men over 65.[2] Gout is encountered more frequently as age increases with a peak onset in the 60s. Osteoporosis is a common problem that occurs more frequently in women than men by a ratio of two to one. It has been estimated to affect 15 million Americans and is more frequent in whites than blacks.[3]

Uncommon Problems

There are many uncommon problems in the musculoskeletal system that affect elders.

Palymyalgia rheumatism is a relatively new syndrome that occurs mostly in patients over 60. Those affected develop symmetrical pain and stiffness of the shoulders and, to a lesser degree, of the hips. Other areas such as the cervical, lumbar, and limbs are occasionally involved. Stiffness is most evident at night while symptoms diminish in daytime hours. It is usually accompanied by a weight loss of 10–20 lb and a markedly elevated erythrocyte sedimentation rate. It is thought that the condition relates to giant cell arthritis, and a few patients show involvement of the temporal arteries. The condition is dramatically reversed by oral steroids. Early treatment will prevent the small but devastating chance of blindness.[4]

Dermatomyositis occurs, presenting with its polymyositis and the characteristic rash. It is often associated with malignant disease in elders.[4]

Carpal tunnel syndrome does appear in elders, although it is more insidious and more likely to be secondary to an old injury, rheumatoid arthritis, myxedema, or myelomatosis. Conservative treatment with splinting and steroid injection can be helpful, but surgery is still the best treatment. In elders, it may be necessary to accept that the median nerve is permanently damaged and surgery not helpful.[4]

Paget's disease occurs with excess bone resorption and excess bone deposition characterizing the disease. Twenty percent of patients are asymptomatic, but bone pain in the lumbar vertebrae, sacrum, pelvis, and skull are the common symptoms. Treatment is largely unsuccessful and is aimed primarily at relief of pain.[4]

Medical and Surgical Emergencies

Polymyalgia rheumatica can be considered an emergent condition because treatment prevents the possibility of blindness due to temporal arteristis. Also an urgent problem in need of immediate relief is gout with its excrutiating pain. (See description of gout on page 222.)

Infections in joints are urgent. The most common organism is staphylococcus; its enzymes destroy cartilage quickly. Knees are most frequently involved, but hips, ankles, shoulders, elbows, and wrists are likely areas as well. Joint infections in elders may not be easy to diagnose as many have ongoing, treated rhematoid arthritis, making it easy to assume the problem is just a worsening of the known disease. Any unexamined swelling should be investigated and treated thoroughly with systemic therapy if infection is discovered.

DIAGNOSIS AND TREATMENT OF COMMON PROBLEMS

Degenerative Osteoarthritis

The prevalence of osteoarthritis increases with age, but many people with x-ray evidence of relatively advanced disease have few or no complaints, while frequently patients with minimal changes on x-ray have relatively severe pain. Some physicians term those cases associated with inflammatory aspects as osteoarthritis and those without inflammatory symptoms or complaints as osteoarthrosis.

The pathologic changes are an exaggerated manifestation of the aging process. The cause, however, is not completely understood. Certainly the wear and tear of mechanical factors—such as obesity and repetitive activity—probably do play a major part in the development of this condition, but most likely biochemical abnormalities are also contributing factors. The infrequent occurrence of osteoarthritis in weight-bearing joints, such as the ankle, and the common occurrence of it in the distal finger joints, questions wear and tear as the only cause.[4]

There is a gradual thinning and breakdown of the joint cartilage with bony sclerosis, marginal spurring or eburnation of bone with the development of subarticular bone cysts. With the distortion of the joints that occurs, there is further breakdown of the joint itself.[5]

DATA BASE

The patient usually presents with overall good health, but with the gradual onset of discomfort related to joints involved with loss of motion. The involvement is usually asymmetric with the knee being the most common joint afflicted. Other frequent sites are distal interphalangeal joints (DIPs), proximal interphalangeal joints (PIPs), spine, hips, and first metacarpal and first metatarsal joints.

On history, the patient may offer such complaints as: "My knee gives out while walking," "It is hard to climb stairs," "It is hard to get up from a chair," "It is difficult to tie my shoes," "I have a dull ache in my hip (or buttocks)." Others will mention bothersome stiffness.

Symptoms may develop acutely with swelling, redness, and pain (often severe) of the joint involved. Often a history of some unusual activity or strain exists. There is usually limitation of passive motion of the joint involved, with pain elicited at extremes of the motion with crepitus. The joint is tender, and frequently there is evidence of effusion. In the hip, limitation of abduction and internal rotation are usual, with pain elicited when the range is passively increased. The DIPs may have Herberden's nodes—hard swellings on the dorsal surfaces. Quadriceps wasting is rather common when the knee is involved.

Low back pain is a very common complaint among the elderly. Although much of this may be related to chronic strain secondary to postural changes, the osteoarthritic changes in the spine do seem to aggravate or prolong disability. Frequently the pain is localized to the lumbosacral level of the low back, but in many patients there is radiation of the pain into the buttocks and down the posterior thigh—similar to that seen with nerve root irritation from disc herniation. With the narrowing of the disc spaces and hypertrophic overgrowth of bone (spur formation) of osteoarithritis, there is impingement on the foraminal canal, causing some pressure or inflammation of the associated nerve roots. This is likely to cause pain similar to disc herniations.

LAB VALUES

Laboratory values are usually normal, but occasionally there is a relatively elevated Erythrocyte Sedimentation Rate (ESR, Sed Rate). This perhaps is related to inflammatory changes and, as the inflammation subsides, the ESR returns to normal.

MANAGEMENT

Degenerative changes are irreversible. The aim of treatment is therefore toward the relief of symptoms and improvement of joint function and activity. Physiotherapy, weight loss, external support, anti-inflammatory and analgesic drugs, and rest are the general treatment. The use of appropriate analgesic medications or anti-inflammatory medications should be combined with active exercise. As with all drug therapy in elders, "start low, go slow" is an extremely important fact to keep in mind. Aspirin remains the best and safest analgesic with anti-inflammatory qualities, but must be prescribed on a regular dosage schedule of 10–15 grains, four times daily to act effectively. If stomach upset occurs this can be treated with antacids. This is preferable to the enteric-coated tablets that do not seem to be as effective. Some patients will develop GI bleeding with the use of aspirin, so stools should be monitored for occult blood when the patient is on this medication regularly.

Other nonsteroidal, antiinflammatory agents such as indomethacin (Indocin), naproxen (Naprosyn), fenoprofen calcium (Nalfon), tolmetin sodium (Tolectin), ibuprofen (Motrin), have proven helpful with many patients. The response to these varies and can be determined by a trial period of two to three weeks.

Other agents helpful for pain relief are acetaminophen (Tylenol), ethoheptazine citrate (Lactarin), or textrapropoxyphene hydrochloride (Darvon).[6] It should be kept in mind that aspirin and some of the antiinflammatory agents (Indocin, Butazolidin) enhance the effect of Coumadin, so precautions must be observed when used in patients taking Coumadin.

The exercise routine is to improve the range of motion of the involved joints while improving the strength of the muscles responsible for movement and joint support. A wider range of movement distributes forces over a larger area of articular surface and helps break the vicious circle—painful joint, muscle inhibition, muscle atrophy, impaired joint stability—that leads to a worsening of the joint diseases. The family can be most helpful in keeping the patient active and ambulatory, as well as in encouraging exercise routines to develop muscle power and joint motion.

The Knee. Elevation of the extended legs while in the sitting position will add some tone and strength to the quadriceps muscle, which is the major muscle involved in stability of the knee. If more strengthening of this muscle is necessary, simple weight lifting of 3 to 10 pounds can be easily worked into the schedule, using a gallon plastic container with the appropriate amount of water as weight. It is important to start with small weights and to increase gradually as tolerated by the patient.

The Low Back. When the low back is involved, developing strength in the abdominal muscles is of help in stabilizing the support of the back. This can be done by isometric contraction of the abdominal muscles while in the supine position. A sit-up is more helpful if it can be performed. It is wise to have the knees and hips flexed for the sit-up to relax the iliopsoas muscle and to prevent hyperextension of the low back.

Physical therapy that applies heat to the areas of involvement with hot packs, radiant heat diathermy, and ultrasound can be very successful when coupled with passive and active muscle-building activity.[1] Occasionally, the use of traction *for involvement* of the low back or the cervical spine, and the above routine, adds to the improvement of the patient's symptoms. During the acute "flare up" of low back pain, short-term use of elastic bracing is of help. This must be combined with a muscle-building program to prevent further muscle atrophy, which would lead to increased strain and disability.

Hips. An orthopedic surgeon is an important team member in the management of the patient who is having fairly constant pain in one of the major weight-bearing joints, or whose joint motion has become restricted to the point of making ambulation difficult. Total hip replacement has added improved function and quality of living for those with advanced joint breakdown. This procedure is utilized when pain has become a constant companion or when limitation of joint motion is so restricted as to prevent adequate mobility. With appropriate selection and preparation for surgery, it is often successful. Although often difficult to convince, the elderly do quite well when selection is appropriate and they are well prepared for surgery. Weight reduction is also a major consideration of importance when any of the weight-bearing joints are involved.

Rheumatoid Arthritis

Rheumatoid arthritis is a chronic disease. The joints are usually involved symmetrically and marked by inflammatory changes in the synovial membranes, articular structures with atrophy, and rarefaction of the bones.[7]

The natural course of the disease results in progressive destruction of articular and periarticular structures, leading to deformity and ankylosis. The usual joints involved are the proximal interphalangeal (fingers and toes), metacarpophalangeal, metatarsophalangeal, wrists, ankles, knees, elbows, and shoulders.

DATA BASE

The onset may be abrupt with simultaneous inflammation in multiple joints or insidious with progressive joint involvement. The onset of the disease is usually between the ages of 35–45, with women affected two to three times more frequently than men. The disease may, however, occur in the later years with about equal frequency in both sexes.[1] If the onset is in the 70s or 80s, it may be more explosive, have more systemic involvement and widespread muscle pain than in younger patients.[4]

Tenderness of the inflamed joints is the most sensitive physical sign, with synovial thickening the most specific physical finding. Morning stiffness lasting one or more hours, or noted after periods of inactivity, is one of the chief complaints. This is associated with obvious joint swelling and pain. The joints are usually noted to be warm and red. The disease can be quite variable in terms of progress and joint destruction. In some cases, very minimal joint destruction and deformity result, while in others the process is severe and widespread.

The disease is a generalized systemic illness and is frequently associated with increased fatigability, malaise, and low-grade fever.[6] Anorexia, weight loss, depression and slowly developing anemia may also be noted. Deformities may occur early in the course of the disease—such as flexion contractures and ulnar deviation of the fingers at the metacarpophalangeal joints.

When the disease first begins after the age of 60, there seems to be less involvement of the wrists and ankles. The x-ray changes are more severe, but there appears to be less deformity. There also seem to be less systemic features of weight loss, lymph node and splenic enlargement, as well as morning stiffness, than in the younger age group with this disease. The older patients also responded better than the young to gold therapy.

LAB VALUES

The sedimentation rate is elevated in approximately 90 percent of cases, with an elevated titre of rheumatoid factor noted in approximately 80 percent of cases. The anemia is usually normochromic or slightly hypochromic and normocytic, which is characteristic of most chronic disease states. There is some overlap with other collagen diseases, so that about 10–20 percent may have positive antinuclear antibodies and/or lupus erythematosus cells present on smear.[6]

X-rays of involved joints show periarticular demineralization and soft tissue swelling in the early stages, with erosion of marginal bone, loss of cartilage, and eventually deformities noted as the disease progresses.[6] The rate of x-ray deterioration is variable as is the clinical course of the disease.

TREATMENT

The management of rheumatoid disease is one of the most difficult for the clinician, particularly with elders. It requires the team approach, with constant psychological support and encouragement. A consultation from a rheumatologist is often helpful in establishing a care plan to be carried out by the primary care clinician. Goals of therapy include: (1) decrease of pain, swelling and discomfort; (2) develop optimum function for individual joints and the entire body; (3) keep drug toxicity to a minimum; and (4) avoid unnecessary costs.

Since many of the patients coming into the older years will have gross deformities due to joint destruction from the early onset of this disease, the use of appropriate splinting and support will aid these people in their daily activities. Physical and occupational therapy can be utilized to advantage in helping these patients care for themselves as much as possible. Keeping joints as mobile as possible with maintenance of muscle tone through regular physical therapy—while advising and developing utensils for feeding, combing hair, putting on shoes, etc.—is carried out by the occupational therapist and is essential to elders with debilitating chronic disease.

For the acute disease, treatment revolves around the use of antirheumatic, antiinflammatory medications in conjunction with physical and occupational therapy. Support and splinting must be utilized to maintain joints in their normal relaxed positions and to prevent some of the destruction of ligaments and tendons seen as the joints are destroyed. Such therapy also helps to prevent the development of muscle contractures that make ambulation more difficult.

Aspirin or salicylates are the mainstay of therapy and should be the first drugs used in treatment. The dosage for effective relief is variable, ranging from 40 g (8 aspirin tabs) to 80 g (16 aspirin tabs) per day. To be effective, serum levels of salicylate should range from 15–30 mg% and should be checked with blood drawn approximately two hours following aspirin ingestion. Failure of aspirin therapy is frequently related to noncompliance, which can be monitored by careful history and at times by following the serum levels. Side effects of aspirin are gastrointestinal irritation with occasional bleeding and tinnitus. Other forms of salicylate may be

considered, although some authorities feel that enteric-coated aspirin is not as effective. Monitoring hemoglobin levels is important with long-term use.

The past decade has provided a proliferation of nonsteroidal, antiinflammatory agents that have proven helpful in the treatment of this disease. These agents have some analgesic effect while the antiinflammation effects a reduction of joint swelling, lowering in the sedimentation rate, and diminishes the morning joint stiffness. There are many drugs available—such as indomethacin (Indocin), ibuprofen (Motrin), naproxen (Naprosyn), tolmetin sodium (Tolectin), etc. These agents are advised in those patients who have not responded to aspirin therapy. Exton Smith and Oversteal suggest the use of rapid-acting preparations in the morning and late afternoon, with a long-acting preparation at night.[5] In contrast to younger patients, pain in older persons may not serve as a guide for recommending activity. Often the severe destructive changes cause pain that would seem to indicate the inevitable loss of function. It often subsides after a week or two and ease of function returns.[4]

When these measures give no improvement, gold therapy [gold sodium thiomalate (Myochrysine)] may be useful. Gold therapy seems to work better on those patients who develop their disease in the later years. This should not be used with those who have hepatic or renal disease, blood dyscrasia, or acute lupus erythematosus. Careful monitoring for toxicity by following the urinalysis and blood count, including platelets, is important. Injections are given at weekly intervals, beginning with 25 mg and increasing to 50 mg weekly until 1000 mg have been given or significant improvement is noted. Fifty mg are then given every three to six weeks as a maintenance regimen, continuing to monitor the urine and blood count and questioning the patient about possible toxic reactions to heavy metal. Pruritis, dermatitis, and stomatitis are the most frequent mild reactions that may be counteracted to some degree with the use of vitamin B$_6$.

Corticosteroids are the most dramatically effective anti-inflammatory drugs for short-term use, but their widespread use during the 1950s has made us aware of the diminishing benefit and complicating side effects with long-term use. As long as they are closely monitored, they may occasionally play a role for short-term use for severe episodes of disease. Intra-articular injection of steroids may, in some cases, help control local synovitis in select joints with relief of symptoms from two to six weeks. Caution relating to overuse of the injected joint must be observed or more joint destruction may result. Although the side effects have decreased the use of steroids in rheumatoid arthritis, Dr. R. Grahame[8] feels there may be a place for daily small doses of prednisone for elderly patients who are unable to move about because of their disease. He suggests dosages up to 7.5 mg daily, with the realization that the dangerous side effects may not become a problem during the lifetime of such elderly patients.

Surgery. Surgery is another modality of treatment. When active synovitis persists despite the use of general and local measures, synovectomy (removal of the inflamed synovial membrane) should be considered. The success of this measure depends to a great degree on the absence of gross destructive change within the joint. Removing the synovium often leads to relief of pain, swelling, and disability. The consultation of a rheumatologist and orthopedic surgeon is necessary in making this decision.

When considerable joint destruction has occurred, stabilization of the joint can be accomplished by arthrodesis (stiffening of the joint). This measure is frequently used in the wrist to give a pain-free, stable joint with beneficial effect on hand function. The ankle can also be stabilized in a similar fashion to aid in continued ambulation.

Replacement arthroplasty has been of great benefit for knee and hip replacement, as well as for small joints of the fingers and hand. This allows for movement and use of the joint, as well as accomplishing freedom from the pain and further destruction of the joint.

As with any chronic disease, a very important aspect of care is education about the disease—not only for the patients themselves, but also for their families and significant friends who share in their support. The management of individual patients will vary, but since there is no known cure for this disease, a realistic approach with the utilization of a team consisting of a primary care physician, rheumatologist, social worker, nurse practitioner–physicians assistant, physical therapist, and occupational therapist has proven to be helpful. Family involvement is optimally desired for care of daily needs, aid in physical therapy routines, and can be extremely helpful and supportive for the frequent episodes of depression.

Gout

Gout is a disorder of metabolism characterized by recurrent attacks of arthritis of peripheral joints that result from deposition of monosodium urate crystals in and about the joints and tendons. The disease primarily involves males with peak onset in the fifth decade. It involves females after menopause with a peak onset in the sixth decade. In a series studied by Grahame and Scott, 11.6 percent of the patients experienced their first attack of gout after the age of 60.[8]

The first metatarsophalangeal joint is the most commonly affected joint, but the metatarsal joints, ankle, knee, wrist, and elbow are other common sites. Over 95 percent of patients with gout have elevated levels of uric acid in their blood. Since uric acid sals have limited solubility in biologic fluids, there is precipitation of crystals into joints and tissues. An inflammatory reaction to the periarticular deposits of crystals accounts for the acute attack, with further deposition leading to joint damage and further disability. A similarly related disease with the same general manifestation is pseudogout, which is evidenced by deposition of crystals of calcium prophosphate dihydrate in the articular cartilage of joints.

DATA BASE

An acute attack of gout usually makes its appearance without warning. It may be precipitated by minor trauma such as ill-fitting shoes or overindulgence in food or alcohol. Occasionally fatigue, infection, or emotional distress may trigger an attack.

Clinical characteristics of the acute attacks are usually dramatic. Normally, they begin suddenly in a joint of the lower extremities and often at night. Within a few hours of onset, the afflicted joint becomes red, swollen, warm, and exquisitely tender. The skin becomes tense and shiny with a dusky red or purplish color. The swelling characteristically extends beyond the anatomic confines of the joint because of the periarticular edema. The intense, extensive swelling, redness, and warmth often resemble septic arthritis or cellulitis. Patients frequently describe the pain as crushing; weight bearing and sometimes even the pressure of bedclothes are intolerable. The attacks usually subside within a few days or weeks, and there is complete restoration of joint function. The patient may be asymptomatic for months or years between attacks. With repeated attacks, there is joint destruction secondary to the urate deposits.

The diagnosis can usually be made both from the rather distinct history and from physical findings. Definitive diagnosis is made, however, by the identification of the urate crystals from joint or tophi aspiration. Many people with no history of gout have elevated uric acid levels so that one cannot make the diagnosis by blood uric acid levels alone. In the young patient, family history is positive in 36 percent, while, with the onset of gout above the age of 60, the family history is positive in only 12 percent. Alcohol consumption and its relation to gout remains controversial. The daily use of alcohol, however, is a common cause of elevation of the uric acid level in the blood. In the presence of chronic gout, x-rays reveal punched-out lesions in the subchondral bone, but this is not specific for the disease.

TREATMENT

Three drugs are commonly used for acute gouty arthritis—colchicine, phenylbutazone (Butazolidin), and indomethacin (Indocin). Colchicine for years was the drug of choice in treating the acute attack. The method has been to give 0.6 mg of colchicine every hour until the symptoms subside or until diarrhea or vomiting occur. Satisfactory response is usually obtained with the use of 8–10 doses. Because of toxicity, no more than 7 mg of the drug should be used in a 48-hour period.

In recent years it has been found that the anti-inflammation agents have been effective in treating the acute attacks. Phenylbutazone 200 mg q6h hours for 48 hours or indomethacin 50 mg q6h hours for 48 hours have been appropriate forms of therapy. Since these drugs do cause gastric irritation, giving them with food is indicated.

After two or three acute attacks, it is appropriate to consider long-term treatment to prevent future attacks. Lowering the level of uric acid can be attained with the use of uricosuric agents such as probenecid (Benemid) on a long-term prophylactic basis. These agents work by causing the kidney to excrete uric acid. These agents should be avoided during an acute attack as they frequently cause an exacerbation of symptoms.

In cases of proven, recurrent gout with kidney involvement, a new agent—allopurinol (Zyloprim)—may be helpful. This prevents the development of uric acid in the body by its action as a zanthine oxidase inhibitor. This agent should not be employed during the acute attack and when first instituted may precipitate an acute attack. This reaction may be prevented by administering indomethacin 25 mg twice daily or colchicine 0.5 mg twice daily along with the allopurinol.

Prosthetic replacement for severely destroyed metatarsophalangeal joints should be kept as a possible option for relief of pain and disability due to limited joint motion.

Acute Muscle Strain

Muscle and ligamentous strain is one of the most common problems causing elders to seek medical care. Muscles in poor tone due to lack of exercise, and those with some atrophy are more vulnerable to strain when unusual or unexpected stress is demanded of them. This can occur following simple activities such as carrying a bag of groceries, stepping unexpectedly off a curb, or merely twisting the body to place a carried load onto a table. More frequently, the acute strain is a result of some unusually heavier activity such as lifting or moving furniture or other items of substantial weight. Minor automobile accidents are also a major cause of muscle and ligamentous strain of the neck and low back, which will be discussed separately.

DATA BASE

The onset of pain following a strain varies according to the severity of the injury. The pain may develop very shortly after the event, but with the less severe injury the pain may not be noticed until 48 hours have elapsed. Frequently the patient has forgotten the activity that caused the strain. Specific questioning about tasks performed around the home or any unusual activity that may account for the symptoms is often necessary to obtain the history of the injury event. Having the patient discuss their activities for three days prior to the office visit will frequently lead to the elusive injury event. Eliciting a detailed account of the mechanics of the activity in question will help in understanding the specific strain involved.

The localization of the pain is determined by the muscle group involved in the injury. The most common area involved is the low back or lumbosacral level of the back. When the upper extremities are utilized for unusual effort, the pectoral muscle area of the chest becomes involved, and pain is frequently localized to the origin of the muscle on the anterior chest wall. Since these muscles are attached to the ribs, even the chest motion of breathing may cause pain in the area of strain. Strain of the muscles of the upper back may cause radiation of the pain around to the anterior chest—often following the intercostal nerve distribution.

The patient complains of dull pain in the area of involvement, which becomes more noticeable on moving about after being at rest or sitting for a prolonged period of time. Some movements become difficult because of the pain elicited when the injured muscles are used. The low back can be most disabling in this regard, making it difficult for the patient to get out of bed during the acute phase.

On physical examination, the muscles involved with the strain are tender to firm palpation and to kneading or pinching between thumb and index finger. Muscle spasm may occur, noted by tightness of the muscles on examination. In general, the more severe the injury the more spasm is noted. Having the patient actively contract the involved muscles against resistance elicits pain. When the origin of the pectoral muscles is involved, this area on the ribs becomes more tender to palpation. Be aware that occasionally a person may fracture a rib while lifting a heavy object.

Low Back Strain. On examining the back, there usually is limitation of the range of motion with a pulling pain noted on flexion, rotation, and frequently on lateral bending as well. Extension of the low back very commonly is painful in the elderly perhaps because of arthritic changes in the facet joints, coupled with some settling of these joints due to decrease in disc spaces. Therefore, noting pain on this motion is not very helpful. With severe back strain, there is occasionally some radiation of pain along the sciatic nerve distribution into the legs. This may be related to the muscle spasm in association with some narrowing of the neural foramen. It is not necessarily due to disc herniation.

X-rays are helpful to determine if there is any new compression fracture of vertebrae, as such fractures in the elderly may occur simply with heavy lifting.

TREATMENT

The important point in treating acute strains is to keep these patients as active as possible during the healing process. Degenerative joint disease (osteoarthritis) is almost universally present in the elderly, and prolonged bedrest or inactivity will cause a stiffening of the facet joints of the back, leading to further disability. Following a strain of the muscle, there is a shortening of the individual muscle fibers, which is a part of the muscle spasm noted. It is felt that much of the pain of the strain may be due to the spasm itself or secondary to possible ischemia caused by the muscle spasm. Allowed to remain, the muscle group will shorten and stiffen in the shortened posture.

The approach to treating the patient with strain is therefore aimed at a reduction of the muscle spasm involved. It must be realized that treatment is modified according to the individual findings based on severity of the injury. In some cases, bedrest will be necessary for a short period of time; for others, some form of simple back support will be helpful; for the majority, an immediate program of muscle stretching and muscle building, worked out with a physical therapist, is the proper approach.

Low Back Strain. The position ideal for treatment when the patient is in bed is the contour position. This can be obtained in the home setting by using a tilted chair under the head of the mattress and by placing some pillows or a suitcase under the knees beneath the mattress. This keeps the back tissues and muscles in the stretched (lengthening or relaxed) position while opening the posterior portion of the vertebral spaces.

When bedrest with or without pelvic traction is used for any period of time, flexion exercises stretching out the tight muscles of the low back is an active and essential part of the treatment program. Without this, there will be more muscle shortening with stiffening of arthritic joints leading to more pain and disability. When pelvic traction is used, the angle of pull should be upwards, rather than straight, to stretch the lower back area and open the posterior portion of the vertebral spaces. Weights of 12–25 lbs are utilized for the traction, geared to the size of the patient and the severity of the strain and muscle spasm. See Fig. 15-1.

Five major exercise routines are of help in the treatment of acute injury or strain of the low back

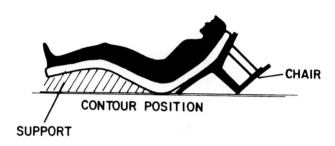

CONTOUR POSITION

SUPPORT

CHAIR

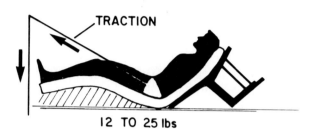

TRACTION

12 TO 25 lbs

Fig. 15-1[9]

and are useful in the prevention of future strain. All exercises are performed with the knees in the flexion, thus preventing the exaggerated extension caused by the use of the iliopsoas muscles when the legs are in extension. The routines are:

1. Stretching of the low back is attained by flexing the knees onto the chest or by dropping the chest onto the knees. This may be performed while lying in bed or on the floor flexing the knees, pulling them to the chest, and causing the body to curl up. The same maneuver may be carried out while seated in a chair by dropping the chest to the knees. See Fig. 15-2.

2. Strengthening of the abdominal muscles is done with sit-ups. Lying on the back with the knees bent, a sit-up is performed by tightening the abdominal muscles and raising the torso to meet the flexed knees. In patients who are unable to perform the sit-up initially, preparation for this

can be accomplished by raising the head and shoulders off the bed by contracting the abdominal muscles and holding this position for a six-second period. This is repeated several times with relaxation in between. After a week of doing this form of "isometric" exercise, the muscles improve in strength so that the individual is able to perform the complete sit-up. See Fig. 15-3.

3. Pelvic tilt: lying on the bed or floor or standing against the wall—with the knees slightly flexed—the abdominal and gluteal (buttocks) muscles are contracted causing a flattening of the small of the back against the bed or wall and effecting a forward tilting of the pelvis under the lumbar spine. See Fig. 15-4.

4. Increasing the strength of the quadriceps muscles of the thigh can be attained by having the patient hold onto a table or chair and move from the squatting to the upright position as illustrated in Fig. 15-5.

5. To strengthen the long back muscles after the acute episode of strain has subsided, simple back arching exercises are performed holding the arch for a period of six seconds. This exercise is contraindicated if there is any pain involved in carrying out this maneuver. In the elderly with arthritic changes in the articular facets, this extension of the back may cause more pain and should be deleted from the regimen. If it can be performed without causing pain, however, it is helpful in strengthening the muscles of the back and in preventing future strain. See Fig. 15-6.

For the relief of muscle spasm, hot packs, ultrasound, diathermy, and even the application of ice packs have been found to be helpful. In addition, muscle stretching is utilized either with intermittent pelvic traction initially or with Williams flexion exercises, which require patient-training, to stretch out the muscles.[9] An elastic back support will frequently help with ambulation by the relief of pain,

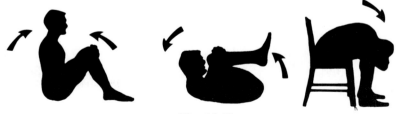

Fig. 15-2[9]

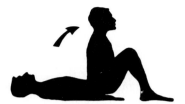

Fig. 15-3[9]

but, with its use, muscle-building exercises must be incorporated to prevent further weakening and atrophy of muscles of the low back.

Drug Therapy. Response to muscle-relaxant drugs for the relief of muscle spasm has been quite variable. Some individuals respond very well to these, while others gain little or no relief. Many of the elderly respond best to the combination of meprobamate and etholeptazine citrate in equagesic. Frequently, one tablet will relieve a good bit of the discomfort. Aspirin may be used along with this, but it is best to avoid narcotic preparations except during a severe acute phase. Many patients will show improvement with the addition of anti-inflammatory agents to the regimen, such as Indocin, Naprosyn, Tolectin, etc. Because the problem is frequently of long-range duration, avoiding use of drugs whenever possible is wise because of the dependent and depressing effects. The use of Valium is not advisable.

It is not unusual for an acute strain to cause an inflammatory reaction in joints involved with osteoarthritis. This makes it somewhat difficult in some cases to separate the cause for the patient's pain, but the overall treatment is basically the same—keeping the patient as mobile as possible, coupled with stretching and muscle-building exercises.

Chronic Ligamentous Strain

Chronic low-back pain secondary to chronic ligamentous strain is directly related to anatomic structure, together with the upright posture; it is aggravated by lack of proper muscle support and poor

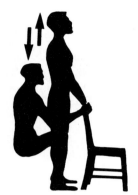

Fig. 15-5[9]

posture habits. This *leads* to our *"leaning"* on the ligaments of the posterior aspect of the spine (posterior longitudinal ligament) that, when under strain, becomes stretched and painful. Much that is labeled as arthritic low-back pain is most likely a chronic ligamentous strain.

TREATMENT

The treatment is aimed at improvement of posture, stretching out the muscles that may be somewhat shortened in the low back, and developing the muscles of the back and abdomen by appropriate muscle-building routines. This will relieve much of the chronic discomfort in the majority of patients and must become part of the daily activities of these patients. See Fig. 15-2–5.

Prevention of muscle strain is much better than having to treat the patient once the strain has occurred. This can be done best through education and an appropriate muscle-building program. Physiotherapists can be most helpful in working with patients to develop good muscle tone. They can also teach methods of lifting and carrying that place less strain on the low back. Using the leg muscles rather than the back for lifting is most important, as is being cautious about the size of the weight that is lifted. When some unusual work is anticipated, engaging in some muscle-building exercises for three or four days in preparation will help to prevent muscle strains.

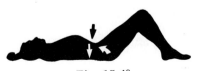

Fig. 15-4[9]

Fig. 15-6[9]

Acute Cervical Strain

The sudden forceful extension and flexion of the cervical spine as a result of automobile accidents, often relatively mild events, leads to a myriad of complaints secondary to the strain of the neck muscles and ligaments. Pain may be mild to severe, may be localized to the posterior aspect of the neck, or may extend down to the mid-upper back, the shoulders, and up the posteriolateral scalp to the top of the head. Headaches beginning at the base of the skull posterially and extending over the entire head is not unusual. Pain and tingling may be noted into the upper extremities as a result of irritation or possible contusion to the nerve roots involved. All motion of the neck is painful—with limitation of range of motion due to the pain and associated muscle spasm. X-ray is important to be sure there is no dislocation or fracture.

TREATMENT

As with other muscle and ligamentous strain, treatment is gauged according to the individual and the severity of the injury. Giving some support to the head and neck to relieve the injured muscles is helpful. This may be done by using a soft cervical collar for a period of time. The neck should be in slight anterior flexion. Many collars are too large, forcing patients to hold their chins high and forcing the neck into extension. This will aggravate the pain. Folding a bath towel lengthwise to a width of about 3 inches and wrapping this around the neck will serve the purpose quite well.

Gentle range of motion activities to keep the muscles stretched out without further injuring the ligaments involved is the aim of treatment. Intermittent cervical traction, diathermy, hot packs, ice applications, and ultrasound are helpful modalities. The length of treatment is dependent upon the severity of the injury and the response of the patient.

It is important for the physician and others treating the patient with cervical strain to maintain an optimistic attitude with continual encouragement while the patient performs the exercises and stretching routines that will eventually decrease the symptoms.

In many patients, using intermittent traction with 5–8 lb in the home setting has been useful in the treatment regimen. It is important that any cervical traction be set up so that there is slight forward flexion of the neck. Most instructions illustrate the patient seated with the head in slight extension, which aggravates the pain in the neck. If the traction is set up on a door, which the patient faces, it allows the patient to move backwards from the door to obtain the comfortable position for the neck in slight forward flexion. See Fig. 15-7.

Other valuable modalities in treatment are the use of antiinflammatory agents, muscle relaxants, and analgesic medication. The antiinflammatory agents have been listed, and, as noted, the response is quite variable. It is only by trial of usage that one can determine their effectiveness. Gastric irritation with occasional blood loss is the most common side effect. With Indocin, dizziness and headaches may also be problems.

Muscle relaxants are also variable in their effects on individual patients. Multiple products are available: Soma, Parafon-Forte, Robaxin, Flexril. Flexril has been found to be helpful for neck injuries with a dosage of 10 mg three or four times daily. One must be aware of the possible arrhythmic actions on the heart in select patients. Analgesics such as aspirin, Tylenol, Darvon, or Zactarin can be used for pain relief.

For treatment of the headaches that are frequently a very annoying part of acute and chronic cervical strain, tricyclic antidepressants (Elavil, Sinequan) as a bedtime medication have been helpful. The dosage is variable and adjusted to the response of the patient. It is wise to begin with low dosages such as 10–20 mg of Elavil, or 25 mg of Sinequan, and to increase the amount gradually as necessary. One needs to be aware of the cardiac and anticholinergic side effects of these drugs.

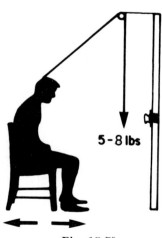

5-8 lbs

Fig. 15-7[9]

Osteoporosis

Osteoporosis is used to refer to a group of disorders characterized by a decreased mass/unit volume of bone with a normal ratio of mineral phase to matrix organic phase. This is characterized by decreased skeletal mass recognized radiologically by declining density of bone, loss of trabeculations, and thinning of the cortexes.[10] There are many causes for local or general osteoporosis. Because the radiologic findings are similar to several other conditions, such disease processes as osteomalacia, hyperparathyroidism, hyperthyroidism, hypercortisonism, multiple myeloma, and neoplastic metastases must be considered. Drugs and toxins such as steroids, Heparin, Dilantin, alchohol, and cigarette smoking have also been known to cause this condition.

The most common form of osteoporosis accompanies aging, is seen particularly in postmenopausal women, and has been termed involutional osteoporosis or osteopenia. It is more common in whites than in blacks. Our discussion will be limited to this form. The cause of this process is most likely multifactorial and is not completely understood. Smaller individuals with smaller muscle mass tend to develop more osteoporosis than those of heavier weight with larger muscle mass. Other factors include dietary intake of calcium, phosphate, and protein; and metabolism of vitamin D or its deficiency. Estrogen hormone or its deficit seems to play some role. Inactivity increases bone loss, and the aging process itself has some causative effect. How all these pieces fit into the picture is not clearly understood at this time.

Most people with osteoporosis are asymptomatic. Early detection is highly desirable to institute therapy and to decrease the incidence of complications such as fractures that cause pain and deformity. Since the trabecular bone is involved in the mineral loss, fractures commonly occur in the weight-bearing vertebrae (lower thoracic or lumbar), femoral neck, and wrist.

Collapse fractures of the vertebrae may occur with lifting and jumping, or with no trauma other than riding on a bumpy road or having to cough while bending over. The resulting pain is acute and localized to the vertebra involved, with local tenderness evidenced. Pain is noted on movement or weight bearing. This acute pain may last for a few days to two or three weeks and is treated supportively by initial rest, accompanied by muscle exten-

sion exercises of the back (back arching). See Fig. 15-6.

It is important to avoid immobilization that aggravates bone loss. Spinal support and bracing, which are poorly tolerated by the elderly, have little place in treatment. Encouraging activities as much as possible during the acute phase, with the institution of muscle-building routines, is of importance. Some patients do gain confidence with the temporary use of a lumbosacral elastic support, which may be used along with mobility and exercises.[1]

When mild back pain is a presenting symptom, there may be a subclinical vertebral fracture responsible for the pain. Extreme forward flexion of the neck frequently will localize the pain to the thoracic vertebra involved. With the gradual vertebral collapse that is part of this process, a person's height will gradually decrease and kyphosis increase.

LAB VALUES

Laboratory data, including serum calcium, phosphorus, alkaline phosphatase, protein electrophoresis, and sedimentation rate, are normal. Should abnormalities be found in these studies, a search for other causes should be undertaken.

Diagnosis is made by x-rays revealing increased radiolucency of bone that is generalized but most noticeable in the trabecular areas of bone. By the time this demineralization is evidenced by x-ray, 30 percent of the bone mineral has been lost.[3] The vertebrae frequently will demonstrate a loss of height on the anterior portion or a "wedging" secondary to gradual collapse.

TREATMENT

By the time osteoporosis has become clinically manifest, it is not possible to restore normal bone mass and structure. The objective is to prevent further bone loss if possible, prevent further fractures and deformities, and improve muscle strength and support to allow the patient to continue daily living activities. Several regimens have been suggested, but at this time there is no real proof that any program is completely effective. There is also much controversy regarding the use of estrogens because of the increased incidence of uterine cancer with its use. Because of the lack of hard data to support any set regimen, it is impossible to delineate a program of treatment clearly. The primary care clinician should consult an orthopedist for suggestions in individual cases.

The best treatment is prevention. Activity and muscle-building programs should be the first line of preventive defense. Since most fractures occur as a result of a fall, encouraging the use of a cane or walker for support in those who are unsteady is of value. The utilization of calcium supplementation earlier in life has been advised,[11] although its effectiveness in prevention is not certain.

Fractures

The osteoporotic changes in bone have an important influence on the incidence of fractures in the elderly. Fractures occur with minimal trauma and with a higher incidence in women. Fractures usually are a result of falls and most often occur near joints at the end of long bones where they are the softest. Fracture of the hip (femoral neck) is the most common fracture in the elderly,[5] and complications from this fracture are one of the leading causes of death in elderly women. Other common fractures include the distal radius (wrist) and fractures of the vertebrae.

In the treatment of fractures in the geriatric patient, it is important to maintain full range of motion of all joints not immobilized in the treatment. It is also important to maintain immobilization only as long as is necessary for appropriate healing so the stiffened joints may again be mobilized to prevent further disability. In many cases, especially if the wrist is involved, it may be more important to retain joint motion than to be concerned about the beauty of the "healed bone."

Wrist Fractures. It has not been unusual in the past to see x-ray evidence of beautiful healing of a collar fracture, while the patient is left with a wrist that is stiffened, painful, and poorly functioning because of prolonged immobilization in plaster casting. With the use of some of the softer "wrap-on" splints, it is possible to maintain good immobilization of the fractured wrist while allowing passive and active motion exercising of the wrist joint after two to three weeks. Some increased deformity at the fracture site may result, but, with more complete range of wrist motion, the patient has greater function of the wrist and hand. The patient presents with pain at the wrist area, usually after a fall, and in most cases obvious deformity is noted. X-rays confirm this fracture.

These fractures can be treated utilizing local anesthetic injection into the fracture site, allowing reduction with minimal pain. The reduction is gen-erally accomplished easily with traction and gentle manipulation as the bone is soft and cancellous. The reduction can usually be maintained by holding the wrist in the position of volar flexion, thus tightening the dorsal tissue over the wrist and fracture site. With the help of an assistant, the fracture can be maintained while the plaster cast material is applied. In the elderly, soft prepared splints may be more appropriate for the treatment of these fractures.

When a plaster cast is used to immobilize a fracture of the wrist, it is important that the metacarpophalangeal joints are free for active motion of the fingers during the period of immobilization. To allow for this mobility, the plaster must not extend beyond the proximal transverse crease in the palm of the hand. Likewise, the wrist should not be brought down into extreme volar flexion, as this may lead to the development of entrapment of the median nerve in the carpal tunnel (carpal tunnel syndrome) as a future complication. Midrange of volar flexion is appropriate with ulnar deviation of the wrist. In patients over 65, plaster should be removed after four weeks with the use of a soft splint to maintain support of the healing fracture and to allow daily exercise to the wrist during the ensuing two weeks. Family members are encouraged to assist the patient with exercise routines.

In a patient with rheumatoid arthritis, the bone is softer with increased circulation, which means fractures occur with less trauma and heal more rapidly when treated. In these individuals, it is extremely important that passive motion of the wrist be started after seven to ten days postfracture, and that routines be set up no later than the end of 14 days to allow daily passive exercises to the wrist. When done carefully, this maneuver causes no pain and does not delay healing of the fractured radius. By the end of four weeks, such patients should be out of the splint, though for protection it should be used for another two weeks for such activities as walking, riding in a car, or sleeping.

Hip Fractures. Thirty years ago, when patients in their 70s suffered a fracture of the hip, the prolonged bedrest necessary for healing resulted in death for many. With the advent of infection control and widespread use of surgery with internal fixation or prosthetic replacement this outlook has totally changed. We have found that the sooner such patients undergo surgery, are again able to move about and be ambulatory, the greater their chances are for leaving the hospital and continuing their independent lifestyle.

Fractures of the hip most often occur as a result of a fall. Patients are unable to stand on their affected leg, and motion of the leg causes pain localized to the hip. In most cases, there is shortening with external rotation of the leg involved. Occasionally, fractures of the neck of the femur may occur without displacement, in which case both extremities would appear normal. Percussion of the trochanter on the side involved is usually painful, but x-rays with comparison of both hips—including lateral views—are necessary to make the definitive diagnosis.

With any disruption of living circumstances, older patients frequently become confused. Suddenly finding themselves in the strange surroundings of a hospital room increases this confusion. Under such circumstances, it is important that their family physician or nurse practitioner, with whom they are well acquainted, be an active participant of the team during their hospital stay.

Attention to bladder and skin care is extremely important to prevent the complication of decubiti during the first several days postoperatively. Rehabilitation is of utmost importance following hip surgery, so the discharge arrangements become extremely important for the rehabilitative period, and the patient should be an integral part of this planning process.

Foot Fractures. One fracture that can be easily treated by the family physician is a fracture of the base of the fifth metatarsal, which occurs when the foot is turned under. As the foot turns into inversion, the attachment of the tendon of the peroneus brevis muscle pulls off the base of the fifth metatarsal. Since this type of injury frequently causes a fracture of the ankle, it is important to check for that injury as well.

Tenderness is localized to the proximal portion of the lateral metatarsal, and an x-ray reveals the fracture. This fracture can be treated by simple immobilization with the use of a zinc oxide (Unna boot) wrap, incorporating soft material as an arch support, and appropriate length tongue blade as support around the fracture site. Three to four weeks of such treatment allow the patient to be up and about without the need for immobilization of the ankle joint in the process. The treatment is geared to the reaction of the patient, and, if neces-

sary, a small plaster shoe may be used for seven to ten days initially.

In the treatment of any fractures in the elderly, it must be recognized that there are individual differences in the rate at which healing occurs. Treatment is therefore always adjusted according to the healing of each patient. For some, this will mean the need for a longer period of immobilization. When this is found to be necessary, it becomes more important to keep joints free of plaster, mobile, and active. It also becomes important to utilize physiotherapy, including whirlpool, heat applications, etc., to aid in the remobilizing of the joints when the plaster is removed.

Shoulder Pain Bursitis—Tendonitis

The most common cause of shoulder pain is a degenerative tendonitis, which is usually nontraumatic in origin. This has been called by names such as bursitis, pericapsulitis, tendonitis, adhesive capsulitis, and, in the extreme case, frozen shoulder.[12]

The shoulder is a rather complex structure with a flat glenoid fossa on which the humeral head rotates through its various motions. The superior portion of the joint is made up of the acromion process and the coracoacromial ligament. In the process of elevation of the humerus, the rotator cuff muscles stabilize and slightly depress the humeral head into the glenoid fossa. In this process, the supraspinatus muscle, which is a flat tendonous-type muscle, must pass under the overlying acromion process. With any swelling or inflammation of the overlying subdeltoid or subacromial bursa, there is some impingement of the supraspinatus muscle as it rides under the acromion process, leading to inflammation of this structure as well.

In the elderly, there is a certain degree of kyphosis of the thoracic spine, which has an effect of bringing the acromion process slightly anterior with resultant lowering of the coracoacromial ligament. As the arm is elevated for most activities in front of the body, there is impingement of the supraspinatus muscle tendon against this ligament and the acromion process. With repeated such trauma, inflammatory changes occur in this muscle tendon, which may lead to calcium deposition noted on x-ray studies.

The patient having such a condition complains of pain on specific shoulder motion when the muscle tendon that is inflamed impinges under the superior hood of the shoulder joint. With repeated use, pain is noted even at rest, and resultant immobilization of the shoulder by the patient rapidly leads to stiffening. If this is not interrupted by appropriate treatment and motion of the joint, a frozen shoulder may result in which all motion of the joint is limited by adhesions.

This process of tendonitis frequently undergoes episodes of acute "flare up" related to the inflammatory process in the muscle tendon involved. In such acute episodes, pain is severe for four to seven days and gradually decreases after that. In many elderly patients, however, there is mild to moderate constant pain that interferes with normal activity as well as sleep.

The patient presents with pain that at times can be specifically localized to one point, while at other times it is rather diffuse around the shoulder and down the lateral aspect of the arm to the elbow. The patient can usually demonstrate the motions leading to an aggravation of the pain. Tenderness is most often localized to the supraspinatus muscle tendon near its attachment to the humeral head. X-rays frequently reveal calcification in this muscle tendon area or in the overlying bursa, but in some cases of inflammation, no abnormalities are noted on x-ray.

In examining the range of motion of the shoulder joint, it is important to place one hand on the scapula as the humerus is elevated with the other hand to determine whether or not there is the normal rhythmic motion of the humerus and scapula. In normal motion of the shoulder, for every 15 degrees of elevation of the humerus, 10 degrees occurs at the glenohumeral joint, and 5 degrees is scapular rotation on the thorax. With adhesions, patients will elevate the shoulder with motion of the scapula and with very little motion of the humerus in the glenoid fossa.

TREATMENT

In treating this condition, it is important that motion of the shoulder be maintained during the acute process. In acute conditions, the pain may be so severe that motion is impossible for a period of three to four days, but no longer time of immobility should be allowed because of the tendency for adhesions and frozen shoulder to occur. Antiinflammatory agents such as Indocin, Tolectin, Naprosyn, etc., along with analgesics—which may include aspirin with codeine during the acute phase—have been found to offer some relief. Injections utilizing steroids such as Kenalog 40 mg, Depo Medrol 40

mg, mixed with Xylocaine have given dramatic relief in many patients following a single injection into the tender point. In others, a series of weekly injections for three to four weeks may be necessary to obtain relief. Physiotherapy has been very beneficial when ice applications, ultrasound, diathermy, and a range of motion exercises are utilized. Early physiotherapy during the acute phase appears to shorten the length of the painful process.

When the patient has delayed coming until three or four days have elapsed and the shoulder is beginning to stiffen, it is important to regain shoulder motion. Codman pendulum exercises, performed with the patient leaning with his or her good elbow on a table or desk and allowing the painful extremity to swing in all directions like a pendulum, can be accomplished even during the acute phase. Help is then given to elevate the humerus to 90 degrees, and passive internal and external rotation is carried out. Having patients climb the wall with their fingers, gradually elevating the humerus, should be performed at least three times a day. It is important to demonstrate these various exercise routines with follow-up visits or physiotherapy evaluations to determine the progress in regaining full motion of this joint. Much of this stage of treatment is under the supervision of a physiotherapist.

For the patient with a frozen shoulder, in which there is very limited to no motion of the humerus in the glenoid fossa, gentle but progressive mobilization under the direction of a physiotherapist is essential. With time and patient perseverance, motion can gradually be regained to full mobility, resulting in a decrease of pain and disability. This process may take about three months.

Range of motion exercises of the shoulder can easily be instituted at home with a minimum of equipment. Using a rope over the top of a door can be utilized to aid in the upward mobilization of both shoulders. Better still is the use of a hook and pulley attached either to the ceiling or wall, and with a rope held on both ends the shoulders can be exercised. See Fig. 15-8.

Internal and external rotation can be enhanced by the use of a hook and pulley in the wall. The patient pulls a weight up and then allows the weight to assist in the motion. The upper arm is elevated and the elbow flexed, both to 90 degrees for these exercises. See Fig. 15-9. Perhaps a simpler method is for the patient to lie on his or her back and

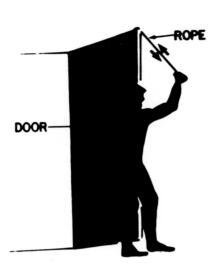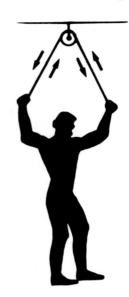

Fig. 15-8[9]

then—with a small weight in hand–to let the weight pull the shoulder either into internal or external rotation. It is helpful to demonstrate these routines to members of the family so they may help the patient with the therapy program.

Other causes of shoulder pain, such as osteoarthritic changes of the cervical spine with some nerve root irritation, are frequently confused with the pain of bursitis—tendonitis. Treatment of this has been considered under the Cervical Strain section of this chapter.

SUMMARY

When treating musculoskeletal conditions in the elderly, the cornerstone of care is aimed at keeping the patient functioning and independent in his or her home environment. The most gratifying and important physical sign to see in the geriatric patient is ambulation. Without walking, true independence cannot be achieved. When disabling conditions occur, appropriate measures must be instituted to help the patient regain as much mobility and independence as possible. Allowing the patient to enter into the planning of appropriate therapeutic regimens will encourage his or her cooperation and effort to attain that goal.

Since many of the disabilities involving this system are a result of injury, prevention and education become extremely important in dealing with the elderly. Frequent review of medication to be sure they are taken as prescribed, as well as alertness to adverse drug interactions, may prevent confusional states that may lead to falls and fractures. Home visits to note and correct or remove hazards unrecognized by the patient may be the most important part of the therapeutic regimen.

HEALTH MAINTENANCE

Prevention and education are the two main ingredients inherent in health maintenance in the elderly.

Exercise routines to improve muscle tone and strength of the back and abdominal muscles can aid in the prevention of acute strains. When a patient is planning some unusual activity that involves lifting or other muscle-straining activity, education and encouragement in some of the muscle-building/conditioning exercises for a few days prior to the event can be most valuable in preventing disabling strain. Such exercise prior to shoveling snow, carrying firewood or other loads is time well spent in the prevention of disability and immobility.

Should a patient require the use of crutches for a period of time, it is important to prepare the home for such use. Removing throw rugs and other items of hazard or obstruction become very important to prevent falls should the crutches slip or become caught while the patient is ambulating. Proper training in the use of crutches is as impor-

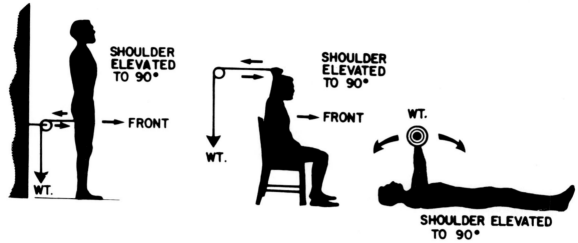

Fig. 15-9[9]

tant as the treatment of the fracture or injury. The physiotherapist can be most helpful in this part of the treatment routine.

Care of the Feet

The importance of ambulation and mobility for general health and well-being in the elderly is readily apparent. It is because of this that footcare becomes an important aspect of the total care of the geriatric patient. A discussion of the various foot conditions is not intended, but some general considerations of care will be noted.

Neglect, abuse, and ill-advised footwear during younger years lead to many of the foot problems and pain in elderly individuals. Hammer toe deformities, bunion formation, metatarsalgia, and other deformities and painful conditions can be traced to some of the shoe styles of the past.

For the elderly, we must not only deal with some of these painful results, but must also be aware of the diminished skin sensation and circulation that easily leads to skin breakdown and infection from ill-fitting shoes. Examination of the feet should be an integral part of every visit to the office to detect developing difficulties before they become serious problems. Examining footwear to determine wear pattern and appropriateness for the patient's present needs should be a part of this routine. Painful bunions and corns can be prevented by relieving pressure caused by tight shoes over the areas of involvement. Appropriate padding between toes,

though it seems to be a simple measure, may relieve pain and foster further ambulation.

Patients with diabetes should be warned about tight shoes that may lead to blisters and infection in tissue already compromised by poor circulation. Such patients should be alerted to the compromise of circulation caused by swelling of the foot confined in tight shoes. Just as serious are shoes that are so loose that rubbing occurs with the same result. Frequent inspection of the feet of such an individual and appropriate nail care are of utmost importance. Trimming of calluses and corns are also important measures to prevent cracking and skin fissures that allow infections.

The elderly should be encouraged to wear slippers or other foot protection when walking in the house to prevent minor and unforeseen trauma. Education on these points should be continuous to help the elderly maintain their mobile independence.

Patient Dignity

Each patient must be approached individually because of the wide variation in physical abilities and capacity. To help each person maintain his or her own sense of dignity, it is important to treat each as a person and not as just another "old person." An individual approach is essential in the maintenance of mental health in the elderly and aids in any course of treatment developed by the primary care clinician.

REFERENCES

1. Brockelhurst JC (ed): Textbook of Geriatric Medicine and Gerontology (ed 2). Edinburgh, Churchill-Livingston, 1978

2. Brewerton D: Rheumatic disease, in Rossman I: Clinical Geriatrics (ed 2). Philadelphia, JB Lippincott, 1979, p 451

3. Lutwak L: Continuing need for dietary calcium throughout life. Geriatrics 29:173, 1974

4. Rossman I: Clinical Geriatrics (ed 2). Philadelphia, JB Lippincott, 1979

5. Smith, Exton AN, Oversteal PW: Geriatrics: Guidelines in Medicine. London, MJP Press Ltd, 1979, vol 1

6. Steinberg FU, Franzill: Cowdry's The Care of the Geriatric Patient (ed 5). St. Louis, CV Mosby Co, 1976.

7. Dorland's Illustrated Medical Dictionary (ed 24). Philadelphia, WB Saunders, 1975

8. Smith NB: Shoulder pain flowsheet. For University of California at Davis Family Nurse Practitioner Program, August 1974

9. Soto-Hall R: The conservative treatment of Low Back Pain. Medical Science, August 1973

10. Robinson D: Osteoporosis and Paget's Disease. New York, Scientific American, Inc, 1980

11. Cailliet R: Low back pain syndrome (ed 2). Philadelphia, FA Davis Co, 1971

16

Hematology

Betty Walraven, F.N.P., M.H.S.
Parveen Malik, M.D.
Donat P. Cyr, M.D.

The hemopoietic system is especially challenging to the clinician due to the scope of the disorders related to the blood and its constituents. In older people, hematologic problems commonly arise in several contexts—with a complex of signs, symptoms, and diseases that span the entire field of medicine. Our appreciation of these principles increases our effectiveness as helpers, as well as the health potential and outcome for patients.

The hematologic disorders commonly seen in the elderly include anemias and lymphoproliferative disorders: leukemia, lymphoma, and multiple myeloma. Hematologic problems less commonly seen include sideroblastic anemia, coagulation defects, Waldenstrom's macroglobulinemia, and idiopathic myelofibrosis. In approaching the older patient with a hematologic problem, it is important to remember that signs and symptoms may be nonspecific or subtle. It requires a most astute clinician to make a diagnosis confirmed by appropriate laboratory studies. The hematologist becomes an integral part of the patient care team for the patient presenting with puzzling symptoms, signs, and perplexing laboratory data. The diagnostic tests and treatment plans for uncommon diseases are best made in conjunction with consultants. The primary health care team should coordinate comprehensive patient care by seeking hematologic consultation expertise for complex patient problems. The hematologist, pathologist, oncologist, and radiotherapist may all have a valuable role in the consulting team.

INCIDENCE OF HEMATOLOGIC PROBLEMS IN THE ELDERLY

LABORATORY NORMALS

It is difficult to evaluate the literature in assessing the prevalence of hematologic disease in older people. One problem is the difference in the criteria for laboratory values used by various authors. Some have postulated that laboratory normal values used in adults may span too narrow a range in the over-70 population. Earney and Earney conducted a study of four hundred relatively "normal" ambulatory nursing home patients and found that the range of geriatric hematologic values was broader at both the higher and lower levels than the standard adult values.[1] (See Table 16-1.) The lab value differences noted in earlier decades between the sexes were negligible in the 70–94 range. Insufficient data are available to assess the hemoglobin values of healthy elders at home and to confirm or refute the above values. Many studies define anemia as below a hemoglobin value of 10 g/100 ml.[2] Let us stress, however, that in practice we consider hemoglobin values in the 10–12 g range to be of clinical concern. There is no convincing evidence that the range of normal values in healthy older adults are lower than in younger adults. Blood value changes over time are probably a more accurate measure of a patient's health status, based on his or her norms. A finding of 13 g of hemoglobin in a man who in

Table 16-1
Hematologic Values Standard Adult Versus "Normal" Ambulatory Nursing
Home Patients Over 70 Years of Age

	Standard Adult	Geriatric Men and Women
Erythrocytes (10^6/cu mm)	4.2–6.2	3.3–5.46
Hemoglobin (g%)	11.5–18.0	10.24–19.04
Hematocrit (vol%)	37–54	31.01–53.29
Leukocytes (10^3/cu mm)	5–10	3.91–11.07
Polymorphonuclear cells (%)	50–65	24.15–70.99
Small lymphocytes (%)	25–40	18.64–64.20
Basophils (%)	0–1	0.00–2.34
Eosinophils (%)	0–4	0.00–3.66
Monocytes (%)	0–8	0.05–8.65

Reprinted from Earney MA, Earney AJ: Geriatric hematology. J Am Geriatr Soc 20: 175, 1972. By permission.

a previous examination had a hemoglobin value of 15 g should be thoroughly investigated. Indeed, a slight change in hemoglobin level or a very mild anemia may be the starting point that triggers a thorough search and discovery of an early and potentially curable malignancy, e.g., silent cancers of the cecum and right colon.

Socioeconomic and cultural differences from one country to the next may compound the confusion about the frequency of hematologic disorders in the geriatric population.. Using anemia as an example, the incidence of anemia seems to range from 5–10 percent in patients living at home. In patients admitted to hospitals, 20–46 percent are anemic, a condition probably related to concomitant disease states.[3–11] The broad general categories of anemias, by etiologic classification, are depicted in Table 16-2.

Anemia

Although anemia is common among the elderly, it is often overlooked because its symptoms develop slowly and insidiously or because there may be no symptoms at all. Usually, symptoms are not noticed early by the patient, as many of them are common to other problems of growing old, i.e., lack of energy, dizziness, increased sensitivity to cold, and dyspnea. All too often these symptoms are dismissed by patients or their families as the concomitants of "old age." Patients on multivitamins with iron and/or folate supplements may actually mask their anemia.

There are multiple factors contributing to the development of anemias in this age group, and many interrelated factors must be kept in mind when considering the etiology of anemias in the elderly. Food quantity and variety often change, related to individual and cultural eccentricities. The expense of iron-rich foods, such as meat, eggs, and green vegetables, coupled with the relative economy of milk, bread, and starches, further contribute to the imbalanced diets and malnutrition. Transportation difficulties limit access to fresh foods and decrease the purchasing power of "shoppers' specials." Thus, canned foods become the staples of many people's diets, especially those of the economically disadvantaged and physically impaired. Physical disabilities such as poor vision, osteoarthritis, and diminishing energy may limit mobility necessary for food preparation. Loss of teeth may result in poor mastication and avoidance of some foods. Stomach or intestinal surgery or disease may impair absorption of iron, essential vitamins, amino acids, and other foods necessary as a source of energy and blood production.

Depression is not uncommon in the elderly, especially those living alone. This can lead to self-neglect and poor nutrition, further contributing to disease states and anemia.

Iron Deficiency Anemia

Iron deficiency is the most common cause of anemia in the elderly. The clinical presentation is dependent upon the severity of the anemia and the causative factor. Signs and symptoms often are a mixture of those caused by the anemia and those caused by the underlying disease.

Table 16-2
Approach to Anemia Etiology in Elders

Impaired RBC Formation	RBC Loss	Accelerated RBC Destruction
Erythropoietic Deficiency	Acute blood loss	Hemolysis
Iron	Chronic blood loss	
Vitamin B$_{12}$		
Folic Acid		
Bone Marrow Dysfunction		
Aplastic and senile hypoplastic anemia		
Infiltration: leukemia, multiple		
myeloma, myelofibrosis, malignancy		
Chronic disease		
"Symptomatic anemias"		

ETIOLOGY

Iron deficiency anemia has many causes. Insufficient intake of iron in the diet, increased demand for iron due to blood loss, and/or defects causing diminished absorption of iron are all possible culprits.

Iron deficiency may develop from an inadequate intake of iron. Nutritional requirements in the elderly actually change very little from adults, except for a notable decrease in caloric needs by 200–300 kcal/day. In women, a decrease in iron needs is evident by nearly 50 percent, from 18–10 mg/day. This change is based mainly on the cessation of the menses.

It must be emphasized that the most common cause of iron deficiency anemia is *blood loss*. Chronic, silent, and often intermittent blood loss almost always is from the gastrointestinal tract. A daily loss of 6–8 ml of blood represents a loss of 3–4 mg of iron, which is the maximum that can be absorbed from food. In time, this amount of blood loss will cause depletion of iron stores, a decrease in serum iron and finally anemia of the hypochromic type. Many gastrointestinal lesions may bleed silently: esophageal varices, hiatus hernia, peptic ulcer, polyps in the stomach or bowel, diverticulosis, vascular anomalies, and hemorrhoids. Chronic gastritis and the chronic ingestion of salicylates, which is not uncommon in the elderly, may cause blood loss and anemia. Perhaps the most rewarding event in clinical practice is to detect—by way of an aggresive pursuit of the cause of iron deficiency anemia—a small, early, and potentially curable malignancy in the gastrointestinal tract. This requires diligent study beginning with the single test of stool guaiac.

Many guaiac tests may be required to detect blood loss since the bleeding may be intermittent.

Radiographic studies with barium often miss a bleeding gastrointestinal lesion. Endoscopic studies may be necessary, and the use of the flexible colonscope in recent years has greatly enhanced our diagnostic capability. In an occasional case, angiography may be required to localize the site of bleeding and to detect vascular anomalies.

Bleeding from hemorrhoids may be the sole cause of anemia. Elderly patients are notoriously reticent to divulge that they bleed with every bowel movement. One must ascertain, however, that no other more serious cause of blood loss exists.

DATA BASE: CLINICAL PRESENTATIONS

The symptoms of anemia are caused by a diminished oxygen-carrying capacity of the blood to the tissues and organs of the body. The relative decrease in physical activities and decline in metabolic rate may enable the elderly anemia patient to tolerate lower hemoglobin levels better. Severity of symptoms and signs is generally dependent more upon the time span in which the anemia develops than upon its severity. Slowly developing anemias, even when moderately severe, allow for volume expansion and cardiovascular adaptation that is often remarkably well tolerated by the patient. In contrast, abrupt onset anemia presents itself dramatically and may be accompanied by cardiovascular collapse and shock.

The anemic patient may complain of weakness, dizziness, shortness of breath, giddiness, headache, increased sensitivity to the cold, faintness, and irritability. Loss of appetite associated with dyspepsia is sometimes seen in these patients. Pallor of the skin, palpitations, tachycardia, and functional systolic murmurs are common. The nails may show changes and develop longitudinal ridging. In iron deficiency of long standing, the nails become flattened and spoon-shaped (koilonychia). There may be atrophy of the mucosa of the tongue leading to a sore, red appearance. The same type of changes may affect the esophageal muscosa leading to a fillamentous web, causing dysphagia, and resulting in Plummer-Vinson syndrome. In severe anemia there may be edema of the ankles, angina pectoris, and myocardial insufficiency leading to heart failure.

MANAGEMENT STRATEGIES

The majority of the patients with iron deficiency suffer from a mild to moderate anemia. The early findings may be minimal. The red blood cells may be slightly microcytic or even normocytic. As the anemia becomes more advanced, hypochromia develops.

Anemia is most commonly diagnosed by a low hemoglobin value in the blood. Alternatively, the hematocrit may be used as a single test to establish the presence of anemia. Red blood cell indices guide the clinician in the initial course of laboratory investigation. In iron deficiency, one expects the mean corpuscular hemoglobin, mean corpuscular volume, and mean corpuscular hemoglobin concentration to be reduced. Iron deficiency is diagnosed when the serum iron is low, and the total iron-binding capacity is increased to the levels of 400–600 μg/100 ml. The transferrin saturation index (ST divided by TIBC) is less than 20. Occasionally in perplexing presentations, especially anemias with more than one deficiency, a bone marrow examination for hemosiderin and stainable iron may be necessary. As previously stressed, the results of these studies can be useless and misleading if not done in reliable laboratories with competent interpreters.

Reticulocytes may be normal or increased. Reticulocyte counts are usually increased in an anemia due to blood loss as bone marrow activity increases in an attempt to compensate for losses. Platelets and white blood cell counts are usually normal.

Treatment for this type of anemia is aimed at correction of the cause. Replacement of the iron deficit and bone marrow stores can be accomplished by iron, either orally or parenterally. The oral route is effective in the majority of patients. Ferrous salts are an economical and readily utilizable source of iron. Parenteral therapy is rarely required and should be used only if intolerance develops to the oral route, if poor absorption in the duodenum occurs, usually from gastrectomy, or when a chronic small or large bowel disease, such as ulcerative colitis or regional ileitus, prevents its oral use. Administration of oral iron should be continued for three to six months after the anemia has been corrected in order to replenish the iron stores in the bone marrow. Ferrous sulfate 200 mg three times a day after meals, or ferrous gluconate 300 mg three times a day after meals, is tolerated by most patients and is sufficient in elemental iron to correct the anemia. Since iron is better absorbed in the fasting state, some authors prefer liquid iron, feosol elixir, 5 cc before meals (5 cc = 45 mg iron). Liquid iron discolors the teeth. Slowly introducing the supplement from once a day to three times a day over two to three weeks will result in fewer gastrointestinal side effects and improved compliance.

When treating any anemia in the elderly, it can be anticipated that the reticulocyte count may take several days longer to respond to treatment than with a younger patient. Thus, patience helps prevent overtreatment of severe anemias by blood transfusion. Transfusion is seldom necessary. Should it become indicated, however, the use of packed red cells should be considered to avoid excessive volume expansion and subsequent cardiovascular insult (Table 16-3), especially in patients with congestive heart failure.

The need for good patient rapport to enhance compliance and facilitate communication cannot be over emphasized. Patients need to understand the reason for various tests and procedures in searching for a source of blood loss. The expected frequency of office visits and laboratory tests should be estimated whenever possible. Dietary sources of iron-rich foods should be reviewed at intervals, i.e., soybean flour, beef, organ meats, clams, peaches, and beans. A weekly diet recall initially and after therapy may provide valuable clues to socioeconomic issues that need further referral or to eccentricities that may be complicating the treatment plan. A review of the effects of some drugs on the gastrointestinal tract, i.e., steroids, aspirin, antiinflammatory medicines, etc., may be necessary with recommendations for concurrent antacid therapy, ingestion with meals, etc. In addition, suggesting oral iron replacement therapy, starting with one tablet per day with a major meal and increasing to three tablets per day over one week, allows for gastroin-

Table 16-3
Indications for Transfusions in Elderly Patients

Hemorrhage or severe blood loss associated with the
following:
  Blood volume of less than 70% of normal
  Persistent pulse rate of 100/min or greater
  Central venous pressure of less than 50 mm
    saline
Hemolytic anemia in hypoplastic bone marrow crises
Aplastic anemia
Chronic anemias associated with:
  Cardiac failure
  Angina pectoris
  Cerebral insufficiency
  Infection
  Hematocrit below 25%
  Hemoglobin concentration below 8 g/100 ml

Reproduced with permission from Baisden CR: Hematologic
problems of the elderly. Hosp Prac 13: 93–104, 1978; and from
Reichel W (ed): The Geriatric Patient. New York, HP Publishing
Co Inc, 1978.

testinal tolerance to occur and decreases side effects,
thus increasing compliance.

Megaloblastic Anemia

The most common causes of macrocytosis are
vitamin B_{12} deficiency, folid acid deficiency, reticulocytosis, liver disease, and chronic alcohol abuse.
Megaloblastic anemia in the elderly generally implies vitamin B_{12} or folate deficiency and is the first
diagnostic thought when considering an elderly
patient whose macrocytic anemia is associated with
an elevated mean corpuscular volume. Pernicious
anemia is almost exclusively a disease of the elderly
and some ethnic groups, with a peak incidence at
aged 60.

ETIOLOGY

The megaloblastic anemias are characterized by
a common biochemical defect of slowed DNA synthesis. Deficiences of either B_{12}, folic acid, or both,
can be caused by inadequate dietary intake, poor
absorption, or increased destruction. Vitamin B_{12}
deficiency is nearly always a result of defective
absorption secondary to a lack of intrinsic factor.
Vitamin B_{12} is found in dairy products, liver, meats,
and fish. It is stored in the liver in quantities
sufficient to provide body needs for up to two years.
Consequently, it is unusual to encounter dietary B_{12}
deficiency. The normal absorption of vitamin B_{12}

from the intestinal tract requires the presence of a
specific protein, intrinsic factor, in the gastric juice
and normal function of the distal ileum where most
of the uptake of vitamin B_{12} occurs. Patients suffering from pernicious anemia lack intrinsic factor and
therefore are unable to absorb B_{12} even if they have
adequate amounts of vitamin B_{12} in their diet.

Pernicious anemia is also associated with achlorhydria and gastric atrophy. The factors leading to
gastric atrophy are not well understood. The relatively high incidence of gastric atrophy in families
suggests that the defect may be genetically determined. In addition, there is evidence that pernicious
anemia is produced by autoantibodies against the
gastric parietal cells. Antibodies directed against
gastric parietal cells are found in a high percentage
of patients suffering from pernicious anemia. Malabsorption of vitamin B_{12} may be caused by gastrectomy, severe chronic gastritis, or intestinal causes—
such as Crohn's disease, ileal resection, anatomical
blind loops, and sprue.

In contrast to the abundant storage of B_{12}, folate
is stored for a period of only two to four months.
Dietary deficiency of folic acid as a cause of megaloblastic anemia is not uncommon in the elderly.
Various malabsorption syndromes also impair absorption of folic acid. Folate is found in nearly all
natural foods, but it is heat labile and is rapidly
destroyed by extensive cooking. Elderly people
whose daily diet does not contain fresh uncooked
fruit or fresh lightly cooked vegetables are at risk
of developing folic acid deficiency. Most of the folic
acid in food is destroyed by cooking at 100 degrees
Fahrenheit for more than twenty minutes. Macrocytic anemia in alcoholics and narcotic addicts is
usually secondary to folic acid deficiency because of
the patient's poor dietary intake. Interference of
DNA synthesis occurs with folic acid deficiency
similar to that of vitamin B_{12} deficiency.

DATA BASE: CLINICAL AND LABORATORY
PRESENTATION

The onset of pernicious anemia is generally insidious. If the classical triad of weakness, glossitis, and
paresthesias are present, the diagnosis is easily
made. Most patients present with one or more of
the symptoms of a gradually developing anemia.
Common complaints are easy fatiguability, weakness, shortness of breath, palpitations, tachycardia,
behavior changes, and headaches. Infrequently,
there may be angina or heart failure. Patients with

vitamin B_{12} deficiency may have a lemon yellow tint due to a combination of pallor from anemia and low-grade icterus from the hemolytic component of this anemia. Gastrointestinal symptoms such as diarrhea and loss of appetite and weight are frequent. Glossitis may appear before the anemia is severe. The tongue may have a "beefy" red appearance. The spleen is palpable in about one-third of patients. Vitamin B_{12} deficiency may cause a symmetrical neuropathy affecting the posterior and lateral columns of the spinal cord, with the lower extremities more commonly affected than the upper. Patients may complain of numbness and tingling in the extremities, or may present with paresthesias, weakness, and difficulty in walking, which may lead to eventual paraplegia. Vitamin B_{12} neuropathy may lead to a loss of vibration sense and deep tendon reflexes. Mental disturbances such as loss of memory and depression may occur.

The hallmark of the anemia of B_{12} or folate deficiency is macrocytosis (MCV above 100 and usually 110 cu mm or greater). The macrocytosis of B_{12} or folate deficiency is accompanied by other features in the blood and marrow that distinguish it from the macrocytosis that may be seen in hemolytic and aplastic anemia. In the latter, the macrocytes are uniform in shape and size. In B_{12} or folate deficiency, the macrocytes are oval in shape and vary considerably in size. Huge macro-ovalocytes are seen if the anemia is severe. Hypersegmentation of the neutrophils is a very early finding. The marrow shows erythroid hyperplasia, and the nucleated red blood cell precursors show nucleocytoplasmic dissociation. The nuclei show a fine sieve-like chromatin pattern. The normal clumping of chromatin in the nucleus lags behind the progressive and normal hemoglobinization of the cytoplasm. The leukocyte precursors are larger than normal and their nuclei assume various bizarre shapes. The platelets are generally reduced in number and may be large in size.

Two points must be emphasized: (1) the morphological features in the blood and marrow do not distinguish B_{12} from folate deficiency; and (2) if the anemia is very mild (Hb 10 g or more), the above-described findings may be very subtle and may be missed. The diagnosis of pernicious anemia has been delayed for several months and even years after the findings of a high MCV was evident.[12]

The most useful test for diagnosing pernicious anemia is the determination of serum vitamin B_{12} level preferably by radioimmunoassay. A low level in a patient with an appropriate clinical picture generally implies a deficiency state. A misleading elevation in serum B_{12} may be caused by previous B_{12} therapy in a patient suffering from pernicious anemia. Serum folate is a less accurate guide to folate stores and is often low before tissue depletion of folate occurs. Other older and less specific laboratory tests are available to aid in the diagnosis of pernicious anemia, including those for histamine fast achlorhydria and the Schilling test that measures radioactive cobalt labeled B_{12} absorbed from the alimentary tract and excreted in the urine. Also, the presence of antiparietal cell and anti-intrinsic factor antibodies can be determined at some laboratories.

MANAGEMENT STRATEGIES

Initial treatment for patients with pernicious anemia consists of giving enough vitamin B_{12} to correct the anemia and replenish stores. Subsequent treatment is aimed at providing lifelong maintenance doses of vitamin B_{12} at regular intervals. In general, B_{12} is given parenterally, 1000 μg weekly for six weeks, when the anemia should be corrected. Then 1000 μg should be given every month, since the liver is able to store B_{12} for prolonged intervals. Due to the lack of known side effects of B_{12} in large doses and due to its inexpensiveness, this dose is recommended even though in excess of body needs.[13] Some mild neurological involvement may be reversible if of short duration. The mechanism for this reversal of symptoms and signs is not known.

In patients suffering from pernicious anemia, there is the rare case in which a correlation between the anemia and a higher incidence of carcinoma of the stomach exists. In a routine follow-up of these patients, it is important to be suspicious of any gastrointestinal symptoms.

Treatment of folic acid deficiency is directed at supplementing the dietary folate. Synthetic folic acid is better utilized than naturally occurring folate. Folate is found in relatively high quantities in bananas, lima beans, liver, and brewer's yeast. It is found to a lesser extent in orange juice, romaine lettuce, egg yolk, cabbage, defatted soybean, and wheat germ. Synthetic folic acid can "mask" a concurrent pernicious anemia. One must be assured that coexisting B_{12} deficiency is not present prior to initiating replacement therapy. This is best done by doing serum B_{12} levels. Giving folate to a patient with pernicious anemia may precipitate or aggravate the neurological syndrome.

The reticulocyte response to therapy begins on

the third-to-fifth day of treatment and reaches a peak on the seventh to tenth day. The patient usually has a feeling of well-being on the third to fifth day of treatment.

PATIENT EDUCATION

Stressing the need for lifelong therapy to prevent progressive neurologic involvement is necessary for patients with pernicious anemia. Specific diet changes usually are of no value since either intrinsic factor is absent or malabsorption is occurring in these patients. Assuming a treatable cause, such as correcting a blind loop, parenteral B12 and dietary changes may be in order. Vitamin B12 is found in relatively high amounts in organ meats, beef, pork, eggs, milk, and milk products.

The need for knowledge about self-injection techniques may be necessary and reasonable for some patients. All need to know how often to expect follow-up visits and laboratory tests. Again, compliance is greatly enhanced when the patient understands the rationale for treatment plans and agrees to a mutual contract with the provider based on the patient's needs and capabilities.

Anemia Associated With Chronic Disease

The second most common anemia in the elderly is the anemia of chronic disease. The underlying disease may be infectious, inflammatory, or neoplastic. More often than not, the underlying disease is obvious and the anemia of secondary importance. Occasionally, an aggressive pursuit for the cause of a mild anemia may lead to an occult malignancy such as renal cell carcinoma. Chronic renal insufficiency, liver disease, and endocrine hypofunction are sometimes overlooked as causes of anemia.

Anemia associated with chronic disease is usually mild normocytic and normochromic. It develops slowly and is usually nonprogressive. The anemia is caused by a combination of a shortened life span of red blood cells and a failure of the bone marrow to respond adequately. Impaired release of iron from the reticuloendothelial system is also present in this disease complex.

The peripheral blood smear is usually normocytic–normochromic but may be normocytic–hypochromic. Serum iron is reduced, and total iron-binding capacity is normal or reduced. The saturation index is normal or only mildly subnormal. Iron stores in the reticuloendothelial cells are increased, and this is reflected in the marrow, which contains

ample or even increased iron. This and a normal transferrin index are decisive features in the differentiation of the anemia of disease from iron deficiency. Treatment is usually not required for correction of anemia, as it is usually mild. The therapy is directed toward the specific underlying disease.

Hypothyroidism is not uncommon in the elderly. Typically, the patient has no complaints. Intolerance to cold, sluggishness, constipation, and slowing of intellectual powers can all be ignored by friends and relatives as part of the aging process. Approximately 30–50 percent of patients with hypothyroidism develop anemia. (The anemia is most commonly normocytic–normochromic but may be macrocytic or hypochromic.) The etiology of the different types of anemia is not clear. The microcytic–hypochromic type of anemia does not respond to thyroid hormone therapy but does respond to iron administration. The macrocytic type of anemia is thought to be due to vitamin B12 or folate deficiency. The normocytic–normochromic type of anemia is a manifestation of hormone deficiency. This type of anemia is usually mild and responds to the treatment of hypothyroidism over a period of several months. The subtle and insidious anemias caused by hypothyroidism need to be considered when approaching the elderly patient.

IDIOPATHIC REFRACTORY SIDEROBLASTIC ANEMIA

This condition is not common but is a disease of older adults. The onset is insidious, and the anemia may remain mild to moderate for several years and is well tolerated by the patients. No treatment is required or effective. In some patients, the anemia may slowly progress to such a degree that the cardiovascular system is compromised, and transfusions of packed red cells may become necessary. The terminal event may be an acute leukemia.

The anemia is normocytic or macrocytic. Hypochromia is almost always present. The transferrin saturation index is increased, and the marrow shows increased iron. The hallmark of this disease is the presence in the marrow of a large number of ringed sideroblasts.

Proliferative Disorders

Why some diseases are more common in the elderly is not known. Changes in the host resistance may be a major factor in the development of some diseases. Leukemia, multiple myeloma, and the lymphomas are more common with advancing age for yet unknown reasons. Factors that influence the activation of these conditions are not understood.

POLYCYTHEMIA

A condition of increased red cells may be encountered in the elderly. Secondary polycythemia (secondary erythrocytosis) is much more common than polycythemia vera, so when presented with an elderly patient with elevated hemoglobin and hematocrit, one should look for contributing causes. Secondary polycythemia is due to increased erythropoiten from conditions resulting in hypoxia, such as pulmonary diseases (emphysema being the most common), as well as from tumors, cysts, adrenocortical steroid androgens, and a variety of chemicals. Stress erythrocytosis consists of a mild to moderate increase in red blood cells and hemoglobin usually seen in anxious, hard-driving men. (See Table 16-4.)

Table 16-4
Causes of Secondary Polycythemia

I. Chronic hypoxia
  A. Chronic lung diseases
    1. Chronic obstructive pulmonary disease (emphysema)
    2. Alveolar-capillary block syndrome
    3. Pulmonary arteriosclerosis
  B. Cardiovascular diseases
    1. Cardiovascular shunts (right to left)
    2. Pulmonary arteriovenous fistulas
  C. Chronic pulmonary congestion
  D. High altitude diseases
  E. Hypoventilation idiopathic and associated with obesity
II. Overstimulation of bone marrow
  A. Hormonal
    1. Adrenal hypercorticism (Cushing's syndrome)
    2. Androgens—virilizing tumors, androgen therapy
  B. Overproduction of erythropoiten
    1. Tumors of kidney, liver, central nervous system, uterus, and ovary.
    2. Renal cysts, rarely hydronephrosis
  C. Chemicals
    1. Cobalt
    2. Shellac
    3. Various alcohols
    4. Nitrites
    5. Sulfonamides
    6. Coal tar derivatives
  D. Stress erythrocytosis

Polycythemia vera is most common in men between the ages of 40 and 70. This is a chronic condition with an inappropriate overproduction of red cells by morphologically normal red cell precursors leading to an absolute increase in circulating red cells in the peripheral blood. Patients with polycythemia vera also have a higher incidence of myelogenous leukemia than the general population.

The symptoms produced are due to the increased viscosity of the blood and from a hemorrhagic tendency. Common complaints are tiredness, headache, dizziness, and blurred vision. Other symptoms due to hyperviscosity and platelet dysfunction can be epistaxis and gastrointestinal hemorrhage. Pruritis is a common symptom. Splenomegaly is present in the majority of patients.

The diagnosis of polycythemia is made when the hematocrit is over 65 or the hemoglobin is above 18 g in men and above 16 g in women. The red cell count is always increased. The platelet count is usually elevated. The bone marrow is hyperplastic, and uric acid elevation, with clinical gout, is common from the increased cell turnover and cell destruction.

CHRONIC LYMPHOCYTIC LEUKEMIA

The most common lymphoproliferative disorder of the elderly and the most common leukemia in the United States is chronic lymphocytic leukemia (CLL). Patients with CLL may be asymptomatic and the initial diagnosis of leukemia is frequently made on a routine physical exam or evaluation of another disorder. The disease progresses slowly and may go on for years on a benign course (Fig. 16-1). An elderly patient with a marked lymphocytosis with or without lymphadenopathy and splenomegaly should be suspect for CLL. A complicating infection may be the first sign of disease.

The laboratory diagnosis of chronic lymphocytic leukemia is made by blood and bone marrow examination. In Wintrobe's series, the median survival time following diagnosis was nine years and longer, if the diagnosis was made prior to the onset of symptoms.[14] With this survival rate and the fairly benign course of CLL, aggressive treatment with antileukemic therapy, with its known hazards and limited value, is not advocated for the majority of patients early in the course of the disease. Only the symptomatic patient with active disease may need antileukemic therapy.

Infection, hemolytic anemia, and generally impaired immune responses should be treated with appropriate adjunctive therapy. Most patients with CLL can be best managed as outpatients by the family practice team.

MULTIPLE MYELOMA

Another disorder in the elderly is the plasma cell dyscrasia, multiple myeloma. The bone marrow is invaded by plasma cells normally involved in antibody production. Patients complain of bone pain and have an increased susceptibility to infections. Multiple myeloma is associated with anemia, hypercalcemia, increased total serum proteins, and impairment of renal function. Radiographs of bones, especially the skull, often show classic lytic lesions. The diagnosis is made by serum and urine protein-electrophoresis, or Bence Jones protein in the urine. Bone marrow examination showing 10 percent or more of plasma cell infiltration is also diagnostic. Appropriate treatment consists of systemic chemotherapy for the generalized disease and irradiation of painful bone lesions, which decreases morbidity and definitely extends the useful life of the patient. The family practice team needs to work in conjunction with the hematologist, oncologist, and radiotherapist in the development of this patient's treatment plan.

WALDENSTROM'S MACROGLOBULINEMIA

A rare disorder seen in the elderly is Waldenstrom's macroglobulinemia. This is a lymphocytic dyscrasia in which the proliferation of these cells produces an excessive amount of IgM. Patients have vague symptoms related mainly to the hyperviscosity of the blood. The diagnosis is made by the characteristic serum protein abnormality and the presence of lymphoid cells in the bone marrow. It must be differentiated from CLL.

CHRONIC MYELOMA MONOCYTIC LEUKEMIA

Chronic myeloma monocytic leukemia (CMML) is another uncommon disease limited to elderly adults. Males are more commonly affected. The onset is insidious and the progress slow, terminating in many cases as an acute myelogenous leukemia. Patients may die of infection or from a concurrent disease common to the elderly before the CMML has evolved to a terminal, acute leukemic process.

The disease may present as a mild anemia with characteristics of a hemolytic anemia (reticulocytosis of about 5 percent and macrocytosis) or an aplastic anemia (reticulocytes less than 2 percent). Early in the course of the disease, the monocytes by absolute

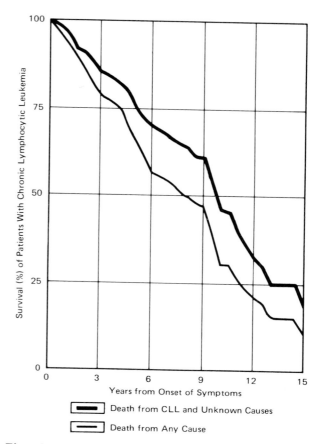

Death from CLL and Unknown Causes

Death from Any Cause

Fig. 16-1. The course of chronic lymphocytic leukemia in the elderly is often quite benign, as indicated by Wintrobe's data on survival time after onset of symptoms in 130 cases. [Reproduced with permission from Baisden CR: Hematologic problems of the elderly. Hosp Prac 13:93–104, 1978; and from Reichel W (ed): The Geriatric Patient. New York, HP Publishing Co Inc, 1978.]

count exceed 800/cu mm. The marrow is essentially normal. As the disease evolves over a period of many months or even years, the monocytes increase in the peripheral blood, the anemia becomes progressively worse, and the marrow shows an increasing number of monocytoid cells, immature myelocytes and myeloblasts.

The clinical course is slow, and the only symptom is weakness or increased fatigability. The spleen and liver may become enlarged. Hemorrhagic manifestations of intercurrent infections may complicate the otherwise benign clinical course.

Treatment is symptomatic and supportive. Antileukemic therapy has no place in the early course of this disease and is of doubtful value in the terminal phase of acute leukemia. The patient will tolerate a mild to moderate anemia for a long time, but in the more advanced stage transfusions of packed red cells may become necessary.[15]

LYMPHOMA

Non-Hodgkin's lymphoma, although existing in all age groups, is increasingly more frequent with advancing age. The presenting symptoms may be a painless enlargement of peripheral lymph nodes. In over 20 percent of patients, however, the presenting initial site of disease is extranodal. The principal sites of initial disease may be in the skin, bone, lungs, or gastrointestinal tract. Even the marrow or spleen may be the primary sites of non-Hodgkin's lymphoma. Patients may manifest systemic symptoms of weight loss, fever, anemia, and night sweats. However, lymphoma may be asymptomatic. Treatment of lymphomas consists of a combination of radiotherapy and chemotherapy. The prognosis has improved in recent years with this adjunctive therapy.

DRUG TOXICITY

Iatrogenic disease in the elderly is not uncommon since unpredictable reactions are more likely to occur in this age group because of the greater drug usage. In hypoplastic bone marrow states, aplastic anemia, or in patients with hemolytic anemia, one should always consider drug toxicity as a working diagnosis and diligently question the patient's history from this perspective. (See Table 16-5).

SENILE PURPURA

Senile purpura is a commonplace condition of easy bruisability—especially on the extensor surfaces and the radial side of the forearms—and is seldom mentioned. It is essentially a benign condition present with aging due to a loss of subcutaneous fat, elastin, and dermal collagen. The purple ecchymotic spots fade to permanent brownish pigmented spots over the span of a few weeks. These may be a source of great anxiety to the elderly patient who often equates the senile purpura with a possible cerebral vascular hemorrhage. The therapy of full explanation and reassurance is very comforting.

HEALTH MAINTENANCE

A primary goal of the family practice team should be to encourage self-care and home care. Emphasis on illness prevention, health maintenance, and pa-

Table 16-5

Drugs Causing Untoward Hematologic Reactions in the Elderly (Ranked in Decreasing Order of Frequency of Side Effect)

Associated With:	
Anemia	Thrombocytopenia
Chloramphenicol	Quinidine
Methyldopa	Gold salts
Penicillin	Ethanol
Diphenylhydantoin	Chlorothiazides
Phenacetin	Diphenylhydantoin
Cephalosporin	Sulfathiazole
derivatives	Rifampin
Chlorpromazine	Quinine
Phenylbutazone	Acetazolamide
Ethanol	Digitoxin
Isoniazid	Acetaminophen
Sulfonamides	Hydroxchloroquine
Quinidine	Chlorpromazine
Quinine	Cephalothin
Para-aminosalicyclic	Phenacetin
acid	Propylthiouracil
Aspirin	Aspirin
	Reserpine
Leukopenia	Meprobamate
Phenothiazines	Promethazine
Thiouracil and	Sulfisoxazole
propylthiouracil	Sulfamethoxazole
Methimazole	Mercurial diuretics
Phenylbutazone	Spironolactone
Sulfonamides	Estrogenic hormones
Chloramphenicol	
Meprobamate	
Penicillin	
Aspirin	
Procainamide	

Reproduced with permission from Baisden CR: Hematologic problems of the elderly. Hosp Prac 13: 93–104, 1978; and from Reichel W (ed): The Geriatric Patient. New York, HP Publishing Co Inc, 1978.

tient education help enhance that goal. (See Table 16-6.)

There are many socioeconomic issues in the elderly that influence the general state of health and, specifically, the hematologic system. A home visit to assess the individual patient's needs may provide essential information to the family practice team. Additionally, family dynamics and support systems are often known to the team. Social workers and public health nurses can also join their resources with the family practice team to help problem-solve the needs of patients. Meals on Wheels, available in

Table 16-6
Health Maintenance—Laboratory Data (Over 60)

Age	60	61	62	63	64	65	66	67	68	69	70	71	72	73	74	75	76	77	78	79	80+
Urine analysis	X		X		X		X		X		X		X		X		X				Every two years
CBC with indices	X	X		X		X	X				X		X		X		X				Every two years
2° pp BS/F BS*	X			X			X			X			X			X			X		Every three years
BUN/Creatinine*	X			X			X			X			X			X			X		Every three years
Stool guaiac	X	X	X	X	X	X	X	X	X	X	X	X	X	X	X	X	X	X	X	X	Every year
FTA/STS*	One Time																				
Pap smear	X	X	X	X	X	X	X	X	X	X	X	X	X	X	X	X	X	X	X	X	Every year
T₄	X			X			X			X			X			X			X		Every three years

*Either test

many communities, can provide warm, balanced meals and social contact for isolated patients. Homemaker services, assisting in shopping and housework, may also be necessary. Many senior citizen groups provide social contact as well as nutritious low-cost hot meals. Since many older people essentially live on tin foods, these services can promote many healthful changes. Social contact may enhance appetite by decreasing the depression so common in the elderly. (See Chapter 20.)

Utilizing the unique skills and training of each team member is a challenge to the family practice team and a bonus for patients. Not only are providers more effective because of high job satisfaction, but collegial relationships enhance professional growth and spur on interest in the never-ending learning process inherent in the practice of medicine. Mid-level practitioners usually have the advantage of taking extra time to develop good patient rapport necessary to assess the socioeconomic and family dynamic issues of patients. Patients have been trained, culturally and by physicians in haste, to think of physician time as very valuable and limited. Thus, they often reglect to mention issues vital to their care. In our experience, mid-level practitioners are not viewed in this manner by patients and therefore are the ideal provider for initial contact with patients. Not only are the dynamics of life style obtained, but health history and physical screening can help better utilize physician time for complex and multisystem diseases.

The team approach to patient care also encourages the development of health maintenance and screening protocols by age and population groups. This allows for the emergence of individual team philosophies of care. The use of consultants is encouraged for secondary and tertiary care. Allowing for terminal care by primary care providers may be a preference of the team, as they may be better able to provide the support of this unique final growth experience for their patient and his or her family.

Senile purpura is a condition that helps remind us of an essential principle of patient care. Those primary care providers who work with elderly patients and their families must keep in mind that the elderly have survived the ravages of economic depression, companion losses, accidents, and atherosclerosis. Their hematologic disorders should neither be overlooked nor overtreated, but managed according to their significance in the balance and harmony of quality living and dignified dying.

REFERENCES

1. Earney MA, Earney AJ: Geriatric hematology. J Am Geriatr Soc 20:174, 1972
2. Davison W: Anemia in the elderly with special reference to iron deficiency. Gerontol Clin 9:393–400, 1967
3. McLennan WJ, Andrews GR, MacLeod C, et al: Anemia in the elderly. QJ Med 42:1, 1973
4. Girdwood RH, Thomson AD, Williamson J: Folate status in the elderly. Bri Med J 2:570, 1967
5. Cough KR, Read AE, McCarthy CG, et al: Megaloblastic anemia due to nutritional deficiency of folic acid. QJ Med 32:243, 1963
6. Read AE, Cough KR, Pardoe JL, et al: Nutritional studies on the entrants to an old people's home,

with particular reference to folic acid deficiency. Bri Med J 5466:843, 1965

7. Varadi S, Elwis A: Megaloblastic anemia due to dietary deficiency. Lancet 1:1162, 1964

8. Forshaw J, Moorhouse EH, Harwood L: Megaloblastic anemia due to dietary deficiency. Lancet 1:275, 1965

9. Hurdle AD, Williams TC: Folic acid deficiency in elderly patients admitted to hospital. Bri Med J 5307:202, 1966

10. Milne JS, Williamson J: Hemoglobia, hematocrit, leukocyte count, and blood grouping in older people. Geriatr 279:118, 1972

11. Evans DM: Hematological aspects of iron deficiency in the elderly. Gerontol Clin (Base I) 13:12, 1971

12. Carmel R: Macrocytosis, mild anemia, and delay in diagnosis of pernicious anemia. Arch Int Med 139:47–50, 1979

13. Schrier SL: Hematology, in Rubenstein E, Federman D (eds): Medicine. New York, Scientific American, 1979, vol 1

14. Wintrobe MM: Clinical Hematology, ed 7. Philadelphia, Lea & Febiger, 1974

15. Miescher PA, Farquet JJ: Chronic Myelomonocytic leukemia in adults. Sem Hematol 11:129–139, 1974

17

Problems of the Ears, Nose, and Throat

Jan McCann, F.N.P., M.H.S.
Jack Rodnick, M.D.
Robert J. Ruben, M.D.

Diseases in the ears, nose, and throat overall do not carry the same morbidity and mortality as diseases in some other systems, yet they can have a profound effect on the quality of life of the elder. The ability to give and receive communication from others can mean the difference between loneliness and social isolation and participation in a vital and active world. As age increases, the number of social contacts, family, and friends decrease. Early detection of communicative problems can profoundly enhance the quality of life.

INCIDENCE OF PROBLEMS OF EARS, NOSE, AND THROAT

A significant loss of hearing occurs in 30–50 percent of persons over the age of 65, and the incidence increases markedly in the late 70s and 80s.[1] The decrease in hearing function is more marked in elderly men. See Fig. 17-1, which shows the hearing threshold at different sound frequencies for men and women of different ages. It has been estimated that 13 percent of the 24 million people over the age of 65 in 1980 will show advanced signs of hearing loss.[2] Hearing loss can be the most devastating to communication of all sensory problems that affect the older person. The sense of hearing not only functions for the abilities to hear and understand what others are saying; it also provides background sounds that contribute to

a sense of orientation, and it may serve as a warning signal for self-protection.

There are many age-related changes in the human ear. The external ear canal undergoes atrophic changes, the walls become thinner, and the cerumen-producing glands decrease their secretions.[3] The tympanic membrane often appears whiter, thicker, and lacks luster.[4] The sclerotic changes in blood vessels may affect the ability of the organ of Corti and the cochlea to function. Loss of hair cells of the organ of Corti results in hearing impairment.[4] The nerves themselves undergo degenerative changes that may contribute to hearing loss.[5] Although there is considerable individual variability, the range and sensitivity of hearing decrease with age.

Nasal tissue atrophies with age, and the olfactory ganglion cells steadily decrease in number. By 75 years of age there is a 68 percent decrease in these cells.[3] In addition to olfactory impairment, taste buds decrease and have a lower threshold of response, thus interfering in the elder's ability to taste and identify food.[6] The mucous membranes of the sinuses atrophy and become less vascular with age, and the atrophic tissues seem to respond less readily to irritating substances.[3]

The overall ability to perceive touch in the mouth is also diminished. The laryngeal cartilages become progressively ossified, and there is a decrease in muscular tonus and strength. These changes, coupled with the decrease in air-force available from the lungs, cause alterations in the voice of the elder.

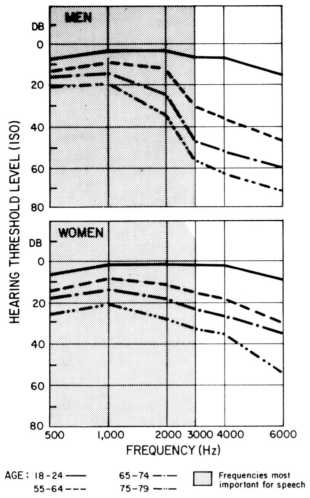

AGE: 18-24 —— 65-74 —·— ☐ Frequencies most
      55-64 - - - 75-79 —··—   important for speech

Fig. 17-1. Decline in hearing with age. [Reprinted from Ruben RJ: Otolaryngologic problems of the old. Hosp Prac 12:73–87, 1977. By permission.]

Typically, the voice range narrows with loss of high tones and decreased ability to sustain a sound. The overall sound of the voice may become monotonous and tremulous.[7]

The common medical problems are occlusion of the external auditory canal by cerumen, external otitis, presbycusis, vertigo, epistaxis, tinnitis, and rhinitis. Other conditions mentioned, but less common, are labrynthitis, Meniere's syndrome, otitis media, otosclerosis, tympanosclerosis, acoustic neuroma, sinusitis, nasopharyngeal tumors, tumors of the larynx and oropharynx, anosmia, and vocal cord abnormalities.

COMMON LAB VALUES

When there is either subjective or objective evidence of a hearing loss, the evaluation should be an audiogram.*

An audiogram measures one's ability to hear pure tones in each ear. It should be performed by someone skilled in its technique and done with a relaxed patient in as quiet a surrounding as possible. Audiometric testing for air conduction is performed by presenting a tone to the ear and noting the lowest decibel level at which the tone is perceived. It is usually done on a range of frequencies from 125 through 8000 Hz. Bone conduction can also be accomplished by placing an oscillator over the mastoid process of one ear while the tones are again presented. A masking noise is given to the ear not being tested, as sound from the mastoid travels to both cochleas.

If the patient has normal hearing, all four curves (air and bone conduction for each ear) should be within 20 db of a zero decibel line. (Fig. 17-1 shows normal audiogram hearing values at different ages.) If the patient has a conductive hearing loss (interference with the middle ear bones), the audiogram will show a bone conduction near the zero decibel level and an air conduction curve lower on the graph (Fig. 17-2). The audiogram of a patient with some neural loss will show both depressed bone and air conduction (Fig. 17-3).

Table 17-1 shows how the threshold of hearing (decibel loss) is related to difficulties in hearing and understanding speech.[8]

Although this is a simplified explanation, additional audiometry tests can, in many instances, be done to measure further one's ability to hear and understand speech, as well as to help localize a lesion causing hearing loss to the eighth nerve or cochlea. Many clinicians do a simple audiogram that only measures air conduction. This is an adequate evaluation only if one is initially confident of the

*Editor's note: A discussion of the Weber and Rinne tests has been omitted at the author's request. Dr. Robert Ruben feels these tests are extremely difficult to administer and require great skill and experience, with the backup of an audiometer. Other authorities feel that these are valuable screening tests for differentiating conductive and neurosensory hearing loss. The tests are described in most texts on physical examination. In addition, the use of the tuning fork is of value in comparing the hearing in the right and left ears of the patient, as well as against the hearing of the examiner.

diagnosis or if one primarily wants to document the extent of hearing loss.

THE DIAGNOSIS AND TREATMENT OF COMMON PROBLEMS

Ears

CERUMEN OCCLUSION

One of the most common and easily treated causes of hearing loss is cerumen that occludes the external auditory canal. The decrease in hearing is usually mild to moderate, but in the presence of other types of hearing loss it may be significant. The patient may also encounter stuffiness and itching in the affected ear.

Cerumen is most easily removed in the office by irrigation of the external canal with a large syringe filled with warm water; this may be preceded (30 minutes) by the instillation of a few drops of a softening agent (such as Cerumenex). A waterpick at low levels of pressure may also be used. If the cerumen is still lodged, the patient may be sent home to instill a softening agent at bedtime and to return in a few days for inspection of results. Irrigation should never be attempted if a perforation in the tympanic membrane is suspected. Evidence of mastoid operation or a history of otorrhea should alert the clinician to this possibility. Once irrigation is completed the canal and tympanic membrane should be examined for any additional abnormalities.

When the clinician is certain pathology of the ear does not exist, the patient can be instructed to treat the problem of cerumen at home. Usually the instillation of a softening agent (such as Debrop or Debrox) into the ear at bedtime, followed by irrigation with warm water in a bulb syringe the next morning, will control the problem. This should be done one to three times a month, depending on the severity of the problem. Elders, like anyone else, should be discouraged from the use of Q-tips, bobby pins, or other sharp objects in the ears.

EXTERNAL OTITIS

External otitis may be viral, fungal, or bacterial. Cerumen impaction may be a predisposing factor. Scalp and skin conditions such as seborrhea, eczema, and contact dermatitis may also predispose to

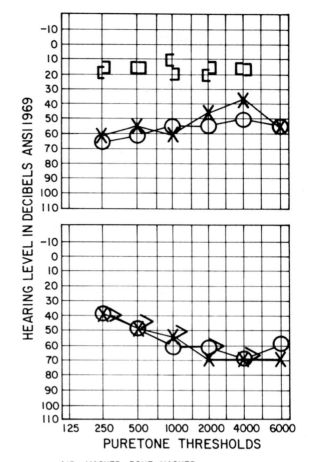

	AIR	MASKED	BONE	MASKED
RIGHT—RED	O	△	<	⊏
LEFT—BLUE	X	□	>	⊐

Fig. 17-2 (top). Typical audiogram pattern in moderate conductive hearing loss.

Fig. 17-3 (bottom). Typical audiogram pattern in moderate neurosensory loss.

external otitis. Bobby pins or other sharp objects used to relieve itching usually result in trauma to the canal, and secondary infection is often the outcome. Infection may also occur without trauma as decreased cerumen and decreased circulation to the area compromise the normal protective mechanisms.

External otitis commonly presents with discharge, itching, edema, and pain. It is usually unilateral, but may be bilateral. In the elder, fever and enlargement of the lymph nodes is usually absent. The ear is acutely inflamed, edematous, and painful to ex-

Table 17-1
Threshold of Hearing Loss in Relation to Hearing and Understanding Speech

Threshold Loss (db)	Characterization	Effect
0–15 (in poorer ear)	Normal	No difficulties
15–30 (in better ear)	Near normal	Difficulty with faint speech
30–45 (in better ear)	Mild impairment	Difficulty with normal speech
45–60 (in better ear)	Moderate impairment	Difficulty with loud speech
60–90 (in better ear)	Severe impairment	Can understand only amplified speech
90 or more (in better ear)	Profound impairment	Difficulty with amplified speech

From Consumer Reports, Consumers Union of US Inc, Mt Vernon, New York, June 1976, p 348.

ternal manipulation. Purulent discharge may be present.

Before treatment is initiated, a culture of the discharge should be taken. This condition usually responds well to the instillation of Burrow's solution for 24 hours, then Cortisporin otitic drops—three to four times a day in the affected ear for seven to ten days. Many patients will also need to have the ear cleansed gently with suction (or "a suction tip") after the first two to three days of medication. Any patient not helped by this therapy should be referred to an otolaryngologist for further work-up as the otitis externa may be caused by other ear conditions such as tympanomastoiditis.

In elderly diabetics, otitis externa may become a runaway disease that may progress to osteomyelitis or meningitis. It should therefore be watched very carefully and treated aggressively.[9]

When dryness and itching are predisposing factors to scratching, ear trauma, and infection, a few drops of a heavy oil (such as mineral oil) can be instilled in each ear two to three times per week to prevent this problem.

OTITIS MEDIA

This condition is not as common in the elderly population as it is in the young. It is usually preceded by a respiratory infection or influenza. The patient will complain of ear pain, stuffiness, and a hearing loss. As in many other infections in this age group, fever is usually absent. Middle ear infection may be an indication of more serious problems such as diabetes, tumors, or cancer.[4]

Cholesteatoma, the sequela of childhood infections, may be seen. These need evaluation for treatment by an otolaryngologist. This is important as cholesteatomas can erode the ossicles and extend into the mastoid air cells.[9]

Treatment of choice for otitis media is penicillin VK 250 mg for ten days with concomitant use of a decongestant during this time, if there is nasal stuffiness. The patient should be reexamined in a week to evaluate effectiveness of the treatment. This condition should be watched closely in elderly diabetics.

A variant of chronic otitis media is tympanosclerosis. Repeated infections and scarring of the tympanic membrane can produce stapes fixation or total ossicular fixation, resulting in a conductive hearing loss. The tympanic membrane in these patients will appear thickened with whitish scar tissue and a distorted light reflex. Patients with tympanomastoiditis cannot be effectively treated with surgery; a hearing aid is the treatment of choice.

PRESBYCUSIS AND OTHER CAUSES
OF HEARING LOSS

The bilateral neurosensory hearing loss that occurs gradually with advancing age has been termed presbycusis. It is thought to be the result of the atrophy of the hair cells and/or the ganglion cells and the cochlear.[2] Sensitivity for high frequency sounds diminishes first and most severely, followed later by a decrease in sensitivity to middle and low frequency sounds. Concurrent with these changes is the gradual inability to descriminate speech. Presbycusis may also be accompanied by tinnitus.[10]

The patient or family will usually report hearing loss or difficulty understanding speech. In some cases, the problem is not noticed until the older person begins to withdraw from social encounters. Difficulty in hearing or understanding conversation can also result in increased irritability in the elder. It is not uncommon for patients with this communication problem to be considered "senile" or "confused" by family and friends.

Physical exam reveals a normal-looking ear, and simple gross hearing tests, such as the whisper or watch-tick, may reveal generally decreased hearing or may be normal. The audiogram may vary in degree but will usually show a bilateral high frequency loss. To date, there is no effective medical or surgical treatment.[5]

In some patients, presbycusis may be compounded by other treatable disorders and may present as both a conductive and a neurosensory loss.

Other sensorineural hearing loss problems can mimic presbycusis. Several drugs have ototoxic effects and their removal may greatly improve the patient's hearing.[5] A list of some commonly used drugs that can cause ototoxicity are listed in Table 17-2. Caution is indicated with the use of all these agents, especially for aminoglycoside antibiotics. Ototoxicity is dose-related and dosages for many of these agents is controversial.

One of the most widely used drugs in elders is aspirin. Patients on relatively high doses of 1.5–2 g/day for arthritis may experience a neurosensory loss. This is usually reversed when aspirin is substituted with other antiinflammatory agents. Removal of the other offending drugs, however, rarely reverses the neurosensory loss. See Table 17-2.

Chronic sound trauma can cause hearing loss in elders. These patients may present with a general hearing loss or may report difficulty communicating in noisy environments. Elders should be questioned as to type of work or hobbies. Jobs in loud industrial environments, such as work involving metal crafts, boilermakers, firearms, or heavy machinery, should be suspect. The hearing loss is symmetrical, frequently associated with tinnitus and has a characteristic pattern on the audiogram.[11]

Hearing aids may help these patients, but the best treatment is prevention and reduction of further noise exposure. Ear plugs and hearing muffs can be used if patients must continue in noisy environments. (It should be thoroughly documented if sound trauma from previous or present working situations is suspected, as the patient may be eligible for compensation by employers.)

Because of the multiple causality of hearing loss in the elder, a thorough evaluation for treatable causes must be done before the diagnosis of presbycusis is made. Patients should have a detailed history and complete physical exam, as well as audiometric testing, both to determine the cause and to evaluate for hearing rehabilitation. See Table 17-3.

Management. Management of presbycusis is a major medical problem in our society as our awareness of the effects of sensory deprivation on the elderly population increases. Rehabilitation requires a broad, multifaceted approach, which must in turn be individualized.

Several patients can be helped with the use of hearing aids, but many elders have been sold such devices when no amplification was needed. See Table 17-4. Many times alterations in the environ-

Table 17-2

Medications Known to Produce Cochlear and Vestibular Toxicity, Causing Symptoms of Hearing Loss, Tinnitus, or "Dizziness"

Medications of Potential Ototoxicity	Medications Associated With Dizziness
Aminoglycoside antibiotics	Antihypertensives
Gentamycin	Barbiturates
Kanamycin	CNS depressants
Neomycin	Estrogens
Streptomycin	Phenothiazines
Viomycin	Phenylbutazone
Amikacin	
Tobramycin	
Other antibiotics	
Viomycin	
Polymixins	
Diuretics	
Furosemide	
Ethacrynic Acid	
Others	
Salicylates	Novocaine
Quinine	Caffeine
Quinidine	Ergot
Chloroquine	Atropine

Table 17-3

Common Causes of Hearing Loss in the Elderly

Conductive	Neurosensory
Cerumen	Presbycusis
External otitis	Ototoxicity
Otitis media	Acoustic neuroma
Otosclerosis	Noise induced
Tympanosclerosis	Birth defect
Foreign body	Paget's disease
Paget's disease	

ment and training in lip or speech reading can vastly improve hearing. See Table 17-5. It cannot be emphasized enough that hearing is critical to both the communication and social environment of elders, and every attempt to help patients operate at their maximum level of function should be made. This usually involves work with other household members and families to educate them in maximizing hearing.

TINNITUS

Tinnitus is an auditory sensation originating within the patient and subjectively noted only by him or her. It may or may not be of ear origin. Significant

Table 17-4
What You Should Know About a Hearing Aid

Nearly 600,000, Americans buy a hearing aid each year. Many more could use one, but don't—some for vanity reasons, some for lack of information, some because the aids don't help, and many because of the cost.

Aids are purchased through hearing aid dealers who are not professionally trained. The audiologist or physician may or may not refer people to a specific dealer. It is best not to go to a dealer first as the HEW Task Force found that of those who did, 85 percent were found "capable of being helped" by an aid. In contrast, other statistics show that only 45 percent of persons who contact audiologists are diagnosed as needing a hearing aid. It is best to view dealers as tradesmen there to sell a product, not to diagnose hearing problems.

Four styles of aids are in widespread use: First, the "in-the-ear" type. It is very tiny and can't provide powerful amplification, and it is for cases of mild to moderate loss. The most common types are the "behind-the-ear" and those contained in eyeglass frames. These two types can be used for moderate to severe hearing loss. People with profound hearing loss may need, on occasion, to wear a body aid. There are "behind-the-ear" aids, however, that can also be used for these severely impaired patients.

Hearing aids can compensate for specific kinds of hearing loss by amplifying certain frequencies more than others. The microphone placed on the opposite side of the head from the receiver reduces noise. Most people find that the quality of the sound is more "brassy" than normal, and it is difficult to tune out distracting background noise.

There is no model of aid that can completely compensate for any type of hearing loss. The audiogram cannot be directly translated into a certain type of hearing aid, and a dealer cannot relate it to product specifications. Therefore, going to different dealers will likely mean different aid recommendations and a wide selection of choices. Besides fitting the earpiece (often needing a mold of the ear canal), a dealer shows you how to operate and take care of the aid. You should insist that the aid be bought on a trial basis or rented for a month and be refundable if you aren't satisfied.

A hearing aid is basically no different from the amplifier in a small transistor radio. Why should it cost $350–500? It has been estimated by a HEW Task Force that the parts in a hearing aid cost $30; the manufacturer sells the aid to a dealer for between $80 and $140. There are few manufacturers who produce a wide array of models and about 8,000 dealers. Dealers not only are subject to pressure from manufacturers, but in addition the low volume makes it necessary to sell those few at high prices.

Financial assistance is limited. Many dealers may provide a small discount if their full range of services is not needed. Medicare provides assistance for diagnosis and treatment of problems leading to ear surgery, *not* for the diagnosis or purchase of a hearing aid. Many states, through departments of vocational rehabilitation, provide assistance for those whose hearing problems handicap their employment. Veterans can obtain free diagnosis and hearing aids from the Veterans Administration. In addition, the VA rates hearing aids on their performance. A copy of a recent report can be obtained from the Superintendent of Documents, US Government Printing Office, Washington, DC 20402. The June 1976 issue of *Consumer Reports* has an excellent article on How to Buy a Hearing Aid and a summary of the 1976 VA ratings of hearing aids.

Table 17-5
Communication With People Who Are Hard of Hearing

Hard of hearing persons will understand more clearly if the following considerations are kept in mind:

1. Talk at a moderate rate.
2. Keep your voice at about the same volume throughout each sentence.
3. Always speak as clearly and accurately as possible.
4. Do not over-articulate.
5. Pronounce every name with care. Make a reference to the name for easier understanding, e.g., "Joan, the girl from the office."
6. Change to a new subject at a slower rate, making sure the person follows the change to the new subject.
7. Do not attempt to converse when you have something in your mouth, and do not cover your mouth with your hand.
8. Talk in a normal tone of voice. Shouting does not help.
9. Address the listener directly. Do not turn away in the middle of a remark or story. Make sure the listener can easily see your face.
10. Use longer phrases that are more explanatory, rather than short ones.
11. Reduce background noises—turn off the radio or TV.
12. Recognize that hard of hearing people hear and understand less when they are tired or ill.

Additional Tips for the Environment
1. Use a telephone buzzer or amplifier.
2. Use a loud door buzzer.
3. Use a radio and TV earphone attachments.

tinnitus is usually accompanied with a hearing loss. Its mechanisms are unknown, but it is regularly accompanied by such problems as otosclerosis, Meniere's disease, noise-induced hearing loss, and presbycusis. It occurs in both conductive and neurosensory hearing loss.[5]

Tinnitus occasionally is described as a to and fro sound in a large seashell. This is usually associated with the pulse and is frequently noted with obstructive ear problems that can be treated, such as cerumen impaction or middle ear fluid. With the exception of this to and fro tinnitus, the nature of the sound heard in not diagnostic. Common sounds are ringing, roaring, clicking, humming, and whistling.

There is no specific medical or surgical therapy for tinnitus. It is important to identify any underlying cause and, if possible, to treat it. If the tinnitus is secondary to hearing loss, it will often become less of a problem with the passage of time. However, it

may return at times of fatigue, stress, or respiratory infection. Reassurance that tinnitus represents an auditory paresthesia may help in relieving anxieties.

For a majority of people, tinnitus is most bothersome when ambient noises are lower at night, and it may keep them awake. The use of a small bedside radio may sufficiently overshadow tinnitus so that patients can fall asleep. Occasionally a small amount of sedation is helpful.

In a few cases, a properly fitted hearing aid will provide sufficient ambient environmental noise to mask the tinnitus. Recent efforts to relieve troublesome tinnitus include relaxation training by biofeedback.[5]

LABYRINTHITIS

Dizziness is a common problem for the geriatric patient. True vertigo and dizziness (dysequilibrium) must be distinguished. Due to the multiplicity and potential severity of causes for this symptom in the elderly patient, a thorough evaluation is essential for any patient presenting with dizziness or vertigo. The evaluation must include a complete history with care given to the detailed description of the complaint, any related localizing ear or neurological signs or symptoms, and a careful past history. Special care should be given to the cardiovascular, ocular, and nervous systems during the physical exam. Laboratory tests may include serum glucose, seriologic tests, and complete blood count.

Vertigo is a symptom of dysfunction of the vestibular system, which includes the peripheral, labyrinthine, retrolabyrinthine, and vestibular system (CNS). Dizziness may come from a wide variety of causes including anemia, neuropathies, arteriosclerosis, cardiac arrhythmias, and endocrine disorders. Dizziness is more diffuse and is often more frustrating to work up. A particular concern in the geriatric patient is vertebrobasilar artery insufficiency. (See Chapter 9 for the section on Dizziness.)

Vertigo can be caused by problems of the inner ear. With vertigo, patients feel the room is moving or whirling when their eyes are open and can still feel movement when their eyes are closed. If patients do not feel whirling or motion, then the problem is probably not in the nervous system or ear. Further questions that help define the cause of vertigo include asking if tinnitus is present or if the vertigo is continuous or paroxysmal. Tinnitus suggests disorders of the ear. Continuous vertigo points to a CNS cause and paroxysmal vertigo to an ear disease.

An inner ear problem is suggested when the

patient has nausea and vomiting with vertigo and no other symptoms of CNS disease, or unilateral tinnitus and hearing loss with acute vertigo, and or if the vertigo is brought on or intensified by position. If the diagnosis is unclear, further studies are indicated, such as calorics or other labyrinthine testing, and this is an appropriate ENT referral.

Vestibular neuronitis as a cause of vertigo is more common than Meniere's disease. Hearing loss, if any, is usually mild, and there is no tinnitus. The vertigo builds up over a one to three day period, but may take three to six weeks to subside. A standard treatment for the relief of vertigo is meclizine 12.5–25 mg three or four times a day. Complications are unusual (unless the etiology is bacterial, 2° to a cholesteatoma, otitis media, or trauma).

MENIERE'S SYNDROME

The etiology of Meniere's syndrome is unknown. It occurs usually in adulthood and is episodic. This condition is not likely to have its onset in the elder years, but symptoms may persist for years, and it should be considered in the work-up of a patient with unilateral neurosensory hearing loss, tinnitus, or vertigo. This triad of symptoms characterizes Meniere's syndrome, although they may not all occur simultaneously. Typically, the patient notes a sensation of fullness in one ear, hearing loss of some degree, and tinnitus in that ear. Later, disabling vertigo appears. The interval between onset of ear symptoms and vertigo can be as long as months or as short as a few minutes. The vertigo is objective and rotary, to one side or the other. It is usually accompanied with nausea and vomiting. The attacks may be several weeks or months apart; over a period of years the condition tends to wear itself out as the patient's hearing and vestibular function are lost. Tinnitus and vertigo may persist, however, even after most of the hearing is gone.[10]

Treatment of this condition has generally been unsatisfactory and controversial. Regimens vary from low-salt diets to antivertigo drugs. Dimenhydrinate 50 mg four times a day orally or by rectal suppository may give relief of symptoms. Meclizine 12.5–25 mg orally four times a day may be equally as effective. There is no treatment available to stop the progression of the disease. Depending on the severity of the loss in the affected ear and the hearing ability of the other ear, these patients may do quite well with a hearing aid. Surgical intervention may be considered on the inner ear to alleviate disabling symptoms in some patients.[10]

OTOSCLEROSIS

Although otosclerosis tends to be a condition of younger ears (second through fourth decades), its effects on hearing may not develop fully until later years. This disease is inherited and is an autosomal dominant with a variable penetration.

Otosclerosis is a growth of dystrophic bone within the labyrinthine capsule. When it involves the area of the oval window and stapes footplate, it becomes clinically significant. This results in fixation of the stapes footplate and a conductive hearing loss.

The patient will complain of a unilateral hearing loss and frequently tinnitus, rumbling, or other disturbing sounds. Audiogram shows conductive loss for low tones and an air-bone gap, in which the air conduction curve is 40–50 db below the bone conduction curve. Speech discrimination remains good. Treatment for otosclerosis is stapedectomy and, with this procedure, the restoration for hearing is good. If surgical intervention is not advisable, these patients do well with hearing aids.[9]

Paget's disease, although less common, should be ruled out in an elder with gradual hearing loss. This condition can be demonstrated on x-ray by demineralization of bone and in the serum by an increase in the alkaline phosphate level.[12]

ACOUSTIC NEUROMA

This tumor of the eighth cranial nerve is not common but should be considered in a patient with progressive unilateral high-tone hearing loss, tinnitus, and disequilibrium. Signs of increased intercranial pressure including headaches, swollen optic disc, and involvement of the fifth and seventh cranial nerves, as well as the eighth, will appear as the lesion grows.[10] The treatment is surgical removal, and this invariably results in total hearing loss on the affected side. Early recognition and referral of this condition is important to avoid complications of tumor enlargement, and particularly involvement of the seventh nerve.

Nose

RHINITIS

Acute rhinitis and upper respiratory viral infections are less common in the older population. When they do occur, however, they should be treated promptly, as the likelihood of progression to bronchitis or pneumonia in debilitated elders is higher.[13]

A chronic mild rhinitis is frequently seen in the elderly. This may be vasomotor in origin or secondary to atrophic changes.[13] If no obvious cause is found, administration of an oral antihistamine at night is usually successful (such as Benadryl, 25–50 mg) in alleviating symptoms.

More frequently, the older patient has problems with nasal dryness. The nose will have the appearance of dry, thin mucosa, and whitish crusts may be present. Minor bleeding or spotting may be associated. This may be due to pollution or low household humidity, especially in winter. The patient or family can help to relieve this condition by using a humidifier or vaporizer in the home and particularly in the patient's bedroom at night. Application of a little vasoline daily to the nasal vestibule will also aid in reducing the symptoms.

EPISTAXIS

Nosebleeds are a common and potentially life-threatening problem for the older person. Both anterior and posterior bleeds occur in the elderly, but the likelihood of a posterior bleed is greater than in a younger person.

Anterior nosebleeds arise from the anterior-posterior portion of the nasal septum (Kiesselbach's plexus), are usually less severe, and are more easily visualized and treated. The cause of an anterior bleed in an elderly person is generally related to atrophy of the mucosa, nasal trauma, or acute or chronic inflammation.

Posterior nosebleeds are seen more frequently in elders, and the bleeding is usually severe. The bleeds arise from the larger vessels in the posterior portion of the nose and are usually caused by a rupture in one of the vessels. Possible etiologies include acute or chronic inflammation, neoplasm of the nose or nasopharynx, hypertension, and diseases of the blood.[14]

Any nosebleed is a very frightening experience for the patient and family members involved. Even a rather minor episode may bleed profusely for a short time and cause extreme anxiety. A calm, assured, deliberate, and supportive manner by the health professional is essential. The examination and treatment procedure will be less traumatic for both the patient and the clinician if the anxiety level can be decreased.

A brief history should be obtained from either the patient or family member and should include the following information:

1. Previous bleeding episodes
2. Recent nasal trauma
3. Whether the bleeding is primarily down the throat or out the front of the nose
4. Duration and frequency
5. History of a bleeding tendency or disorder
6. Family history of bleeding disorders
7. Other diseases: hypertension, diabetes, liver disease
8. Anticoagulant medication or other drugs (such as ASA or Butazoladin)

Treatment. At the outset, it is essential for the clinician to get a clear appreciation of the amount and speed of blood loss and to determine if the bleeding is primarily anterior or posterior. The location of the bleeding vessel can be assessed rapidly by having the patient sit erect without bending his or her head forward. If the site is anterior, most of the blood will come out of the nose anteriorly. If the site is posterior, as much blood will be seen in the pharynx as is seen coming from the nose anteriorly.

If the vital signs are normal, the patient should be seated erect in a chair or in a semi-Fowler's position. Both the patient and the clinician should be adequately draped. It is essential that a good light source be available, such as that provided by a head mirror, and that suction equipment is at hand. If the bleeding is not profuse and appears to be from an anterior site, the nose can be cleared of clots with an angulated sucker, the site located, and a cotton ball impregnated with hydrogen peroxide or aqueous epinephrine 1:1000 placed into the nostril. Firm pressure should then be applied for several minutes and the cotton ball removed. If the bleeding persists, the nose should be packed anteriorly with a small amount of oxycel covering the bleeding spot, and this should be gently reinforced with a small amount of one-half inch vaseline gauze. The nose need not be packed to the point of pain or to the point where one can see distortion of the external nose. This will usually stop most simple anterior bleeds. A nasal speculum and boyonet forceps are needed. The anterior pack should be left in place for 24–48 hours.

A posterior pack followed by an anterior pack should be inserted when the bleeding is from the posterior portion of the nose. Posterior nasal packing is more involved and requires someone who is adept at the procedure. Hospitalization is always required. Posterior packing subjects the patient to a significant increase in mortality due to hypoxia. All elders with posterior packs should have a continuous ECG monitoring.

SINUSITIS

Sinusitis occurs less frequently in elders than in younger persons. A sinus infection, when it occurs, usually follows an upper respiratory infection. It may also be due to dental infection, trauma, tumor, or to alterations in blood supply.[13]

Symptoms may include pain over the affected sinus, swelling, purulent nasal discharge, and fever. Severity of symptoms in an elderly person does not necessarily indicate severity of the disease. Radiographs of the sinuses will show clouding in the involved area.

Differential diagnosis should include allergic sinusitis as well as bacterial sinusitis and tumors of the sinuses.

Treatment of infection consists of a culture of the nasal passage and an appropriate antibiotic therapy. Vascoconstriction of the nasal mucosa to allow drainage of the sinuses is also advised. Ephedrine, 1 percent in normal saline, 3–5 drops in each nostril every four hours is effective for this purpose. Any nasal spray or nose drops should not be used more than four to seven days to prevent the "rebound effect." Analgesia is frequently necessary and the drug selected carefully with consideration given to the frequent side effects in the elderly.

NASOPHARYNGEAL TUMOR

Signs of nasal obstruction or facial pain, especially unilateral, should alert the clinician to investigate the possibility of a tumor in the nose. Concomitant signs of nasal obstruction and fluid in the middle ear may indicate a malignancy in the nasopharynx. A chronic unilateral nasal discharge should also be evaluated for possible tumor.[15]

ANOSMIA

Although rare, anosmia (or the total loss of the sense of smell) may occur in the elderly and is more commonly seen in chronic heavy smokers. Normally, the sense of smell decreases with age, but, when patients complain of a complete lack of the ability to smell, an evaluation should be done to rule out treatable causes. Possible etiologies are:

1. Airway obstruction (allergy, polyps or tumor)
2. Mucosal destruction (atrophic rhinitis, senile atrophy or toxic chemical poisons)
3. Intracranial lesions (tumors or vascular abnormalities)[14]

The patient can be tested by using the strong odors of coffee and ammonia. If an organic etiology is present, the smell of coffee and ammonia will not be detected, but ammonia will cause a burning or tingling sensation.[9]

When no local cause can be found, a thorough neurological exam should be done and further brain and vascular studies considered. If no treatable cause is found, patients and families should be counseled on nutritional ways to deal with the problem. Since the sense of smell is directly related to the ability to taste food, elders may lose interest in eating. Varying the texture, consistency, and temperature of foods, as well as the eye appeal, will help encourage eating in patients with this problem.

Throat

HOARSENESS

Although hoarseness is a symptom, not a diagnosis, it is an early symptom of laryngeal cancer. As such it must be evaluated thoroughly. Any patient with hoarseness that has persisted for more than two weeks should have an examination that thoroughly visualizes the vocal cords.

TUMORS OF THE OROPHARYNX

Oral tumors are more common in people over the age of 50 and especially in the person who is or has been a heavy smoker or drinker. There are frequently no symptoms. An enlarged firm irregular node may be noticed in the neck if the tumor is cancerous and has metastasized. Common sites are the lateral borders of the tongue and the floor of the mouth. If the tonsils are still present, they should also be carefully examined. A complete oral exam in an elder always involves the removal of the dentures and palpation of any suspicious looking area. If leukoplakia, ulcerations, or masses are present, the patient should be referred to an otolaryngologist for further evaluation.

DYSPHAGIA

This symptom in an elderly person may be due to muscular incoordination in the esophageal muscle that occurs with aging or is brought on secondarily as the result of a stroke. Another cause to consider is a tumor of the larynx or upper esophagus. For a more detailed discussion of this problem, refer to Chapter 14.

HEALTH MAINTENANCE

Routine evaluation of the ears, nose, and throat in an elderly patient should be included in the regular history and physical exam. Patients should be questioned about their hearing function, as well as about the presence of symptoms such as vertigo, tinnitus, ear discharge, lack of smell, hoarseness, or dysphagia. Physical exam of the ears should include otoscopic exam and gross hearing tests with the whisper test. Routine audiograms are not indicated unless there is a complaint of hearing loss. The nose exam includes visualization into the nasal vestibule, noting the mucosa and presence of any lesions. The mouth should be without dentures, and it, as well as the throat, should be visualized for lesions.

Loss of hearing occurs with age. Elders need to be educated on the normal aging changes in not only their ears, but in their nose and throat as well. It is likely that the most bothersome problem will be hearing loss, however. Many elders will consider a hearing aid and should be encouraged to use it when needed.

REFERENCES

1. Von Leden H: Speech and hearing problems in the geriatric patient. J Am Geriatr Soc 25:422–426, 1977
2. Corso JF: Presbycusis, hearing aids and aging. Audiol 16:146–163, 1977
3. Rossman I: Clinical geriatrics. Philadelphia, JP Lippincott, 1977, p 248
4. Brocklehurst, JC: Special senses: the aging auditory system, in Fisch L: Textbook of Geriatric Medicine and Gerontology. New York, Churchill-Livingston, 1978, pp 280–281
5. Goodhill V: Ear Diseases, Deafness, and Dizziness. New York: Harper & Row, 1979, pp 719–721
6. Schiffman S: Food recognition by the elderly. J Gerontol 32:586–592, 1977
7. Meyerson M: The effects of aging on communication. J Gerontol 31:29–38, 1976
8. Consumer Reports, Consumers Union of US Inc, Mt Vernon, New York, June 1976, pp 346–355
9. DeWeese DD, Saunders WH: Textbook of Otolaryngology, ed 5. St Louis, CV Mosby Co, 1977, p 335
10. Ausband JR: Ear, Nose and Throat Disorders: A Practitioner's Guide. Flushing, New York, Medical Examination Publishing Co, 1974, pp 39, 42
11. Hull RH: Hearing impairment among aging persons. Lincoln, Nebraska, Cliffs Notes Inc, 1977, pp 1–83
12. Ruben RJ: Otolaryngologic problems of the old. Hosp Prac 12:73–87, 1977
13. Goldstein R, Hersperger WS, et al: Otorhinolaryngologic aspects, in Wilson FB, Senturia BH (eds): The Care of the Geriatric Patient. St Louis, CV Mosby Co, 1971, pp 335–337
14. Ballenger JJ (ed): Diseases of the Nose, Throat and Ear, ed 12. Philadelphia, Lea & Febiger, 1977, p 124

RECOMMENDED RESOURCES

For Professionals and General Public on Where to Seek Help for Hearing Problems:

Academy of Rehabilitative Audiology, National Technical Institute for the Deaf, One Lomb Memorial Drive, Rochester, New York 14623

Acoustical Society of America, 335 E. 45th Street, New York, New York 10017

Alexander Graham Bell Association for the Deaf Inc, 3417 Volta Place, NW, Washington DC 20007

American Deafness and Rehabilitation Association, 814 Thayer Avenue, Silver Spring, Maryland 20910

American Speech and Hearing Association, 10801 Rockville Pike, Rockville, Maryland 20852

Center for Deafness, 600 Waukegan Road, Glenview, Illinois 60025

National and World Center for Education and Information on Deafness, Gallaudet College, Kendall Greens, Washington DC 20002

18

Problems of the Eyes

Elizabeth A. Taisch, F.N.P., M.H.S.
Dennis A. Taisch, M.D.
Henry S. Metz, M.D.

Good vision throughout life is a precious asset. The physiological changes of aging result only in slightly decreasing visual acuity. As other physical capabilities decline with age, vision becomes an important source of satisfaction in maintaining contact with the world.

Diminution of keenness of sight is common and often accepted as inevitable by many elders. This acceptance often prevents them from seeking advice for a pathological and possible remedial problem.

Physiological changes of aging affect all anatomical structures of the eye. This may cause a variety of symptoms or signs. See Table 18-1. Aging affects visual functions, all of which decrease with increasing age. See Table 18-2.

INCIDENCE OF EYE PROBLEMS

Although patients generally do not die from diseases of the eye, a decrease in visual function profoundly affects the quality of life. Presbyopia is the most common problem and is almost universally present to some degree. The most common primary ocular disease is the cataract or lens opacity. At least some degree of lens opacification exists in 95 percent of persons over 65 years of age. Cataracts are present to a disabling degree in 5 percent of the elderly. It is estimated that between 5–10 million individuals become visually disabled each year because of cataracts. They are rare before 50 years of age, except in diabetics who may develop cataracts

in middle age rather than old age. Approximately 300,000–400,000 cataract extractions are performed annually in the United States. Patients who refuse surgery for operable cataracts constitute the second largest group of blind persons in the United States.[1]

The second most common eye problem is glaucoma which occurs in about 5–10 percent of elders.[2] The overall frequency increases gradually from the age of 40. It is estimated that there are 800,000 cases of undiscovered glaucoma in the United States today. Open angle glaucoma accounts for 60–70 percent of glaucomas. Glaucoma is a major cause of blindness in the United States.[3]

Macular degeneration is another common cause of visual loss in elders, beginning about the sixth decade. When it occurs with a reduction in vision, the incidence is about 5–10 percent of those over 65 years of age. Ophthalmoscopic changes of macular pigmentation or depigmentation occur in approximately 30 percent of elders.[4,6]

Two percent of patients having cataract surgery will experience a retinal detachment in that eye. Retinal detachment is also more common in patients with myopic eyes and in men. It is bilateral in 25 percent of the cases.[5]

Diabetic retinopathy is the leading cause of blindness in the United States and affects 50,000 persons. The incidence of diabetic retinopathy is increasing as a result of improved medical diabetic management that has lengthened the life span of diabetics. Approximately 2 percent of all diabetics become blind from retinopathy.[1]

Table 18-1
Physiologic Aging Changes of the Eye

	Anatomical/Physiologic Changes	Signs or Symptoms
Lids	Loss of orbital fat	Eyes appear deep in orbits
	Atrophy of elastic tissue	Wrinkling of lids
	Decrease in muscle tone	Ptosis
		Ectropion
		Entropion
Lacrimal Apparatus	Atrophy of glandular tissue	Decrease in tear secretion
		Dry eyes
Conjunctiva	Becomes thin/friable	Pinguecula
		Pterygium
Cornea	Decrease of endothelial cells (endothelial degeneration)	Decrease in luster/translucency and visual acuity
	Flattens	Astigmatism
Sclera	Fatty deposits	
	Decrease in elasticity	
Iris-pupils	Pupils more constricted	Delayed pupillary reaction with decreased night vision
		More illumination needed for clear vision
Lens	Increase in rigidity	Presbyopia
	Decrease in elasticity	Decrease in accomodation, visual acuity and glare tolerance
	Becomes opacified	
	Enlarges	Acute narrow-angle glaucoma
Fundus	Drusen	Decrease in visual acuity as manifestation of macular or retinal degeneration
	Narrowing vessels	
	Loss of bright macular and foveal light reflex	
	Choroid changes	
	Pigmentation around macula	
Vitreous	Shrinks in size	Floaters
	Becomes more liquid	"Lightning flashes"

Common Lab Values

The measurement of visual acuity is the same for elders as for younger adults. It can be helpful to classify elders as to their visual acuity. Good vision falls in the range of 20/20 to 20/30; fair to adequate vision is 20/40 to 20/70; and poor vision is 20/100 or less. Fair to adequate vision may meet many elders' needs if their activities are limited.[4] The acceptable intraocular pressure range is measured by Schiotz tonometry at 21 mm Hg or less.[3] Elders as a group tend to fall in the higher range.

UNCOMMON PROBLEMS AND URGENT CONDITIONS

The primary care clinician needs to be aware of the uncommon eye problems that occur in the elderly. The major ones would include temporal arteritis, vascular occlusions, and iritis; all except the latter occur in increasing frequency with age. Although relatively uncommon, vascular occlusions of the retina will be discussed.

Table 18-2
Changes in Visual Functions With Aging

- Decrease in visual acuity
- Decrease in peripheral visual fields
- Decrease in light sensitivity
- Decrease in color adaptation
- Decrease in color sensitivity
- Decrease in dark adaptation
- Decrease in depth perception
- Decrease in ability to converge
- Decrease in discrimination
- Decrease in accomodation
- Decrease in recovery from glare

Atherosclerosis (Vascular Occlusions of the Retina)

Amaurosis fugax occurs when small emboli from atheromatous plaques in the internal carotid arteries break off and travel to the retina causing retinal ischemia. Presenting symptoms are unilateral transient loss of vision lasting a few seconds or minutes. Arterial occlusion may be caused by emboli from atheromatous plaques in the aorta or carotids or by atherosclerosis of the central retinal artery or its branches with accompanying vasospasm. The clinical presentation of an occluded central retinal artery is a sudden and painless loss of vision. Occlusion of a branch vessel causes loss of visual field corresponding to the branch affected. On exam, one will see retinal artery stenosis, local edema, or a cherry red macula when the central retinal artery is involved. See Fig. 18-1. This is a true ocular emergency and must be treated within the first six hours. An eye that has its blood supply deprived for more than six hours will generally lose vision permanently. Treatment is directed at reducing the vasospasm and moving the blockage "downstream" to a smaller branch vessel. A simple emergency measure is to have the patient rebreathe into a paper bag, thus increasing carbon dioxide content of inspired air and, it is hoped, dilating the retinal artery, as well as allowing movement of the embolus. Immediate referral to an ophthalmologist is indicated, at which time other measures are initiated.

Venous occlusion may have several causes, including thromboses and external compression of the veins. The main symptom is rapid visual loss. The prognosis, however, is better than with arterial occlusion. Venous occlusion is characterized by large retinal hemorrhages in a single area, if a branch is affected, or over the entire retina, if the central vein is involved. See Fig. 18-2. Immediate referral

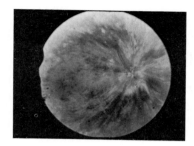

Fig. 18-2. Central retinal vein occlusion.

is indicated, and treatment with anticoagulants may be considered.

Temporal Arteritis (Giant Cell Arteritis)

Temporal arteritis is another relatively uncommon problem, though it occurs primarily in patients over 65 years of age. It is characterized by weight loss, malaise, fever, and severe headaches. Physical findings include prominent and tender temporal arteries with nodularity and erythema. Sudden loss of vision may occur. An elevation of the sedimentation rate and alkaline phosphatase, along with a temporal artery biopsy, assist in the diagnosis. Corticosteroids are indicated for management. Immediate referral to an ophthalmologist is indicated.

Eye Injuries

Eye injuries also occur in the elderly, and their management is similar to that of adults. These include foreign body, lacerations, hyphema, intraocular foreign body, and chemical injuries. Proper referral is indicated with the exception of a simple foreign body. Loss of vision is another true ocular emergency that necessitates referral.

Sudden painful loss of vision should alert the practitioner to consider the possibilities of angle closure glaucoma, retrobulbar neuritis, or optic neuritis. With sudden painless loss of vision, one must consider the possibilities of central retinal artery occlusion, central retinal vein occlusion, temporal arteritis, retinal detachment, and vitreous hemorrhage.

DIAGNOSIS AND TREATMENT OF COMMON PROBLEMS

The most common eye problems of the elderly fall into four basic pathophysiological groups: refractive errors, external eye problems, primary ocu-

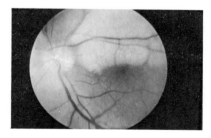

Fig. 18-1. Branch artery occlusion.

lar disease, and secondary systemic disease. (See Table 18-3.)

Symptoms of the various eye problems are similar. Only with a thorough history and physical can they be accurately diagnosed. A careful eye history should also include other aspects of the patient's medical history that might relate the eye disorder to a neurologic, oncologic, cardiovascular, renal or metabolic disorder. The common symptoms and history points are listed in Table 18-4. Specifically, a history of diabetes, hypertension, previous eye problems, surgeries or injuries, and a family history for glaucoma or other eye disease should also be included. The patient's drug history is important, as several drugs may have adverse effects on the eyes. (See Table 18-5.) A knowledge of the patient's daily activity level and home situation is also important.

The primary care clinician should remember that decreased visual function may become manifest in

Table 18-3
Common Eye Problems of the Elderly

I. Refractive errors
   A.   Myopia
   B.   Hyperopia
   C.   Astigmatism
   D.   Presbyopia
II. External eye problems
   A.   Lids
      1.   Ectropion/entropion
      2.   Tumors of the lid
      3.   Inflammations
      4.   Senile ptosis
      5.   Dermatochalasis
   B.   Lacrimal apparatus
      1.   Dry eyes
      2.   Tearing
   C.   Conjunctiva
      1.   Conjunctivitis
      2.   Red eye
   D.   Cornea
      1.   Arcus senilis
III. Primary eye disease
   A.   Cataracts
   B.   Glaucoma (open angle)
   C.   Macular degeneration
   D.   Retinal detachment
IV. Secondary eye disease
   A.   Diabetic retinopathy
   B.   Vascular disease
      1.   Arteriolar sclerosis

Table 18-4
Symptoms of Eye Disease and History to Elicit

I.   Disturbances of vision
   A.   Unilateral/bilateral, improvement with corrective lenses, transient/permanent, onset gradual/sudden, near/distance vision or both, normal vision with visual phenomena (floaters)
   B.   Color vision
   C.   Peripheral vision
   D.   Dark adaptation
   E.   Irridescent vision (halos)
   F.   Diplopia
   G.   Floaters
II.   Pain
   A.   Superficial foreign body sensation
   B.   Deep pain within eye
   C.   Headache
   D.   Burning, itching, "tired" eyes
   E.   Photophobia
III.   Abnormal secretion from eyes
   A.   Tearing
   B.   Mucous/pus
   C.   Dry eyes
IV.   Physical signs described by patient as symptoms
   A.   Red eye
   B.   New growths
   C.   Abnormal position, eyes/lids
   D.   Protrusion globe
   E.   Wide/narrow palpebral fissure
   F.   Abnormal pupils

a number of ways, e.g., a decline of attention, loss of interest in a task or environment, anxiety, defensiveness, and decreasing confidence or morale. A sense of isolation may exist.

Physical Examination

A systematic eye exam is completed in all eye problems. (See Table 18-6.) With either the Snellen eye chart or the Rosenbaum pocket screener, visual acuity in each eye is tested separately, both with and without glasses. Next, confrontation visual fields test the function of the peripheral field of vision. The examiner and patient sit facing each other at a distance of 1 m. The examiner closes one eye directly opposite the patient's closed eye. With the examiner's hand midway between the patient and him or herself, the examiner brings the hand slowly inward from the periphery with extended fingers. The patient states when he or she is able to see and count the extended fingers. If both have a normal

Table 18-5
Potential Ocular Complications of Some Systemic Drugs

Classification of Drug	Potential Adverse Effect
Corticosteroids—systemic	Subcapsular cataracts Increasing intraocular pressure Glaucoma
Phenothiazine derivatives	
Chlorpromazine HCL (Thorazine)	Significant retinopathy Pigmentary deposits of the lens, cornea and conjunctiva
Thioridazine HCL (Mellaril)	Significant retinopathy Loss of visual acuity
Antibacterials	
Ethambutol HCL (Myambutol)	Decrease in visual acuity Optic neuritis
Chloramphenicol, streptomycin, Sulfonamides, INH	Optic atrophy
Antimalarials	
Hydroxychloroquine sulfate (Plaquenil)	Corneal deposits Visual field defects Retinopathy
Chloroquine (Aralen)	Corneal deposits Visual field defects Retinopathy
Anticholinergics	Mydriasis Increase in intraocular pressure (contraindicated in patients with narrow angle glaucoma)

visual field, the patient and examiner should be able to see and count the number of fingers at the same time. Each eye is tested separately in its circumference. It is important to remember that this is a gross screening test for visual fields, and more sophisticated methods such as a tangent screen and a perimeter are available to the ophthalmologist.

Screening for extraocular muscle problems in the elderly is important as palsies may develop from stroke or diabetes. The *extraocular* muscles are tested for range of motion by having the patient follow the examiner's finger up, down, right, left, and on both diagonals. To test oculomotor alignment the corneal light reflex method is also useful and involves holding a penlight about 13 inches in front of the patient's eyes. Normally, the image reflected

back from the cornea is approximately in the center of each pupil, when the patient looks at the light.

The eyes must be tested for alignment. An "ortho" (straight) position as opposed to an "eso" (inward) or an "exo" (outward) deviation are three alignments seen. Almost everyone's eyes tend to drift either inward or outwards. Our desire for single vision, however, helps keep our eyes locked on target. To test whether the "lock" is working correctly, the patient reads letters at a distance of 20 feet. The examiner watches the left eye for movement as he or she covers the right eye. If the left eye must swing in or out to find the target, it is out of alignment. If there is no movement, then the practitioner knows the eye is not grossly deviated full time (a condition known as tropia). Thus, this is a *screening* test for gross, full-time deviation.

The funduscopic examination begins with an estimation of the clarity of the media. Beginning with the anterior segment, including the cornea and lens, look for opacities. Cataracts can be detected by using a plus lens with the ophthalmoscope, often outlining the cataract against the red reflex of the fundus. Visualization of the retina is very important although difficult at times with elders. The pupils should be dilated if necessary to complete the exam. Dilating agents such as mydriacyl 1 percent or 2.5 percent Neo-Synephrine can be used.

Table 18-6
Physical Exam of Eyes

I. Visual acuity
II. Visual fields by confrontation method
III. External eye exams
    A. Lids/lashes
    B. Conjunctiva/sclera
    C. Cornea/anterior chamber
    D. Iris/pupillary reflexes (direct and indirect)
    E. Extraocular muscles
IV. Tonometry
V. Funduscopy
    A. Cornea
    B. Anterior chamber
    C. Lens
    D. Vitreous
    E. Retina
        1. Optic disc
        2. Optic cup
        3. Retinal vessels
        4. Retinal background
        5. Macula

Clinical testing of intraocular pressure is carried out by means of indentation tonometry such as with Schiotz tonometer.

Refractive Errors

Refractive errors cause a decrease in visual acuity and include myopia, hyperopia, astigmatism and presbyopia. Of these, the first three may occur at any time in life, although their incidence tends to increase wth age. The refractive error that is seen almost universally with aging is presbyopia.

PRESBYOPIA

Presbyopia results from decreasing accommodation or a decrease in the eye's ability to focus on objects at varying distances. With aging, the lens nucleus becomes harder and less elastic and is unable to respond to the ciliary muscle, resulting in a gradual loss of accommodation. At age 10, the eye has about 14 diopters of accommodation for near/far focusing, yet only two diopters remain at age 50. Accommodation loss occurs in everyone, regardless of their refractive error. As a result, most patients can read without difficulty until age 40. At this time, reading glasses are frequently required. Focusing ability continues to decrease until approximately aged 65–70, at which time it is stabilized and subsequently changes very little.

The chief symptom of presbyopia is an inability to see near work distinctly, especially small print and in dim illumination. The individual has to hold objects farther and farther away to see them clearly. Ocular discomfort and headaches often occur. When the newspaper has to be held at arms' length to be read, the individual will usually seek relief. Presbyopia is not farsightedness, but solely an accommodative problem superimposed on whatever refractive error already exists. Treatment consists of convex lens (spectacles) added to the correction for distant vision. Bifocals or trifocals are frequently prescribed so that the patient does not require a separate pair of glasses for near, intermediate, and far distances. Reading glasses that correct only the presbyopia are indicated if distance correction is not required. They may take the form of separate reading glasses, bifocals with clear glass on the upper portion, or "half-frame lenses." One of the new innovations in bifocals has been the bifocals without lines. Many older people prefer these, as they feel that the bifocals with a line are reflective of their age, and prefer an alternative.

External Eye Problems

CHANGES IN LIDS AND LACRIMAL APPARATUS

Ectropion–Entropion. The most common findings in the lids of the elderly are loss of orbital fat, atrophy of the elastic tissue, and decreased muscle tone. These changes cause the eyes to sink deeper into the orbits, as well as wrinkling and looseness of the lids and ptosis. Ectropion is a common occurrence and is a result of the laxity of supporting lid structures. See Fig. 18-3. The lid margin becomes everted and results in exposure of the conjunctiva, tearing, and increased incidence of chronic infection. Surgery is the treatment of choice, although palliative measures can be successful. Training the patient and family members to wipe tears in an up- and inward motion and to use artificial tears hourly (or as needed for patient comfort) may delay the progression of symptoms but does not cure the ectropion.

Entropion is the inversion of the lid margin, is often intermittent in the early stages, and is the result of laxity of the lid structures. See Fig. 18-4. The presenting symptoms are a gritty, sandy feeling, or foreign body sensation in the eye and tearing caused by the lashes rubbing on the cornea. Adhesive strips may be used to evert the lid as temporary relief. Surgery is usually required.

Tumors of the lid. Benign tumors of the lids are common in old age and include senile keratosis, pedunculated papillomas, horns, and keratin cysts. Xanthelasma—soft, yellowish, slightly raised plaques– are an accumulation of lipid material often found at the inner portion of the lids. This condition can occur with lipid abnormalities but more commonly occurs spontaneously. If troublesome or unsightly, these benign growths can be removed. The most common malignant neoplasm of the lids is basal cell carcinoma, which usually involves the

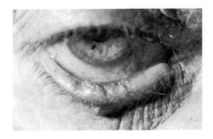

Fig. 18-3. Chalazion; ectropion.

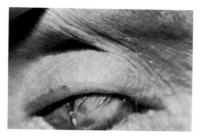

Fig. 18-4. Ectropion—upper lid. Trichiasis—upper lid.

lower lid. See Fig. 18-5. Squamous cell cancer may also occur on the lids, though it is much less common. Surgery or cryotherapy for these malignant lesions is indicated.

Lid inflammation. The incidence of inflammations of the glands in the eyelids (hordeolum, chalazion) is similar to that in younger people, whereas the incidence of certain types of lid margin inflammation (blepharitis) appears to be higher.

Blepharitis occurs in several forms—angular, squamous, ulcerative, or allergic—with presenting symptoms of itching, burning, and irritation of the lid margins. Angular blepharitis, or inflammation of the angles of the lids, can be associated with angular conjunctivitis and is more common in the elderly. In the elderly person, these conditions result from wrinkling of the skin, which favors the collection of moisture and tears and predisposes to infection.

A few brief comments on antibiotic therapy are necessary before discussing appropriate treatment. It is important to remember that the treatment choice of an antibiotic varies with each patient, depending on a patient's known allergic history, concurrent infections, and medication. One particular problem to consider in prescribing topical ocular antibiotics is the high incidence of neomycin sensitivity. This is particularly troublesome to the practitioner as there are numerous "combination" products available that contain neomycin, which may be highly sensitizing.

For angular blepharitis, a brief course of conservative antibiotic therapy, such as erythromycin ointment applied to the lids three to four times a day, may be helpful. Referral to an ophthalmologist is indicated if this is a persistent problem.

Squamous blepharitis is associated with seborrheic dermatitis and is another common problem of the elderly, especially in males. It is often associated with hyperemia of the lid margins, scaling and flaking of the skin surrounding the lashes. Treatment is directed mainly toward correction of the seborrheic dermatitis with cleansing shampoos such as 2.5 selenium sulfide (Selsun). Local hygiene twice daily to cleanse the scales from the lid margins with moistened Q-tips and baby shampoo is recommended, and often the family can be involved in the treatment. Steroid application to areas of inflammation on the face is also helpful. Frequently, this is a long process that often takes months. Older persons and their families therefore need to be encouraged to be diligent in the treatment.

Ulcerative blepharitis is an uncommon chronic infectious process often presenting with redness, inflammation, suppurative lesions, and loss of lashes. Treatment involves the use of topical antibiotics such as chloramphenicol or sulfonamides.

Inflammation of the glands in the eyelids such as hordeolum (sty) or an acute chalazion is best treated by hot compresses applied at frequent intervals for ten minutes. Frequently, an antibiotic ointment is applied on the lid margin to prevent involvement of adjacent glands. A noninfected chalazion, when small and asymptomatic, can be observed, though excision by an ophthalmologist may be indicated if it enlarges or persists. See Fig. 18-3.

Senile ptosis. Relaxation of the skin of the upper lid, weakness of the levator muscle and herniation of orbital fat into subcutaneous tissue can cause senile ptosis. Surgical intervention may be necessary.

Dermatochalasis. This is a condition causing loss of elasticity of the skin of the upper lid so that it hangs as a fold over the lid margin. Treatment is usually not required, unless the skin fold covers the pupillary area and interferes with vision. Surgical excision of the excess skin may then be indicated.

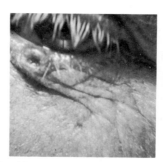

Fig. 18-5. Basal cell carcinoma.

Dry eyes and tearing. Decreased tear secretion due to atrophy of glandular tissue commonly occurs with aging. The eyes feel dry, burn, and have a constant foreign body sensation. It may be difficult to diagnose this condition as the eye may appear wet with tearing due to ectropion, reflex tearing, or stenosis of the puncta. This tearing is to be contrasted with actual overproduction, which may have several causes that include lacrimal gland inflammation; lesions of lids, cornea, conjunctiva, and iris; glaucoma; and retinal stimulation by glare and excessive light. Tear formation is measured clinically by the Schirmer test. Insert a strip of Whatman No. 41 filter paper folded so a 5 mm portion can be placed over the lower lid. Instruct the patient to close his or her eyes for four minutes. Normally, tears will moisten the paper to a distance of 10 mm. A result of less than 5 mm of wetting is considered positive for decreased tearing. Management of inadequate tear production is the instillation of artificial tears, or 0.5 percent methylcellulose as often as needed for comfort. Management of the overproduction of tears is aimed at the underlying problem.

CONJUNCTIVA

Conjunctiva, pinguecula pterygium. In elders, the conjunctiva becomes thinner and more friable. A pinguecula, or benign degenerative growth of the conjunctiva, presents as a yellowish-white, raised oval mass on either side of the cornea on the conjunctiva. They become increasingly common as one ages. A pterygium is a degenerative lesion consisting of a fold of conjunctiva at the limbus encroaching on to the cornea. It appears whitish-pink and is usually raised. It usually is found on the nasal conjunctiva, and surgical excision is required if it interferes with vision or causes significant discomfort. See Fig. 18-6.

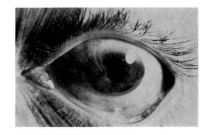

Fig. 18-6. Pterygium.

Conjunctivitis—red eye. Conjunctivitis is the most common red eye problem in elders and is caused by bacterial, viral, and allergic conditions. Symptoms include conjunctival hyperemia, discharge, and crusting. The diagnosis and management of conjunctivitis is the same in elders as it is in younger adults.

Any red eye should be carefully evaluated to distinguish three major categories: (1) blepharoconjunctivitis, which the provider should be able to manage; (2) vision-threatening disorders, which should be referred promptly to an ophthalmologist; and (3) systemic diseases causing redness of the eyes. The red eye should be approached systematically by obtaining a thorough history and physical with particular attention to the following points: visual loss, photophobia, and headaches; measurement of visual acuity; clinical notation of the pattern of hyperemia, type of discharge, lacrimation, opacities of media; appearance of cornea and anterior chamber; pupil size and reaction; and intraocular pressure. A thorough discussion of red eye is beyond the scope of this chapter. Refer to Table 18-7 for a synopsis of the differential diagnosis of the red eye.

CORNEA

Cornea—arcus senilis. Changes of the cornea associated with aging include loss of luster and translucency, loss of endothelial cells, and a decrease in sensitivity. Arcus senilis is a very common degenerative change of the cornea and is characterized by the deposition of fatty substances near the periphery of the cornea, separated from the limbus by a clear margin of cornea. Initially, it appears white, progressing to yellow as the individual grows older. Arcus senilis increases in size with age, is more common in males, has no pathological significance, and does not interfere with vision. Studies show that arcus senilis may be associated with arteriosclerosis and familial hypercholesterolemia.[6]

Primary Eye Disease

Primary eye diseases that are most common in the elderly include cataracts, glaucoma, macular degeneration, and retinal detachment.

CATARACTS

The most common disability in the aging eye is the formation of a cataract or lens opacity. Normally, the lens of the eye is a uniquely clear and transpar-

Table 18-7
Differential Diagnosis of Red Eye

Signs and Symptoms	Acute Glaucoma	Acute Conjunctivitis	Acute Iridocyclitis	Corneal Abrasion and Foreign Body
Incidence	Uncommon	Extremely common	Common	Common
Pain	Usually severe	Minimal or none	Moderate to severe	Moderate to severe
Photophobia	Minimal to moderate	Usually none	Severe	None to minimal
Vision	Usually markedly decreased	Normal	Usually slightly decreased but may be markedly decreased	Variable
Discharge	None	Moderate to copious	None	Watery
Cornea	Steamy	Clear	Usually clear	Irregular cornea light reflex
Anterior chamber depth	Shallow	Normal	Normal	Normal
Pupil	Dilated and fixed	Normal	Smaller than opposite side and sluggish	Normal
Conjunctival injection	Circum corneal injection	Diffuse injection located near fornices	Circum corneal injection	Diffuse injection
Intraocular pressure	Elevated	Normal	Normal, increased or decreased	Normal
Emergency treatment	Miotics, refer to ophthalmologist	Antibiotic drops	Mydriatic drops, steroids, antibiotics, refer to an ophthalmologist	Removal of foreign body; antibiotic drops
Prognosis	Blindness without proper therapy	Self-limited	Serious without proper therapy	Serious without proper therapy

ent structure. Growth continues throughout life, with newer fibers laid down around older fibers that migrate towards the center, forming a dense central nucleus. As the lens ages, the fibers lose their transparency and assume a yellow or yellow-brown color, referred to as a nuclear sclerosis. The lens progressively loses both its water content and elasticity and enlarges, with changes becoming clinically manifest after age 40. Changes of the lens interfere with the transmission and refraction of light, causing decreased accommodation, depth perception, and glare tolerance. At least some degree of lens opacification exists in 95 percent of persons over 65 years of age. These opacities appear gray or white by direct illumination. See Figs. 18-7 and 18-8.

Although the main symptom is a gradual decrease of vision, some patients may report a more rapid loss of acuity over a period of weeks or months. It is rarely associated with pain or inflammation of the eye.

The term senescent or senile cataracts indicates primary cataracts that develop in older persons. Ninety percent of all cataracts fall into this category. There is no known etiology, though the patient's medical history sometimes reveals a postive family history for this condition. Nuclear sclerosis is the most common cataract type. In nuclear cataracts, intitially there is often marked increase in the refractive power of the lens, resulting in the patient's renewed ability to read at near distances without glasses, despite a decrease in distance acuity. The "improvement" is transient. Another type of cataract formation is the cortical cataract, characterized

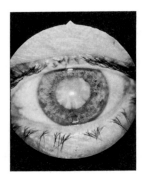

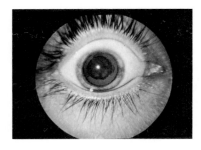

Fig. 18-7 (Top).   Mature cataract.
Fig. 18-8 (Bottom).   Cataract.

by opaque peripheral spokes in the lens cortex. A third type is the posterior subcapsular cataract. Patients who complain of glare from light distortion or "halos" with night driving may have posterior subcapsular cataracts. Even though specific complaints of decreased color vision are not common, patients do experience a "yellowing" of vision.

Currently, there is no therapeutic measure available that will affect the formation or progression of cataracts. The treatment, surgical extraction, is successful in 95–98 percent of the cases. With new surgical techniques, newer suture material, and local anesthesia, ambulation is possible on the first postoperative day. Only on rare occasions need surgery be withheld because of age or associated disease. Surgery is indicated when: (1) the decreasing vision interferes with an individual's ability to read, write, sew, or carry out what the patient feels to be a necessary activity; (2) the increased size of the lens threatens to cause a secondary glaucoma; or (3) when a mature cataract begins to break down, causing inflammation within the eye. "Vision" here refers to the best corrected vision. With surgical removal of the lens, the aphakic patient has lost

one-third of the focusing power in that eye, and this power must be replaced. A relatively thick eyeglass lens is one way to replace the power. The magnifying effect of this spectacle lens, however, produces a retinal image 25 percent larger than the normal fellow eye, and diplopia results. A contact lens can help the situation with the retinal image then being only 8 percent larger. Not all patients, however, can tolerate or physically manage contacts. New extended-wear contact lenses, which need removal and cleaning only once a month (with fulltime wear between cleaning), have recently been approved. These may prove very beneficial to the elderly and their families, who may have difficulty manipulating contacts.

A new and still controversial technique, the implantation of an artificial plastic lens at the time of cataract extraction, is under nationwide investigation. The advantages of intraocular lenses over aphakic glasses and contacts include full visual fields, 24-hour wear, little or no magnification of images, better depth perception, binocular vision when only one cataract has been removed, and absence of discomfort or inconvenience. They are especially helpful in elderly patients who would have trouble inserting contacts. The major disadvantage of intraocular lenses is that they are foreign bodies and may have unanticipated long-term side effects. Complication rates are slightly higher than for simple cataract extraction. The complications that can occur include chronic iritis, secondary glaucoma, corneal edema, endophthalmitis, and displacement of the implant.

GLAUCOMA

Glaucoma is a disease in which increased intraocular pressure can result in irreversible blindness through progressive loss of the field of vision due to optic nerve damage. It is the third major cause of blindness in the United States. Every provider should be familiar with the implications of the disease and be able to screen for it because of its prevalence and potential to cause blindness.

The etiology of various types of glaucoma is different, but the basic defect is some impairment in the outflow of aqueous humor from the eye. Aqueous humor is formed in the ciliary processes of the posterior chamber and flows through the pupil into the anterior chamber. The outflow is at the angle of the anterior chamber through the trabecular meshwork, Schlemm's canal, and into the scleral veins that drain the eye. Impairment of aqueous outflow causes an elevation of intraocular pressure that is transmitted hydraulically to all areas of the eyeball, including the optic nerve and retinal vessels, and may cause irreversible changes such as optic atrophy and loss of visual field and vision. Glaucoma can be congenital, primary, or can occur secondary to trauma or other intraocular diseases. The two types of primary glaucoma are open angle glaucoma and angle closure glaucoma, both types increasing in incidence with age. Of the two, chronic simple glaucoma is much more prevalent, comprising greater than 90 percent of the primary glaucomas.

Open angle glaucoma. This is the most common of all glaucomas. It is also referred to as wide angle, chronic simple, or glaucoma simplex. One-third of patients with chronic open angle glaucoma have a positive family history. It is characterized by a slow, insidious rise in pressure apparently due to an abnormality in the trabecular meshwork. Subjectively, the patient is symptom free. Glaucoma is painless, and the loss of side vision may go unnoticed for a long time. The endstage glaucoma patient has marked tunnel vision. Primary care clinicians should screen for glaucoma by checking intraocular pressure routinely, along with performing visual field studies and ophthalmoscopy for optic nerve changes at a routine exam.

The routine measurement of intraocular pressure is done in most offices with the Schiotz tonometer. The scale reading is converted to millimeters of mercury; the range of normal varies from 12–21 mm Hg. Pressure between 21–25 mm Hg is considered suspicious of early glaucoma. Any pressure above 25 mm Hg is abnormal. One must be cautious about such absolute limits. A Schiotz tonometer may give misleading readings such as in patients with abnormal curvature of the cornea or high degrees of myopia or in patients who squeeze their eyes. Patients with normal pressure—but evidence of cupping, pallor of the disc, or a visual field defect—could have a rare low-tension glaucoma. On the other hand, a patient with high pressure—but no evidence of cupping, pallor, or visual field loss—may have the entity known as ocular hypertension. Thus, measurement of intraocular pressure alone is not sufficient to make or eliminate a diagnosis of glaucoma, but it is a useful screening procedure.

In glaucoma, the funduscopic exam reveals that the ratio of cup to disc usually exceeds 0.5, and a difference of more than 0.2 between the two eyes suggests glaucoma.

Management of open angle glaucoma should be done by an ophthalmologist. It includes the use of several topical agents to improve the aqueous outflow. Pilocarpine drops 1–4 percent are the traditional medication. They may be used alone or in combination with epinephrine compounds. A new promising addition is the beta blocker Timolol, which has minimal side effects compared to other traditional glaucoma medications. Systemic carbonic anhydrase inhibitors (acetazolamide) may be used to reduce the secretion of aqueous humor. A new method of administering medication called an "Ocusert" involves placing a medicated polymer membrane containing pilocarpine into the conjunctival sac. The medication is released uniformly for a week. This method has certain advantages; however the cost is several times that of pilocarpine drops. Surgical intervention may be necessary only if the drugs are ineffective in maintaining a lower pressure. The need for surgery has decreased as medical therapy has improved.

Major problems in the treatment of glaucoma involve patient compliance. Often, patients do not appreciate the severity of the disease as initially it may be symptom free. Most eye drops have to be inserted three to four times a day for the remainder of their lives and are often associated with irritation or burning, discomfort, and visual blurring, Thus, the management of disease may seem worse than the disease process. The primary care clinician should be aware both of the glaucoma medications their patients are on and of all potential side effects and should provide continual encouragement to comply with the treatment.

Narrow angle or angle closure glaucoma. This is caused by an anatomic defect in the angle of the anterior chamber. The narrowing between the iris and the trabecular structure is often suggested on physical exam by a shallow anterior chamber. One can see the decreased distance between the posterior surface of the cornea and the anterior surface of the iris by obliquely shining a penlight on the anterior chamber of the eye. This area can be studied directly by an ophthalmologist with a gonioscope, a special prism contact lens that is placed on an anesthetized eye. Both eyes are usually involved, although one eye may present symptoms two to five years before the fellow eye. Patients can go for years and may be asymptomatic, but, with the gradual increase in size of the lens that occurs with aging, patients may have their first sustained attack.

Clinically, a typical angle closure attack occurs unilaterally—in a darkened place that causes dilation of the pupil, with emotional stress, or precipitated by the use of mydriatic drugs. The patient may present with a sudden onset of severe ocular and facial pain, nausea and vomiting, abdominal pain, decreased vision or a halo or rainbow vision. On physical exam, the cornea is edematous and cloudy, the pupil fixed in middilation, and the conjunctival vessels are injected. Intraocular pressure is elevated. In some patients, the attack may be subacute characterized by mild ocular pain, headaches and halos around light resulting from corneal edema. Immediate referral is indicated. Surgical intervention is indicated following medical therapy to decrease intraocular pressure. Many ophthalmologists believe that patients with subacute attacks should be operated on to prevent an acute attack.[4] Some ophthalmologists are now studying the effect of laser iridotomy as a possible alternative to peripheral iridectomy.[1]

MACULAR DEGENERATION

Another common cause of visual loss in the elderly is senescent macular degeneration. The macular area is completely devoid of retinal circulation and derives its nutrition from the underlying capillary layer of the choroid. This makes the macula particularly vulnerable to arteriosclerotic changes in the capillary layer of the choroid. There are several forms of macular degeneration including atropic, exudative, and hemorrhagic. The disease begins about the sixth decade and is almost always bilateral but often presents in one eye initially. It occurs with a reduction in vision in about 5–10 percent of those over 65 years of age.

Patients complain of a slow, progressive impairment of central vision characterized by a gray shadow in their central field of view. They can see well at the shadow's border but cannot make out details straight ahead. This loss of sharp, clear, central vision is very frustrating, especially to those who depend on their vision for their occupations or avocations. Ophthalmoscopic changes include a subtle migration of pigment around the fovea centralis that progresses to clumping of the pigment and some white scarring. See Fig. 18-9. Medical therapy is ineffective. Some patients can obtain improved

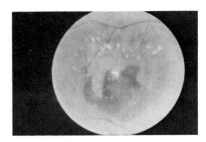

Fig. 18-9. Disciform macular degeneration with hemorrhage.

vision with telescopic lenses, special magnifying lenses, and similar optical aids. Patients should be offered these visual aids, although the number of patients who obtain satisfaction is quite small. The patient can also learn to look just to the side of objects, but many older individuals find this task of visual relearning most difficult. Patients must be reassured that this condition will not lead to total blindness, that they will be able to take care of themselves and lead useful lives. Use of the argon laser will occasionally improve vision.

Drusen (colloid or hyaline bodies) occurs almost universally with aging, especially in the peripheral eyegrounds. Drusen are usually small, yellow, round spots and can be quite large. They usually occur in the macular area of elderly patients and are generally a benign degenerative change. See Fig. 18-10.

RETINAL DETACHMENT

The vitreous body shrinks and becomes more liquid as a person ages. Vitreous condensations or "floaters" may form. Shrinking of the vitreous body can cause traction on the retina at points of adhe-

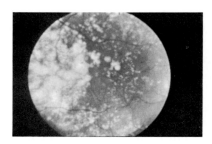

Fig. 18-10. Drusen of fundus.

sion, causing "lightning flashes." This traction in turn can cause tears of the retina that lead to retinal detachment. Although retinal detachments may occur in all age groups, the factor that most predisposes to retinal detachment is the surgical removal of a cataract from the eye. This is seen most commonly in the elderly. Immediate referral to an ophthalmologist is indicated.

Secondary Eye Disease

Secondary eye disease includes retinopathy and vascular disease such as arteriolar sclerosis and atherosclerosis.

DIABETIC RETINOPATHY

The retinopathy changes of diabetes can be divided into: (1) background retinopathy as characterized by microaneurysms, deep and superficial hemorrhages, hard exudates, cotton wool patches and/or macular edema see Fig. 18-11; and (2) a process called neovascularization or proliferative retinopathy characterized by new vessel formation, retinal and vitreous hemorrhages, and fibrous tissue proliferation with subsequent retina detachment.

In general, prognosis for vision is good if only background or nonproliferative retinopathy is present. If proliferative retinopathy is present, the prognosis is considerably worse, and loss of vision may be abrupt.

Currently, there is no uniformly satisfactory treatment of diabetic retinopathy. Good control of diabetes in the first years of the disease may delay onset or minimize the amount of retinopathy but seems to have little or no effect on the established condition. Over the last decade, photocoagulation using the argon laser or xenon photocoagulator has

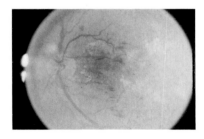

Fig. 18-11. Diabetic retinopathy.

offered some therapeutic success in earlier and moderate stages.[1]

VASCULAR DISEASE

The ocular fundus is the only place in the body that one can directly observe small arteries, arterioles, and the accompanying veins. It is important to note that the retinal arterial tree is arteriolar in nature with the exception of the central retinal artery and its large branches near the disc. Arteriosclerosis is a generalized term that includes several different types of degenerative disease of the arterial tree, anywhere in the body, only two of which occur in retinal vessels. The first is arteriolar sclerosis, the other atherosclerosis.

Arteriolar sclerosis. Arteriolar sclerosis is a result of hypertension, which causes changes and damage to the vessel walls. Changes occurring in the arterioles' include increase in arteriole light reflex, arteriovenous compression, copper wire and silver arteries. The literature contains much about the fundus changes of hypertension and arteriosclerosis.[1,7]

Blindness

Half of all blind people are over 65 years of age. Early detection of eye problems leading to prompt treatment is essential, as half of all cases of blindness can be prevented.

Generally, a person is considered legally blind when with lenses, his or her best visual acuity in the good eye is 20/200 or less, or when his or her visual field is restricted to 20 degrees or less. Visual acuity more than 20/200, but less than 20/70, is not considered legally blind, though the individual may be eligible for some services. Total blindness is defined as no light perception.

In the United States, the leading causes of blindness in the elderly are glaucoma, unoperated cataracts, and diabetic retinopathy.

A multitude of services and resources are available to the blind. A newly blinded person (i.e., from diabetic retinopathy) may benefit greatly from the program of a rehabilitation center. Rehabilitation programs teach independent functioning in areas such as orientation and mobility, personal and home management skills for daily living, communication skills, vocational and avocational skills. Psychological and social services may also be available to help the newly blinded person and his or her family adjust to living with blindness.[8,9,10]

Diabetics often have special needs and requirements. Peripheral neuropathy may interfere with mobility, and impaired touch can make certain skills such as braille difficult to learn. Large-dot braille and special syringes are some of the many available resources. Family involvement and awareness are important. A mobility instructor must be sensitive to the special needs of a person blind from diabetes.

The newly blinded individual must deal with the reactions of society in addition to those of his or her family. The family may often deny the blindness or become overprotective. They may not be aware of the degree of independence achieved by a rehabilitated blind person, which is the goal of the program.

HEALTH MAINTENANCE

We often take for granted our ability to see until some changes in our vision occur that remind us of its value. Health maintenance of our eyes is important throughout life. Injuries can be prevented, and many eye problems can be successfully treated if diagnosed early.

Through eye care, one can preserve the gift of sight. Routine eye examination, including visual acuity and tonometry, should be done every one to two years after the age of 35–40 to check for glaucoma, presbyopia, and other problems. Intraocular pressure checks for glaucoma should be performed every two years or annually if there is a family history of glaucoma.

Diabetic patients may require special monitoring. Every diabetic patient with visual symptoms should seek consultation from an ophthalmologist. Routine eye examination by an ophthalmologist is recommended at least annually for the elderly who had a juvenile onset of diabetes, as this group is in a relatively high risk group to develop proliferative changes. This also applies to any patients whose diabetes is of long duration. After 25 years, for example, nearly 90 percent of patients will have some evidence of change in blood vessels that could be called diabetic retinopathy.[11]

Simple precautions to avoid eye injury certainly applies to elders, especially if one has vision in only one eye. Safety goggles at home, work, or in sports can protect the eyes against flying objects and against penetration from sharp objects, e.g., those encountered in gardening (tools, plants, etc.), as well as from harsh sprays and fumes.

Knowing what to do in the event of an injury is important. One should seek medical attention for a foreign body unless positive that it is a minor irritant such as dust or dirt.

Simple eye care tips to promote wellness should be taught. Proper use of prescribed eye medications include reading the label and following directions exactly. Teach proper instillation of eye drops by pulling down the lower lid, applying ointment or drops inside the lower lid, and keeping the container away from the lid. Avoid over-the-counter remedies, as they are often unnecessary for healthy eyes. Impact-resistant glasses can protect against injury in a person with useful vision only in one eye. Proper lighting and reading glasses, as appropriate, are also important.

Eye warning signs that should require prompt medical attention should be discussed with the patient and family. See Table 18-8.

Low Vision

The primary care provider should be knowledgeable in assisting individuals and their families when there is a visual impairment.

The term "low vision" refers to a person who cannot read without a magnifier or other similar visual aid. Many of these people are classified as legally blind. Such a severe visual impairment has a profound impact on several aspects of a person's life. Many major medical centers and agencies servicing the visually handicapped have low vision clinics or services that include comprehensive visual rehabilitation. Low vision clinics: (1) evaluate how the individual functions in the home or work situation; (2) evaluate the nature of the medical eye problem and prescribe the appropriate visual aid, both optical and nonoptical; (3) review the impact of the prescribed aid on the individual's performance and

Table 18-8
Eye Warning Signs That Require Prompt Medical Attention

1. Persistent pain
2. Unusual sensitivity to light
3. Seeing rainbows or halos around lights
4. Persistent seeing of "flashing lights"
5. *Any* sudden visual disturbance
6. Loss of vision
7. Red eye

family situation; and (4) recommend other available community services. Specific instruction is provided for each patient, including various reading techniques, aids for daily living, and aids for mobility. Counseling services are recommended as needed. Many services exist to assist people with decreased vision and are often available through the American Foundation for the Blind or low vision clinic resources.[9,10,12,13]

Low-vision aids such as magnifiers or telescopic devices recommended by the ophthalmologist can be obtained from agencies for the blind even if the person is not legally blind. Magnifiers are used for near vision acuity, whereas telescopic devices are available for distant acuity. Lighting must be adequate for these magnifiers. Electric illumination magnifiers are available.

Stove, refrigerator, telephone, and thermostat dials adapted to assist with touch are available. Simple devices such as an envelope addressor, letter writing aids, signature guides, felt tip pens, use of a penlight at restaurants for menu reading, use of a simple magnifying glass, and use of a door viewer to expand field of view can be most helpful. A yellow acetate sheet placed over reading material can cut down glare, and reversing black and white on printed pages can assist with reading. Many self-care techniques used by the blind can also be used for those with decreased vision. These techniques encourage the use of tactile cues. A few examples include: identification of coins by size, edge texture, and thickness; folding bills according to their value; and notching keys.

Large-print cookbooks, checkbooks, newspapers, books, and other reading devices are available. Large, dull-black type on matte-white paper to avoid glare can be helpful on prescriptions. Many games are available for the blind or partially sighted. Arranging food and utensils in the same places with each meal, using drawer dividers, arranging clothes in order in the closet all can assist the patient. Family members need to be instructed in these and similar matters.

A high-intensity light source lamp for reading is very useful. Many of these devices can be of little cost to the individual.[9,10]

Community Resources Differ

Services available might include "Newspaper for the Blind" (radio show), lending library for talking books, magazines and tapes (such as the Library of Congress), public transportation privileges, Department of Motor Vehicles parking permit, schools and universities with special visual-handicapped programs, rebate on insurance policies, and tax exemptions.

Environmental Modifications

It is evident from discussing the age-related physiological and pathological changes affecting visual function in the elderly, that modification must be made in their environments to compensate for loss in visual functions. These factors need to be considered when developing institutional and other environments for the elderly so as to optimize visual performance.

Special housing needs should be considered. A simple but often overlooked factor is adequate lighting in all areas of the home or building, to compensate for the decrease in light sensitivity. Often a portable, high-intensity lamp can be most useful. The light source should be constant and without flicker. Lighting should be from yellowish sources rather than bluish "cool" sources that cause lenticular glare.

Railings or guiderails offer tactile input when the accommodation process is slow and the depth perception decreased. Painting the first and last stair can aid with depth perception; painting a bright color on the edge of the step can aid visual acuity. Avoidance of low-hanging objects is helpful because of the decrease in visual field. The use of transitional lights in hallways can help with the dark adaptation problem of entering a dark building or home from the sunlight. Also, allowing more time when switching from reading light to dark surfaces is helpful. Strong color contrast can be helpful with elevator and floor numbers. Highly polished surfaces or high-gloss paints should be avoided as they produce glare.

A decrease in vision can occur with the physiological changes that the elderly undergo. Modifications can be made in the environment of the elderly that can provide optimum conditions to assist with visual function. It is essential that health care providers be sensitive to, and aware of, the needs and fears of the elderly regarding visual loss. Individuals with severe loss should be evaluated for visual aids through specialized low vision clinics in hospitals or eye institutes. A small improvement in a patient's vision can be a very meaningful event in his or her life. A family or primary care provider is in an excellent position to intervene.

CONCLUSION

The aging process in most individuals causes a slow but steady decrease in visual acuity. The cause of many of these conditions can be discovered by thorough and appropriate examination. The ophthalmologist should be called upon for evaluation in many situations. The health care provider must be familiar with the process of aging and conditions that affect the eye. Since some of these conditions begin in the younger individual, the importance of early recognition and management for the maintenance of optimum visual acuity can not be overemphasized.

REFERENCES

1. Newell FW: Ophthalmology Principles and Concepts. St Louis, The CV Mosby Co, 1978
2. Kornzweig A: Visual loss in the elderly, in Reichel W (ed): The Geriatric Patient. New York, HP Publishing Co Inc, 1978, p 141–150
3. Paton D, Craig JA: Glaucomas: diagnosis and management. Clin Sym 28: 3–47, 1976
4. Kornzweig A: The eye in old age, in Rossman I (ed): Clinical Geriatrics. Philadelphia, JB Lippincott Co, 1971, pp 229–245
5. Scheie HG, Albert DM: Adler's Textbook of Ophthalmology. Philadelphia, WB Saunders Inc, 1969
6. Miller D: Ophthalmology: The Essentials. Boston, Houghton Mifflin, 1979
7. Kweskin S, Aitken P, Henkind P, Mamelok A: The eye: a window to many diagnoses. Pat Care 13: 50–79, 1979
8. Blindness and Diabetes (pamphlet). New York, American Foundation for the Blind, 1975
9. Products for People with Vision Problems. New York, American Foundation for the Blind, 1979
10. Directory of Low Vision Aids Facilities in the United States. New York, National Society for the Prevention of Blindness Inc, 1973–1974
11. Fine SL: Some plain talk on diabetic retinopathy. The National Society for the Prevention of Blindness Inc, Sight-Saving Rev 46: 3–9, 1976
12. The Aging Eye: Facts on Eye Care for Older Persons. New York, National Society for the Prevention of Blindness Inc, 1978
13. Macular Degeneration. New York, National Society for the Prevention of Blindness Inc, 1979

RECOMMENDED RESOURCES

Cohen K, Hyndiuk R: Ocular emergencies. Am Fam Phys 18: 178–184, 1978

Corso JF: Sensory processes and age effects in normal adults. J Gerontol 26: 90–105, 1971

Cristarella M: Visual functions of the elderly. Am J Occ Ther 13: 432–440, 1977

Gardiner PA: Visual difficulty in old age. Brit Med J 1: 105–106, 1979

Harvey AM, Johns RJ, Owens AH, et al: Opthalmology in medicine, in Harvey AM (ed): The Principles and Practice of Medicine. New York, Appleton-Century Crofts, 1976, p 1763

Jones M, Tippett T, Assessment of the red eye. Nurse Pract 5: 10–15, 1980

Marmor M: The eye and vision in the elderly, Geriat 32: 63–67, 1977

Monk C: Primary care for ocular emergencies, Heal Pract Physi Assist 3: 34–39, 1979

Palumbo PJ, Munoz JM: Diabetic retinopathy, Am Fam Phys 14: 60–63, 1976

Paton D, Craig JA: Cataracts–development, diagnosis, management. Clin Sump 26: 2–32, 1974

Rai GS, Elias-Jones A: The corneal reflex in elderly patients. J Am Geriatr Soc 27: 317–318, 1979

Stokoc NL: Eye problems. Primary Care 220: 723–732, 1978

Soll DB: Emergency care of eye injuries. Bull Am Coll Surg 61: 15–17, 1976

Waring GO: The red eye: diagnosis and therapy. Sixth Annual Family Practice Refresher Course, Davis, California, Departments of Family Practice and Postgraduate Medicine, University of California at Davis, August 1978

Patient Education Materials:

American Foundation for the Blind, 15 West 16th Street, New York, New York   10011

- Blindness and Diabetes (pamphlet), 1975

- Catalog of Publications, 1977–1978
- Products for People with Vision Problems, 1979

Audio visual aids. Material on various ophthalmological problems is available for almost all office teaching formats: Softcon Products, Division of Warner-Lambert Co., Morris Plains, New Jersey 07950.

Glaucoma and You, 1965. Alcon Laboratories Inc, 6201 South Freeway, PO Box 1959, Fort Worth, Texas 76101

Glaucoma: Eye Pressure Building up to Blindness, 1975. Alza Pharmaceuticals, 950 Page Mill Road, Palo Alto, California 94301

National Society for the Prevention of Blindness, 79 Madison Avenue, New York, New York 10016

- Catalog, publications, films, 1980
- Directory of Low Vision Aids Facility in the United States
- Free glaucoma tests
- Pamphlets: The Aging Eye

Cataract
Facts on Eye Care for Older Persons
Glaucoma
Half of all Blindness is Needless
Macular Degeneration
Organization of Glaucoma Screening Programs

- Research, education, etc.

Physicians Art Service Inc, 343-B Serramonte Plaza Office Center, Daly City, California 94015

- Contact lenses
- Eye Safety is a Good Idea (poster)
- I Care—Eye Care at Work, Home and Play
- Seeing Again After Cataract Surgery

Talking books and cassettes. Division for the Blind and Physically Handicapped, Library of Congress, Washington, DC 20542

19

Geriatric Dermatology

Nancy D. Sullivan, F.N.P., M.S.
Rodney S.W. Basler, M.D.

Because of its obvious visibility, the skin has always been, and undoubtedly will continue to be, the principal organ considered in the visual determination of a human's age. Regardless of the condition of the heart, liver, or kidneys, people are judged to have the appearance of being "young" or "old" for their chronologic age depending primarily on the state of preservation of their skin.[1] As is true with the other organ systems, the natural processes operant in the skin that cause structural and functional changes over time are markedly influenced by the degree of care and protection people give their integument throughout life. Specifically, the speed and severity of cutaneous aging is largely dependent on the cummulative effects of sun exposure.[2]

The suggestion that prolonged exposure to sunlight causes damage to the skin, far out of proportion to lapsed time, has been confirmed both by simple observations and detailed histopatholic, as well as biochemical studies.[3] Energy from sunlight penetrating into the dermis brings about alterations in the replacement capabilities and functional characteristics of collagen and elastic fibers. At the same time, the layer of subcutaneous fat is diminished over all parts of the body. The combined effect of these processes is the loss of skin turgor, producing a wrinkled appearance, the hallmark of aging.

The regenerative capacity of the stratum germinativum of the epidermis is also decreased with advancing age. This explains the significant increase in neoplasms of the skin in people over 50 as the supply of normal cells is no longer adequate to replace damaged cells. The process of repair replication is often not active enough to prevent clones of cells with aberrant nucleic acids from rapidly reproducing in a malignant fashion. In addition, reduced regeneration leads to modification of keratinization and a thinning of the stratum corneum. A concomitant decrease of sebaceous gland activity contributes to the dryness and tendency toward flaking of this layer, which gives rise to the clinical picture of xerosis in the elderly with its associated pruritus and, indirectly, to the eczemas and neurodermatitis.

The altered function of internal systems generates certain cutaneous problems seen almost exclusively in an aging population. Reduced circulation to the extremities and diminished elasticity within the venous network may cause edema and the typical stasis dermatitis and ulceration of the lower legs. Diminished arterial flow may also result in ulceration or more serious problems such as infarction and gangrene. The flow of nutrients to the skin may be further compromised by chronic pressure brought about by neurological defects or general debility that give rise to decubitus ulcers. The immune response becomes less competent in defending the skin from proliferation of externally and internally latent organisms. For this reason, herpes zoster and superficial Candida infections show increased incidence with advancing age. The inescapable reality of nature is that all systems of each organism begin a programmed demise when the individual has outlived his or her biologic ability to replenish the species.

In dealing with patients whose problems are for the most part a consequence of the diminished capacity of their bodies' organ systems to maintain previous levels of integrity, special understanding and concern are necessary. The patient requires continued reassurance that many of the aggravating changes are normal and to be expected. Patience and tolerance must be stressed as response to treatment will be slowed by sluggish repair mechanisms, as in the case of stasis ulcers. Regardless of the relative seriousness of any condition or the predictability of its occurrence, the practitioner is obligated to instill a feeling of confidence in the patient—that with proper care, his or her body is still capable of some level of restoration.

INCIDENCE OF DERMATOLOGICAL PROBLEMS

Skin problems are very common in the elderly and in the hospitalized geriatric population; as many as 98 percent can be expected to have identifiable skin disease.[4] Besides those conditions which characteristically appear at a later age, many problems persist from earlier life. An example is psoriasis, which is found in about 1 percent of the young adult population and is also present in about 1 percent of the senior population.[4] Most epidermologic studies deal with conditions such as climate, occupation, complexion, sex, and race rather than age. Consequently, very little data exclusive to this group is available.

The most commonly treated skin problems in the elderly are pruritus, eczema, keratoses, venous leg ulcers, basal cell and squamous cell carcinoma;[4] although the prevalence of the latter two is significantly higher in white than in black populations. Approximately 90 percent of those over 80 years of age will have senile angiomas or senile lentigines, while xerosis will be found in 40–80 percent of the elderly.

Common Problems

In the aging process, hair changes include both graying and thinning. It has been estimated that over half the population will experience 50 percent of their body hair turning gray by the age of 50 years.[4] Graying usually begins at the temples and then extends towards the vertex. Axillary hair graying is more common in men than in women and may not even occur. By the fourth decade of life, body hair has reached its full distribution pattern, and from then on there is a progressive loss of hair in the reverse order of its development. The trunk hair is the first to become finer, followed by the

axillary and pubic regions. Leg hair becomes sparse, and eyebrow, ear, and nasal hair becomes coarser and longer in both sexes over 60 years. Both men and women will experience scalp thinning and recession. Clinicians may find women more frequently concerned over scalp hair loss, and the patients may fear that some underlying problem is the cause. Reassuring patients that hair thinning is a normal aging process might alleviate these fears of undetected disease. It is not, however, likely to reduce concerns regarding the cosmetic effect of hair loss. Generally, the thinning of scalp hair in women is limited and does not result in baldness, and this reassurance may be of benefit.

Another common complaint and concern of the elderly is senile lentigo, better known as liver spots. Senile lentigo occurs on the exposed surfaces of the skin, while senile angiomas occur on the protected areas of the skin. These lesions may be found singly or in combination on the vast majority of the elderly population. With aging, the dermal capillaries become fragile, dilated, and are subject to frequent subcutaneous hemorrhages. The patient needs to be reassured that there is no disease process and generally no treatment necessary.

Uncommon Problems

Certain dermatoses occur predominantly in the elderly segment of the population but are seen so infrequently as to be considered uncommon or even rare. Among the vesiculo-bullous diseases, the incidence of bullous pemphigoid increases with age with a slight predilection for women. In this condition, tense, large bullae are seen on a nonerythematous base, especially over the lower abdomen, groin, and inner aspect of the thigh. Treatment may consist of potent topical steroids alone in mild to moderate cases, and, in more severe cases, in conjunction with systemic steroids. A variant of this disease is cicatricial or benign mucous membrane pemphigoid, which is also seen mainly after the age of 60. Chronic involvement of the eye in this entity may lead to scarring and ultimately to blindness.

Some cutaneous abnormalities that appear more frequently in the elderly are characterized by atrophy and scarring and often are difficult to differentiate clinically. Lichen sclerosis et atrophicus is seen among older patients and presents as thinned areas of atrophic skin with "cigarette paper" texture. The areas are usually hypopigmented and show telangiectasis. Women are affected ten times more often than men, commonly being afflicted in the genital area where the condition is referred to as kranrosis vulvae. No specific treatment is available for this problem, and close intermittent examination is indicated because of a somewhat increased risk of malignant transformation.

Another cutaneous manifestation that warrants a complete examination because of its association with malignancy in the aged is dermatomyositis. In adults over 40, as high as one-third of all patients with dermatomyositis have an underlying neoplasm. Clinically, a soreness and weakness of the proximal muscles is accompanied by a violaceous eruption showing telangiectasis and, later, calcinosis. A purplish discoloration of the eyelids is diagonstically very helpful when present. Periungual telangiectasis is often one of the first cutaneous signs. Treatment is generally unrewarding except in those cases in which a removable underlying cause is ascertained.

DIAGNOSIS AND TREATMENT OF COMMON PROBLEMS

Pruritus

Most clinicians agree that pruritus is the most common dermatologic complaint of the elderly. The causes for pruritus are myriad but may be divided into two distinct catagories: generalized and localized. The nervous network of the skin is capable of transmitting several sensations including itch, pain, touch, heat, cold, and pressure. The itch and pain sensations are both carried by the C fibers and become discernable depending upon multiple factors. These nerve endings are found in the papillary dermis and lower epidermis.[4] Itching is produced when several pain points are weakly and repetitively stimulated simultaneously. Once itching has been produced, the pain threshold is lowered due to this activation.[5] When a second stimulus, scratching, is applied, the itching usually ceases momentarily.

Different areas of the skin are more susceptible to itching than others. The most sensitive areas to pruritic stimuli are the inguinal region, anogenital area, popliteal and clavicular fossa, the neck, upper arm, and forearm. The least susceptible areas are the knuckle of the thumb, tip of the nose, and the sole of the foot.[5] The intensity of pruritus varies from individual to individual as does response and may become increased or dimminished as part of

the aging process. Many people experience an increase in pruritus with stress, anxiety, or overstimulation. Most agree that it is especially severe just prior to falling asleep, when other incoming stimuli are decreased.[6]

Generalized Pruritus Without Lesions

Generalized pruritus may occur without skin lesions and is frequently a symptom of an internal problem such as malignancy, uremia or diabetes mellitus. Certain drugs are known to cause pruritus without lesions, including tetracycline, alcohol, and opium derivatives.[7] It is also possible that generalized pruritus without skin lesions may be a manifestation of a psychiatric disturbance. However, to proceed with treatment as if this complaint were solely of emotional origin would be a dangerous assumption. A careful and thorough review of systems and of all medications is pertinent. If the history reveals a suspect medication, discontinuance of the drug is the obvious first step of treatment. At least two weeks must elapse before reevaluation, because that much time may be required for the body to clear the medication. If pruritus persists beyond two weeks, evaluation is necessary. The application of a topical medication containing menthol or phenol in a lubricating base may be helpful. Antihistamines are usually given, but dosage must be scaled down in older patients to prevent oversedation. In extreme cases, the use of systemic steroids may be justified to bring about rapid relief of symptoms.

As previously mentioned, the elderly may indeed have a systemic problem that is asymptomatic except for the presenting complaint of itching. For this reason, the following screening blood tests should be considered: liver panel, blood urea nitrogen, alkaline phosphatase, thyroid panel, fasting blood sugar, complete blood count, and sedimentation rate. Successful treatment of underlying systemic problems will often result in immediate cessation of the pruritus.

For a more extensive, but not all-inclusive, list of causes for generalized pruritus without skin lesions, see Table 19-1 and 2.

Generalized Pruritus With Lesions

The most common cause of pruritus in the aged is xerosis. With aging, the epidemis has a decreased ability to retain water, which, combined with envi-

Table 19-1
Internal Causes of Generalized Pruritus Without
Lesions

Diabetes mellitus
Chronic renal disease (uremia)
Hyperthyroidism
Malignancy
    (especially Hodgkin's disease, lymphoma, abdominal
    cancer)
Leukemia
Hepatic biliary obstruction
Iron deficiency anemia
Leprosy
Polycythemia
Psychiatric disturbances

ronmental factors creating low humidity, increases the risk of dry skin in the elderly. An arid environment—whether occurring naturally such as in deserts or from dry cold winds or induced artifically as with central heating or air conditioning—contributes significantly to dry skin. In order to control the environment, the patient could indeed move to coastal areas where the humidity is higher. However, placing a humidifier or vaporizer in the more frequently used areas seems to be an easier and far less expensive course of action. See Table 19-3.

Pruritus hiemalis is a term used to describe pruritic dry skin that occurs during the fall and winter months. Typically, xerosis is first seen in nonhair bearing areas of skin such as around the waist and the lower legs but, in more severe cases, can become diffuse (Fig. 19-1). The patient usually complains of a tight immobile sensation and an increasing amount of scales, as well as static electricity. Pruritus is most intense when first going to bed.

Xerosis is mainly treated by lubricating the skin. It is true that bathing will hydrate the stratum corneum, however, after the water evaporates, the skin will become even dryer due to reduction of natural oils. Reducing the amount of bathing may be of some benefit, and it is critical to lubricate the

Table 19-2
Drug-induced Causes of Generalized Pruritus Without
Lesions

Antibiotics (tetracycline, penicillin, sulphonamides,
    chloromycetin)
Alcohol
Gold
Opium derivatives
Arsenic

Table 19-3
Causes of Generalized Pruritus With Lesions

Xerosis (asteatotic eczema)
Nummular eczema
Infestations (see Table 19-4)
Seborrheic dermatitis
Psoriasis
Lichen planus
Miliaria
Drug-induced eruptions
    (Including: urticaria, erythema multiforme, erthyema
    nodosum, vasculitis, exfoliative, pigmentation,
    lichenoid, eczematous)

skin immediately with an ointment after leaving the bath. Aquaphor, which is 95 percent petrolatum, is effective and inexpensive. The patient needs to be instructed that bathing in extremely hot water or using detergent soaps will further aggravate the dryness. Oil-based soaps such as Dove and Caress are recommended if soap is used. An alternative to soaps is the use of mineral oil added to the bath water (e.g., Alpha Keri or Lubath). It is important to remember when recommending the use of lubricants in bath water that there is an increased risk of injury from slipping and falling in the tub, and this risk must be weighed. Topical applications twice a day of petrolatum, Keri lotion, Eucerin, Nivea oil or cream trap the skin moisture and are of great therapeutic value.

The anogenital area is among the most common localized sites for pruritus. As mentioned previously, this region is among the most sensitive areas to pruritic stimuli. Infections and infestations must be ruled out and, if present, treated appropriately. Infestation causes of pruritus are scabies, roundworm, pediculosis capitis, pediculosis carporis, and pediculosis pubis. Other causes to be considered are poor hygiene and allergic reactions to toilet tissue, detergents, or synthetic underwear. Poor hygiene is remedied by the obvious—patient compliance that will be best achieved through understanding the skin and its needs. Often, toilet tissue that is either abrasive or dyed may be a cause for itching. The patient may be demonstrating a primary irritant reaction or an allergic response to the chemical used in producing a decorative tissue. In these instances, the patient should switch to an all white tissue that is soft.

Detergents and soaps are also a cause for anogenital pruritus. The detergents can become trapped in this region simply because of the difficulty in

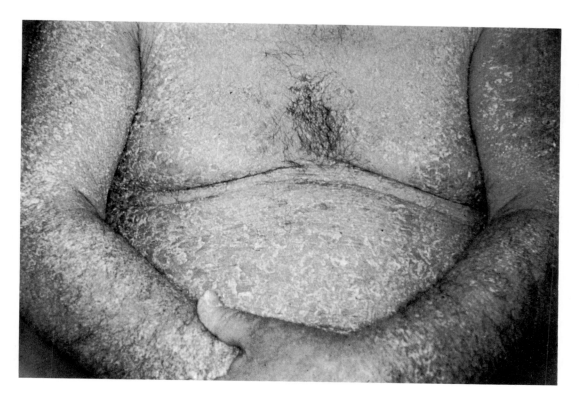

Fig.19-1. Severe xerosis.

thorough rinsing; natural occlusion adds to the irritation. The elderly need to be reminded to switch to a bland soap such as one of those previously mentioned and to rinse the perianal region thoroughly after cleansing.

Underwear made from synthetic material does not absorb as well as cotton. Perspiration that is not absorbed and lies on the skin not only increases the pruritic sensation, but also acts as an irritant to the skin and may promote maceration, which leads to fungal growth and infection. Elderly patients should be encouraged to use 100 percent cotton underwear that will absorb moisture.

Eczema

Eczematous conditions are said to be found in 25 percent of the elderly living at home, and the most common site is on the lower legs.[8] For the most part, eczema is mild and easily treated. Unless symptoms are severe, however, the elderly may not seek treatment until a secondary infection has occurred. Even with appropriate treatment, the elder-

ly skin may remain sensitive for months and experience relapses. Treatment should be tapered gradually and other factors such as nutrition, hygiene, drugs, and contact irritants considered to ensure treatment success.

Nummular eczema is a common form of eczema in the elderly and presents in the primary form as highly pruritic coin-shaped vesicular plaques on the extremities. Secondary lesions may show lichenification and have superficial bacterial infection. Recurrences are the rule with special predilection for sites of previous activity. The history may be positive for atopic eczema, asthma, or hayfever.

The elderly should be instructed to avoid excess bathing with soap. Topical use of hydrocortisone ointment 1 percent and an occulusive dressing is the first step in treatment. If there is no response, stronger fluorinated steroids may be used. For those resistant cases, a coal tar solution of 3–10 percent added to the topical steriod treatment may be beneficial, although often objectionable because of staining and odor. In the past, Depo-Testosterone injections were given in resistant cases; however, this is contraindicated when treating the elderly due to the increased stress these injections place on the cardiovascular system.

Contact dermatitis is easily recognized when there is an unusual pattern of distribution and the lesions are well marginated and erythematous with papules and vesicles. In the elderly, however, there may be a depressed inflammatory response and the lesions may be scattered, generalized, and persistant. A thorough history is mandatory in order to eliminate the offending agent. Perhaps the most common error in diagnosing and treating contact allergies is the misconception that products used for a long time cannot be the offending allergens. In fact, the longer a substance has been used, the more likely it is to be the sensitizing offender, and every chemical that the patient comes in contact with must be considered as a potential allergen. (See Table 19-4 for a partial list of common allergens.)

Treatment consists first of removing the allergen from the patient's environment. A topical steriod such as hydrocortizone ointment 1 percent applied three times a day is often sufficient treatment. Weeping and oozing lesions can be treated with tap water or Burow solution compresses. On occasion, systemic steroids are required. The elderly need to be told that the skin may remain sensitive and inflamed for weeks or even months in spite of treatment. During this time, the elderly should avoid further trauma, such as overcleansing, until the skin returns to normal.

Neurodermatitis usually presents as a pruritic patch of dermatitis that may lichenified. It is commonly found on the posterior neck of menopausal women and on the anterior shins in both sexes. This lesion begins as a small patch that may have

been an insect bite or other minor irritation and develops into a dermatitis because of the constant irritation of scratching. The history will reveal an increase in pruritus when the patient is nervous, tired, or upset.

The treatment is directed towards controlling the itching. Hydrocortozine ointment 1 percent applied four times a day may be sufficient. However, a fluorinated steroid cream under an occlusive dressing of Saran Wrap left on for 8–12 hours per day may be desired initially. During severe bouts of itching, ice cold boric acid packs may be applied for 15 minutes as necessary. One tablespoon of boric acid crystals to one quart of ice cold water will achieve the desired solution. Undoubtedly, the most important factor is to break the itch-scratch-itch cycle, for once scratching is eliminated, the lesion will clear without further treatment.

Seborrheic dermatitis is one of the skin conditions that often begins early in life and persists into old age, frequently with increased severity. The most common sites of occurrence for this erythematous eruption with a browny-white scale are the scalp, central portion of the face, perioral region, retroauricular skin fold, and the mid chest. Symptoms are usually more aggravating during the fall and winter months. Adequate treatment of the scalp may simply consist of shampooing with a sebolytic shampoo such as Ionil, Sebulex or Zincon. Tar-containing shampoos should not be used on light gray or white hair because of the risk of imparting an objectionable yellow tint to the hair. Pure hydrocortisone 1 percent may be used on the facial areas and is usually adequate to control the eruption. Fluorinated steroids must be avoided because of their potential to produce atrophy in facial skin, especially in the elderly.

Table 19-4
Contact Allergens

Rubber additives (especially shoes)
Glues (in clothing and shoes)
Nickel
Cosmetic ingredients (dyes, preservatives, perfumes)
Plants (poison ivy, poison oak, ragweed, chrysanthemum)
Clothing (permanent press garments)
Dry cleaning agents
Laundry products
Hand and body soaps
Topical medications (neomycin, ethylenediamine)

Infections

Herpes zoster occurs most commonly between the fifth and seventh decade of life and is often associated with underlying diseases such as Hodgkin's or lymphomas. Clinically, herpes zoster is easily recognized once the grouped papulovesicular lesions appear in the area of distribution of a cutaneous nerve (Fig. 19-2). Pain may precede the skin lesions by 24–48 hours and even mimic cholecystitis or angina. The pain may be associated with malaise and fever. In over 50 percent of the patients over 70 years of age, postherpetic neuralgia occurs, and

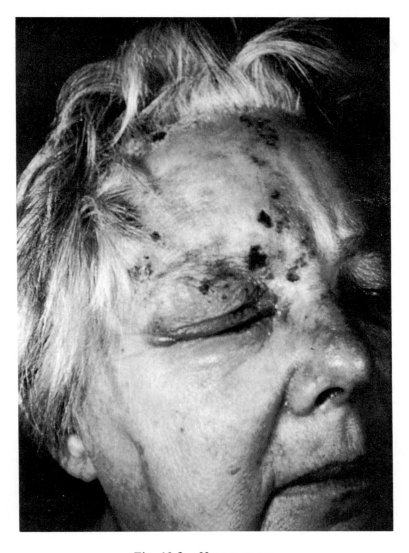

Fig. 19-2. Herpes zoster.

occasionally complications such as foot drop or neurogenic bladder dysfunction are seen.

There is no specific treatment for herpes zoster. Calamine lotion or phenal lotions may be helpful during the early stages. Postherpetic neuralgia may be treated with sedatives, analgesics, or even neurosurgery; however, no one treatment is recognized as constantly helpful. There are some advocates for using cortisone therapy during the acute stage in order to prevent herpetic neuralgia in the elderly, but this remains controversial because of the risk of producing a disseminated herpes infection. The

suggested treatment is up to 80 mg prednisone per day initially, tapering the dosage over a three-week period.

Fungal and yeast infections are quite common in the elderly and are, on occasion, the first sign of an underlying systemic problem such as diabetes mellitus or lymphomas. The classic clinical appearance of erythematious, well-marginated circinate papules and plaques in a scattered distribution, is almost diagnostic and can be confirmed by microscopic examination of a potassium hydroxide preparation. If there is no underlying disease, topical clotrimazole or miconazole applied three times a day is usually sufficient treatment. When candidal pustules are present, topical treatment often fails unless the patient debrides these lesions daily. Resistant yeast infections of the mouth or perineal area may require both systemic and topical nystatin.

Ulcerations of the Skin

Cutaneous ulcerations can generally be classified into three basic catagories: those that are secondary to externally applied trauma, those that result from one of the bullous diseases, and those that are due to an insufficient supply of nutrients to the skin. The latter of these groups is the one seen most commonly in geriatric-age patients and can be further divided into venous, arterial, and decubitus ulcers. In venous or stasis ulcers, the hydrostatic pressure, increasing as a result of inadequate venous return from the extremities, causes edema, thereby preventing adequate nutrition to maintain cutaneous integrity. Repeated cycles of ulceration and healing may result in marked scarring and constriction of the extremity (Fig. 19-3). In ulceration due to compromised arterial vasculature, the blood supply is directly compromised, and in decubitus ulcers the compression of vessels from chronic pressure is responsible for the nutrient deficit.

As with all disease, the first approach to the problem of cutaneous ulceration is an awareness by the patient of appropriate measures of prevention. Stasis ulcers may often be prevented by encouraging elderly patients to elevate their feet during all times of rest and by the application of occlusive wraps or elastic stockings at the first sign of peripheral edema. Ulceration may be postponed by early treatment of stasis dermatitis, which further robs the skin of nutrients by maintaining an inflammatory state in the dermis-diminishing lymphatic drainage. For this reason, patients should be instructed to watch for the early signs and symptoms of this problem, which often presents as a tawny erythema about the ankles. Topical steroids in a moisturizing base such as Aquafor or Eucerin are effective in treating the dermatitis and may be conveniently applied under occlusion if first covered with a plastic wrap. Compromised circulation secondary to arterial insufficiency is harder to improve, short of surgical intervention. In the case of decubitus ulcers, fastidious attention to rotating body weight may prevent or greatly reduce their occurrence even in totally debilitated patients.

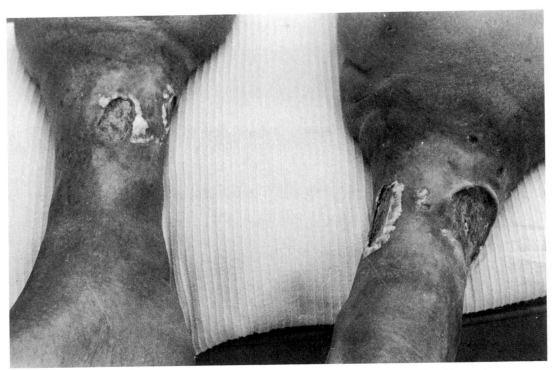

Fig. 19-3.   Ulceration and constriction from chronic venous stasis of lower leg.

Stasis dermatitis becomes clinically apparent only as a late manifestation of chronic venous insufficiency. The first sign of the condition is usually an edema of the lower one-third of the legs so minor as to be clinically inapparent or may be strking. As the hydrostatic pressure increases in the extremity, the skin will often take on a hyperpigmentation and become erythematous and scaling. Significant pruritis may accompany this superficial change, and excoriations are often noted. The initial discoloration due to extravasated erythrocytes is replaced by a deeper brown pigmentation as melanocyte replication within the skin is stimulated and increased amounts of melanin are deposited. Continued excoriation may produce a lichenification of the area that contributes to deeper pigmentation. Finally, if not adequately treated, nearly all stasis dermatitis will evolve into ulceration.

A myriad of treatments have been proposed for stasis ulcers, but all are dependent on the basic necessity of occluding the involved extremity in such a way as to decrease hydrostatic pressure. This is most successfully carried out by using an elastic wrap first applied to the very distal end of the foot and continued proximally to extend above the knee. Care should be taken to ensure that there are no improper overlaps of the material which might cause further constriction. The other essential ingredient in the successful resolution of cutaneous ulcers of all types is patience. Granulation tissue may be very slow to form, and, in most cases, epithelium will migrate from the periphery at a distressingly slow rate. A positive attitude and continued encouragement of the patient are indispensible. Careful attention to the patient's nutrition, especially protein intake, is another important adjunct to therapy.

Regardless of the medication used within the stasis ulcer, it is fundamental to improve the microdrainage of the area by decreasing the surrounding dermatitis by the use of topical steroids. These medications may be applied two to three times per day in most instances for maximal effect. Ointment preparations have the advantage of a moisturizing effect and may be preferable in treating the elderly.

The ulcer itself can be approached using one of the basic axioms of dermatology: "if it is wet, dry it; if it is dry, wet it." Ulcers that show obvious purulent exudate should be cultured, although the superficial infecting organism may be playing a very minor role in the maintenance of the ulcer. Obvious signs of cellulitis—such as fever, lymphangitis, or lymph-adenopathy—are, of course, indications for the use of the appropriate systemic antibiotics. Compresses made from a 3–5 percent Burow solution and changed every two to four hours will often bring about satisfactory drying of draining lesions in three to five days. The combination of equal parts of Gelfoam powder and Neosporin powder has a similar action and is preferred by some clinicians. Debridement of exudate is effectively obtained with a minimum of patient discomfort by having the extremity in a whirlpool, but it may also be achieved by gently cleansing the lesion with peroxide or antibacterial soap if a whirlpool is not available. The capillary action of dextranomer (Debrisan) has a very beneficial drying and antibiotic effect and is often useful in weeping ulcers. A simple compress using tap water and an antibacterial soap, such as pHiso Hex, are simple means of promoting drying of the lesion.

As previously mentioned, the key to treatment is decreasing hydrostatic pressure through elevation of the extremities and occlusion, and this point must be stressed to patients continually so that they may contribute to their own improvement. If this is being successfully carried out, the actual ingredients placed within an ulcer are of secondary importance. Once the ulcer is no longer actively suppurating, there are a myriad of various formulations, each of which has gained favor with individual clinicians and may be used to prevent suprainfection, as well as to promote granulation in a chronic stasis ulcer. The simple application of an antibiotic ointment, such as Neosporin, is favored by some. If a neomycin sensitivity is present or is a consideration, other antibiotics such as erythromycin, gentamycin, tetracycline, or chloramphenicol ointment may be used. Ingredients traditionally considered to be effective in promoting granulation may be used separately or compounded with the antiobiotics. Examples of such ingredients include zinc oxide paste and Balsam of Peru. Benzoyl peroxide in a 10–20 percent concentration is believed to have both an antibiotic and granulation promoting effect. Insulin has been reported to be beneficial when placed directly into healing ulcers. It is sometimes used in combination with glucose, in which case the two are added to the ulcer simultaneously. Alternatively, glucose may be used by itself, either in a 50 percent aqueous solution or as a 50 percent concentration in Aquaphor.

While attempts should be made to increase pressure around stasis ulcers, the exact opposite is true with decubitus ulcers. It is essential that no body weight be allowed to compress the vasculature in the immediate vicinity of one of these types of ulcers. Continually observant nursing care is a necessity for proper positioning of the patient. When all pressure has been successfully removed, any of the treatment forms already discussed for use within the stasis ulcer may be employed. It is often necessary that necrotic or infected tissue first be removed before treatment can begin. Surgical debridement or the application of a enzyme such as Travase or Elase under damp occlusion will usually be sufficient to remove tissue debris.

In the case of very large decubitus ulcers that have become saccular or tunneling, daily packing is necessary to ensure that healing will progress from the innermost part of the defect to the surface. Roll gauze or Kerlix is very useful for this type of packing. Either of these materials can be soaked in normal saline for a noninfected ulcer or in a solution of 1 percent clindamycin or 1:1000 potassium permanganate if an infection is suspected.

Arterial ulcers are the most difficult and least rewarding type to treat medically. If they are primarily due to an autoimmune vasculitis, as in the case of rheumatoid arthritis, great improvement can be seen in the ulcers with successful treatment of the underlying disease. Serious circulatory compromise can be approached only with extensive revascularization procedures and large areas of cutaneous infarction and necrosis necessitate amputation. The local care of arterial ulcers is essentially the same as that outlined for the other types, with combination ointments containing antibiotics and steroids favored by some practitioners.

Neoplasms

An increased incidence of premalignant and malignant neoplasms of the skin is noted with advancing age. This fact is due in part to the cummulative effect of long-term sun exposure and in part to the inability of the stratum germinativum to replace damaged cells completely. The latter phenomenon had been metaphorically compared to a reserve army unit marching through a hot day.[2] Early in the morning, the fresh troops have no difficulty increasing their pace in an advance to the front to reinforce the lines. As the day progresses, however, fatigue sets in and the poorly functioning front-line soldiers are replaced at a slower and slower rate until finally there are insufficient reserve troops to

meet demand, and the integrity of the line breaks down. The cutaneous equivalent of the "reserve forces" are cells that leave the mitotic cycle for extended periods and then reenter, enhancing regenerative efficiency.[10] Decreased reentry into mitotic cycling has been correlated with advancing age.[11]

The fact that long-term sun exposure is a primary predisposing determinant in the pathogenesis of skin cancer is well documented.[1] Basal cell carcinomas (Fig. 19-4), squamous cell carcinomas, and premalignant actinic keratoses are all neoplasms of epithelial origin, which are formed by the dysplastic proliferation of keratinocytes in response to chronic solar stimulation. These tumors are relatively common. The incidence of actinic keratoses in a farming population was found to be 16.3 percent, and in the same study the incidence rate for basal cell carcinomas was 4.4 percent.[12]

Since the degenerative effect of long-term ultraviolet rays is cummulative over decades, the majority of potential injuries may have taken place by the time a geriatric patient is seen for actinic changes. It is not too late, however, to strongly emphasize protective measures to minimize further damage. The segment of the ultraviolet spectrum that induces actinic injury is localized to wavelengths of 290–320 nm (Fig. 19-5) and corresponds to the sunburn spectrum. These rays can be effectively shielded from the skin by a number of sunscreen preparations, especially those containing 5 percent paraaminobenzoic acid (PABA). Protective garments such as long sleeve shirts and wide-brimmed hats should be encouraged during long periods outdoors.

Certain pigmented neoplasms are also seen predominantly in the elderly. By far the most common example of this group is the seborrheic keratosis (Fig. 19-6), which may appear in widely varying colors, shapes and sizes. Newer lesions are thin and flesh-colored or faintly yellow or tan. In time, they thicken, forming a verrucous surface, and the pigment becomes more intense, often progressing to a dark brown-black coloration. Multiple lesions in various stages of progression are commonly seen on one patient.

Other pigmented lesions are melanocytic in origin. Chronically exposed areas, such as the forehead and dorsum of the hands, develop clones of melanocytes that increase in relative numbers along epidermal ridges giving rise to senile lentigines often referred to as "liver spots." The lentigo maligna or

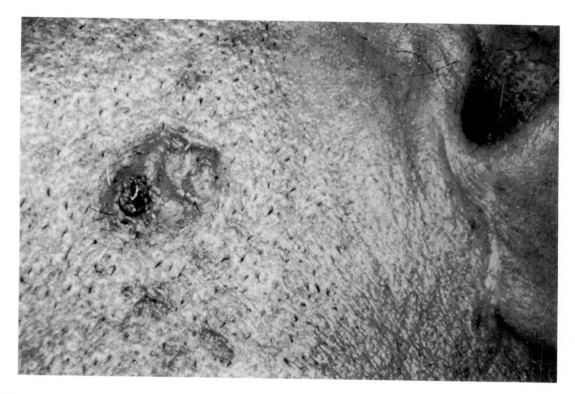

Fig. 19-4. Basal cell carcinoma presenting as pearly papule with rolled border and central depression.

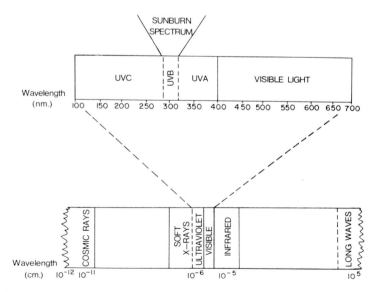

Fig. 19-5. Electromagnetic spectrum showing wavelengths responsible for sunburn and degenerative changes.

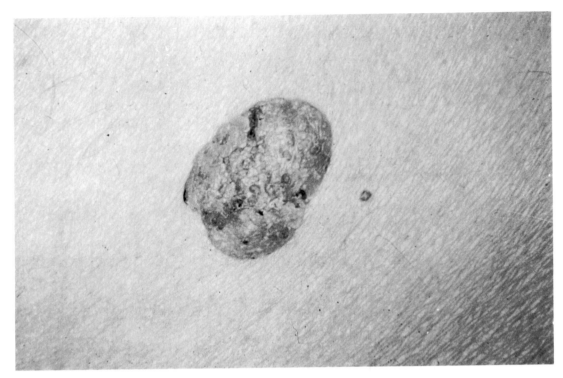

Fig. 19-6. Seborrheic keratosis.

Hutchinson's freckle (Fig. 19-7) contains a typical melanocytes at the dermal-epidermal junction. These usually show a very darkly pigmented center surrounded by a more lightly colored periphery. Both areas will increase with time, and the center may become nodular indicating progression into a lentigo maligna melanoma.

The treatment of all forms of cutaneous neoplasms requires tissue destruction or removal. A noninvasive medical approach to premalignant actinic keratoses employs the antimetabolite, 5-fluorouracil (5FU) applied in a 1, 2, or 5 percent concentration in a cream or gel base to areas showing actinic damage with keratotic papules. Applications are usually made twice each day for three or four weeks on the face and somewhat longer on the hands and arms. It is of prime importance that the patient be informed at the outset of the dramatic nature of the reaction in certain individuals. Intense inflammation usually is seen in the vicinity of each keratoses. Significant erythema is an almost universal response and often cosmetically disfiguring for a time. Patients may complain of extreme discomfort with burning and itching, and isolated lesions may bleed. These reactions usually peak at about

two weeks of treatment, and the patient should be reassured at this point that everything is progressing as expected. When the course of therapy is completed, a topical steroid may be prescribed to diminish inflammation. Within a month, the reaction has usually resolved, giving way to a healthy, new, keratosis-free epithelium.

Among the modes of treatment for individual actinic keratoses, one favored for its ease and speed is the application of liquid nitrogen. This form of cryotherapy may be employed using either a cotton-tipped swab dipped into the liquid and then touched onto the lesion or any one of a number of specially designed units that combine a container with a spray attachment. Individual keratoses are treated until thoroughly frozen as indicated by a white halo of frozen tissue surrounding the lesion. Usually within the course of seven to ten days, each will either blister or form a crust that will gradually slough leaving a normal appearing base. Some of the thicker lesions may be curetted after they have been frozen. This technique is especially useful if a pathologic specimen is desired to rule out with certainty the possibility of an early squamous cell carcinoma. Single keratoses may also be treated by

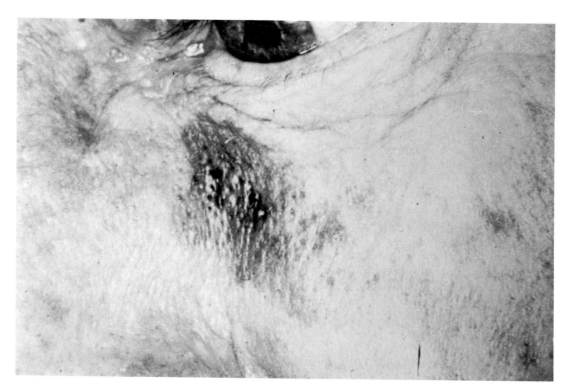

Fig. 19-7. Lentigo maligna on cheek.

injection of a local anesthetic followed by excision, using either a scalpel or curette. Older lesions may be easier to remove if they are first hyfrecated.

Once a lesion has progressed into a malignancy, more aggressive therapy is indicated to ensure total eradication. Basal cell carcinomas are most commonly removed by electrofulguration and curettage because this form of treatment allows the clinician to remove cancerous tissue to the depth of normal tissue by discriminating between the soft, mushy consistency of the cancer and the firmer texture of underlying normal dermis. Once the pliable tissue has been removed, the base and edges of the defect are treated with electric current, either from a monopolar or biopolar source. This procedure causes the complete destruction of a further amount of tissue at the borders of the lesion, allowing for a margin of safety. Electrofulguration and curettage may be alternated a number of times until a totally firm base remains under the site of the previous basal cell carcinoma. It is probable that this form of treatment also diminishes the recurrence rate by stimulating a marked inflammatory cell infiltrate in the tissue adjacent to the treated cancer.

Simple eliptical excision of basal cells is possible in areas such as around the eyes and mouth where redundant skin can easily be approximated to close the defect. This form of treatment has a somewhat higher incidence of recurrence since the borders of the lesion cannot be discriminated using the surgeon's tactile sense. Certain lesions on the other hand may be best suited to cryosurgical techniques in which the lesion and surrounding tissue is physically destroyed by freezing with liquid nitrogen. The use of a thermal couple is recommended to ensure that the depth of the tissue freeze is adequate to surround the carcinoma.

Certain other lesions, such as recurrences following another mode of treatment, lesions around the nose and mouth, and particularly large lesions, may be best approached using therapeutic radiation. This form of therapy has the obvious drawback of requiring expensive equipment and the expertise to use it and will not be available to most practitioners except through referral to a dermatologist or radiation therapist. Besides expense, another shortcoming of x-ray therapy is the fact that treated areas tend to become more noticeable and less cosmetically acceptable with time due to the long-term effects of radiation.

Squamous cell carcinomas (Fig. 19-8) can be approached in most of the same ways as basal cells. It must be remembered, however, that this type of malignancy is more aggressive and runs a higher risk of local spread and distant metastasis. The squamous cell carcinomas that arise in areas of sun damage are somewhat less aggressive than those arising on nonexposed skin, in which cell type and malignant potential simulates those of squamous cell carcinomas of internal organs. Electrofulguration and curettage is usually an adequate form of treatment for squamous cell carcinomas of the skin. It is advisable to obtain a pathologic specimen prior to beginning this form of destructive treatment. Cryosurgery may also be indicated in some instances, and radiation therapy is usually effective with the same limitations as have already been discussed.

Seborrheic keratoses are simple lesions to remove from the skin, and patients will often remove them themselves. However, the base of these lesions must be treated to prevent recurrence. Cryotherapy using liquid nitrogen is especially popular in the treatment of these lesions because of its ease of application and effectiveness. A keratolytic topical cream containing urea and salicylic acid may be applied to each of the lesions for three weeks, after which they can also be easily removed by curettage. Immediate removal can be accomplished by infiltrating the area of the lesion with a local anesthetic and then either by curetting the lesion directly or by first "softening" it with electrocautery.

Lentigines are often too numerous to be worth treating, but may respond either to light cryotherapy with liquid nitrogen or to a bleaching agent such as hydroquinone. Lentigo malignas require treatment to prevent progression into more serious neoplasms. They may be excised with a simple closure, if small, or may be treated with cryosurgery. Any areas within the lesion that show nodular change should be biopsied to rule out a melanoma.

HEALTH MAINTENANCE

The importance of skin care is paramount as the skin is the first-line of defense for the body. For the bedridden or wheelchair-bound elderly, it is even

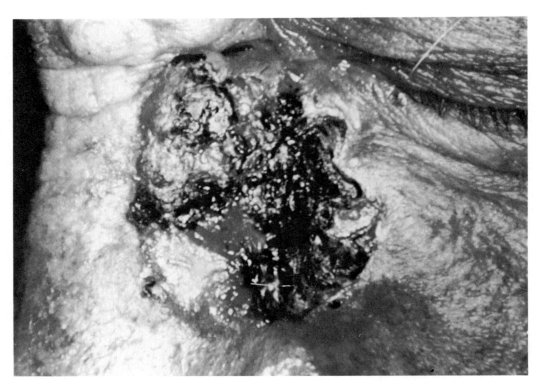

Fig. 19-8. Squamous cell carcinoma with local invasion and extension.

more important to maintain a healthy integumentary system. The elderly who are not ambulatory risk decubateous ulcers. Any person who is taking care of the elderly should be instructed in the importance of aiding circulation to the skin. Frequent repositioning is mandatory every two hours, and the most common mistake is turning the patient from side to side only. For maximum efficiency and health care, the patient should be repositioned every two hours in each of the following positions: supine, right side, prone, left side. After the patient has been turned, that area recently uncovered should be massaged to stimulate circulation. The use of sheepskins, air mattresses, or foam padding underneath the bedridden has proven helpful in reducing skin friction.

In recent years, flotation systems and waterbeds have proven of great benefit in reducing decubateous ulcers. There are numerous sizes and shapes on the market. The newer waterbeds that are the same size as conventional twin beds are the most practical for the bedridden patient. This style of waterbed uses regular standardized bedlinens. However, there are two drawbacks: they are expensive and the head of the bed cannot be elevated.

There are other flotation systems available that are portable and can be placed directly on top of a standard bed. The most common types are air or water filled and come in a variety of sizes ranging from full bed length to small areas designed for the coccyx region. The most economical way of converting a standard bed to a flotation system is to place an air mattress covered by a sheepskin on top of the bed. These other flotation systems, sheepskin, or foam padding may all be found or ordered through a local medical supply house. Waterbeds and air mattresses may be found in local department stores.

Footcare is of utmost importance in the elderly. The circulation to this distal portion of the body is subject to compromise due to aging changes that occur in the cardiovascular and dermatological systems. Consequently, the feet are at an increased risk for stasis ulcer, bacterial invasion, and fungal or yeast infections. The elderly are less agile than the younger population and may experience difficulty in maintaining the same standard of hygiene that they once enjoyed. They may experience shortness of breath while bending over or experience an inability to reach the feet due to pain, decreased musuclar mobility, or dizziness, and, because of these limitations, the feet may not be thoroughly dried after bathing. The feet need to be thoroughly dried in order to reduce the risk of maceration, which may lead to ulceration or infection. The elderly need to have a careful and frequent examination of their feet. Emphasizing the importance of keeping the feet dry may be beneficial. For those who are unable to bend over, however, discussion of the problem is not the solution. For those living with someone else, the solution may be that footcare is done by the other person with both people sitting down and drying the feet for the other. For those who live alone, the use of a hair dryer held 15–18 inches away will dry the feet.

Another potential problem is care of the toenails. For the same reasons that the skin may not be thoroughly dried, the toenails may go unclipped. Long, jagged nail edges can lead to embedding and laceration that in turn can lead to bacterial invasion. The clinician needs to assess the level of self-care of his or her elderly patient. For those who are unable to clip their own nails, a family member or friend can do it for them. Instructing patients to soak their feet for 15 minutes once a day for four days prior to toenail clipping will help to soften the nails, consequently reducing the possibility of injury during the cutting. Also, instructing the patient to cut the nail straight across rather than curving the nail will further reduce the incidence of embedding.

REFERENCES

1. Basler RSW: Damaging effects of sunlight on human skin. Neb Med J 63:377–40, 1978

2. Lynch PJ: Sunlight and aging of the skin. Cutis 18:451–453, 1976

3. Kligman AM: Early destructive effects of sunlight on human skin. JAMA 210:2377–2380, 1969

4. Brocklehurst JC: Textbook of Geriatric Medicine and Gerontology, ed 2. New York, Churchill Livingston, 1978, pp 626–637

5. Roth HL: Pathophysiology and treatment of atopic dermatitis. Int J Derm 16:1163–178, 1977

6. Tindall JP: Skin changes and lesions in our senior citizens. Cutis 18:359–362, 1976

7. Kelly R: Dermatosis in geriatric patients. Austral Fam Phys 6:34–46, 1977

8. Hanifin JM: Eczematous conditions in the elderly: Common and curable. Geriatr 34:29–38, 1979

9. Sauer GC: Manual of Skin Diseases, ed 3. Philadelphia, JB Lippincott, 1973

10. Selmanowitz VJ: Cutaneous changes associated with aging. J Derm Surg Oncol 3:628–634, 1977

11. Gelfant S, Smith JG: Aging: Noncycling cells as an explanation. Science 178:357–361, 1972

12. Zagula MZW, Rosenberg EW, Dashgakian M: Frequency of skin cancer and solar keratosis in a rural southern county as determined by population sampling. Cancer 34:345–349, 1974

RECOMMENDED RESOURCES

Allison RJ, Rist T: Skin infections may be outward signs of inner disorders. Geratr 30:87–95, 1975

Fears TR, Scotto J, Schneiderman MA: Skin cancer, melanoma, and sunlight. Am J Pub Health 66 5:461–464, 1976

Fisher AA: Drug-incuded skin eruptions: Typical treatments for topical problems. Geriatr 34:45–51, 56–64, 1979

Fisher AA: Drug eruptions in geratric patients. Cutis 18:402–409, 1976

Jackson R: Solar and senile skin: Changes caused by aging and habitual exposure to the sun. Geratr 29:106–112, 1972

Knox JM: Common-sense care for aging skin. Geratr 30:59–60, 1975

Lantis LR, Lantis SDH: Allergic dermatosis in the older patient. Geratr 30:75–84, 1975

Lubowe II: Treatment of the aging skin by dermatologic methods. J Am Geratr Soc. 24:25–28, 1976

Montgomery, RM: Foot complaints of the elderly. Cutis 18:462–463, 1976

Ogawa CM: Degenerative skin disorders: Toll of age and sun. Geratr 30:65–69, 1975

Reichel W: The Geriatric Patient. New York, Hospital Practice Publishing Co Inc, 1978, pp 134–140

Rosen T, Rubolph AH: Identifying and treating bacterial and fungal infections of the skin. Geratr 33:71–82, 1978

Rosenblith WA: Sensory Communication. Cambridge, MIT Press, 1964

Rothman S: Physiology and Biochemistry of the Skin. Chicago, University of Chicago Press, 1961

Rudolph RI, Rudolph LP: Intraoral psoriasis vulgaris. Int J Derm 14:101–104, 1975

Tindall JP: Relieving localized and gereralized pruritus. Geriatr 30:85–92, 1975

Thorne EG: Coping with pruritus a common geriatric complaint. Geriatr 33:47–49, 1978

Verbou J: Skin problems in the older patient. Practition 215:612–622, 175

Willis I: Sunlight, aging, and skin cancer. Geriatr 33:33–36, 1978

20

Health Maintenance

Jean Johnson, M.S.N., N.P.
L. Gregory Pawlson, M.D., M.P.H.

Prevention in the elderly population is even more important than in the younger population, given the reduced ability of the body to counteract disease and the often delayed self-recognition of established disease in elder patients. Further, there are a variety of relatively simple measures that can be applied in the geriatric population which can significantly change their susceptibility to disease or injury. It is unfortunate that our educational and service system fails to encourage preventive practices, which often delays identification of problems in the elderly.

Four types of prevention are generally recognized: first is *primary prevention,* which means actions that prevent a disease or injury from occurring. The chronic disease burden of elders could be significantly reduced by appropriate intervention in earlier life; *secondary prevention* refers to the early detection of disease before the patient's reporting symptoms prevent or delay the effects of the disease; less commonly recognized as prevention is *tertiary prevention,* which is aimed at reducing or controlling the established manifestations of a disease and includes *quartian prevention,* aimed at control of complications of a disease.

PRIMARY PREVENTION

Primary prevention is of key importance in ameliorating problems of elders in several areas. These have been summarized in Table 20-1.

General Health and Well-Being

The medical care provider may be the only link with the outside world for some elderly, so it is imperative that we assess our patient's situation in terms of housing, social contacts, physical activity, financial status, and mobility. Even if direct intervention is impossible, empathetic listening may go a long way toward preventing significant mental and physical deterioration.

An area that is often neglected in the elderly patient is the prevention of suicide. Unfortunately, this is an all too common cause of death in elder patients, especially in males. It is often the result of a potentially reversible, undetected depression. Patients who have recently undergone bereavement, loss of job, who are separated from family and friends, and are suffering a recent acute or exacerbated illness should be watched closely for the development of depression and should be treated promptly if it occurs. In many cases, this must be accomplished through outreach programs, since these patients tend not to seek out medical help. The problems of substance abuse, either alcohol or drugs, is regrettably still a problem in the elder population, as is cigarette smoking. In some quarters, there is a feeling that if people have survived to old age despite the abuse of alcohol or cigarettes, they are somehow immune to the development of liver disease or lung cancer. The high incidence of lung cancer in the seventh and eighth decades and deaths from alcoholic liver disease cast considerable doubt upon these beliefs.

Accident Prevention

It is clear that accidents take a heavy toll on elders.[1] Falls, burns, hypo- and hyperthermia, and accidental poisoning (usually by medications) are all threats to the elder. Many of the physiologic and pathophysiologic concomitants of aging can be

Table 20-1
Primary Prevention—Accidents (e.g., Driving, Pedestrian, Inhalation, Fire, Drug
Ingestion, Falls)

Predisposing factors	Intervention
Host	
Impaired olfaction	Counseling on possible effect on appetite and nutritional counseling
Reduction in visual acuity	Detection and correction where possible, escort service, large print signs
Impaired equilibrium and hearing	Hearing aid, escort service when possible, counseling on use of walking aids, lip reading or sign language
Orthostatic hypotension	Counseling on slow, careful rising, review of need for medications contributing to orthostasis
Reduced strength and coordination	Use of handrails, walkers, and provision of exercise and/or plan physical therapy
Slowed reaction time and/or impaired judgement	Counseling on meaning of specific limitations and careful review of with patient
Cardiac arrythmias	Detection and control
Dementia (with wandering)	Environmental control, family counseling
Drug usage (Digitalis, anti-hypertensives, barbiturates, etc.)	Review of drug use, proper storage, and disposal
Stress and depression	Detection and intervention with counseling or medication
Smoking in bed, chair	Smoking prohibition or control
Environment	
Street curbs	Ramps at corners
Insufficient crossing time at stoplights	Increased time at intersection most used by elderly
Poor lighting in hallways, stairs	Increased illumination
High or narrow steps	Handrails
Low chairs and sofas	Redesigned furniture
Gas pilot lights	Electric ignition, safety valves
Throw rugs, slippery floors	Nonskid rugs, treads, wall-to-wall carpeting
Unplanned egress in fire	Planned and practiced escape route

thought of as requiring the elder to live in a more carefully controlled environment. Knowledge and acceptance of these limits can enable the elder person to live a full, rich, and active life without taking needless risks.

Immunizations

All too often, immunization in the elder patient is neglected. There is a need for ongoing tetanus and diphtheria immunizations for all elders, as well as influenza vaccines[2] and, more recently, pneumo-coccal vaccines[3] in elder persons with chronic lung disease or heart disease.

Iatrogenic Disease

One of the greatest problems facing elders, for which primary prevention is clearly possible, is that of iatrogenic disease. Much of this burden results from the inappropriate use of drugs. Diminished kidney and liver reserves and reduced lean body mass are among the factors that make the use of drugs in the geriatric population a challenge even for the most capable physician. Elder patients are often put on potentially lethal drugs, such as digoxin or furosemide, during acute intercurrent illnesses or for conditions such as dependent edema, and are left on these drugs at the initial dose for many years. All too often, the first reminder of this problem is when the patient is admitted to the hospital—confused and in heart block—due to digitalis toxicity or in a state of collapse due to potassium deficiency. Just as great a problem is the inappropriate use of psychotropic drugs in the elders, which can result in needless institutionalization due to confusion or to side effects such as tardive dyskinesis or jaundice. A full discussion of the appropriate use of drugs in elders can be found in Chapter 6. Procedures such as IVPs, sigmoidoscopies, or cardiac catheterization can give rise to devastating complications in the elders. Judicious use of both diagnostic and therapeutic modalities should be a central concern of the physician or other health professionals who care for the elder patient.

SECONDARY PREVENTION

The detection of disease prior to the reporting of symptoms by the patient implies the use of tests, examinations, or other procedures to detect problems in those seemingly well persons who *may* have a disease. Although screening programs have not had much success in the total population, two factors at least should encourage screening in elders. First, the prevalence of chronic disease is much higher in the elder population and, thus, the usefulness or predictive value of a screening test may be greatly enhanced. Secondly, diseases often present in older patients in very subtle or atypical ways, or the early symptoms are ignored by elders who attribute symptoms to "growing old".[4-6] The relationship of the asymptomatic person to the health professional is different from that of a person who comes to us with a self-defined problem; it implies an even more careful adherence to the doctrine of "first, do no harm." A number of criteria have been developed as guidelines in considering the use of screening programs:[7]

- The disease should be prevalent in the population to be screened.
- The natural history of the disease should be

known and the therapy for the condition must improve survival.
- There should be adequate health services and facilities to diagnose and provide treatment.
- The disease under surveillance should be an important public health problem.
- The test and the diagnostic follow-up should be acceptable to the population.
- Long-term beneficial effects must outweigh any long-term detrimental effects.
- There should be a recognizable and detectable latent or early symptomatic stage.
- There should be clearly defined policies that determine which patients with abnormal screening values will be subjected to further diagnostic tests and treatment.
- The cost of case finding, subsequent diagnosis, and treatment should be clearly defined.
- Case finding should be linked carefully to ongoing medical care.
- The sensitivity, specificity, and predicted value of the screening test must be known about the population to which it is applied.

While few tests meet the rigors of all guidelines, it is unfortunate that many tests or examination procedures are applied with little attention to any of the guidelines.

Screening Procedures

Many of the negative conclusions about screening may not be appropriate to the elder population in which the prevalence and natural history of the disease may be different. There are a number of procedures or tests that are already in common usage and that have some rational basis for use in the elder patient. Tables 20-2 and 3 suggest some of those examinations that *appear* to have a net "benefit" in elders. The benefit of some procedures are more doubtful in the elder population as a whole and should perhaps be reserved for high-risk populations. (For example-screening for diabetes, glaucoma, and cancer in persons with family history of these diseases.) For more information about a specific organ system, refer to the section on Health Maintenance in each chapter in Section II.

PREVENTIVE PROGRAMS

A number of factors that appear to be important to the success of a preventive program are:[8-11]

- Programs linked directly to the patient's usual

Table 20-2
Approach to Prevention in the Elderly Outlined by Exam Type

Listed are suggested screening exams for *asymptomatic* elderly patients. Also included are important primary interventions. Specific risks (occupational, genetic, behavioral) or symptoms should result in more extensive evaluation in the area of risk. In terms of the history, physical exam, and patient education, the areas listed are those that require *special* attention in the elderly.

Baseline (initial exam)
  History
    Current problems, past medical history, review of systems, etc.,
      with added attention to:
        mobility-exercise   family support
        social interactions   medication usage
        environment/housing   nutrition
  Physical exam
    Basic exam with added attention to:
        breast   peripheral vascular system
        rectal/prostate   ear (gross hearing and
        extremities (especially feet   nerve versus bone conduction)
          for bunions, callouses, etc.)   eye (visual acuity, cataracts)
        mouth (status of teeth and   mental status (screen for
          gums)   dementia, depression, paranoia)
  Laboratory
    VDRL   hematocrit/hemoglobin
    ECG (if prior exam not   creatinine, BUN
      available)   PPD
    chest x-ray (if prior exam
      not available)
    urine analysis   tonometry*
    PAP smear   audiometry*
    stool guaiac × 3–6   mammography*
                                             cholesterol, triglycerides*
                                             fasting glucose*

  Immunizations
    influenza vaccine*   tetanus–diphtheria (if more than
    pneumococcal vaccine*   1 year since prior immunization)
  Patient education (see also Table 20-1)
    activities   exercise
    nutrition   loss (retirement, bereavement)*
    accident prevention

Follow-up (yearly)
  History—focused on:
    Intercurrent illnesses
    Review of systems (especially diet, exercise, weight loss or
      gain, chest pain, extremity pain, syncope, transit weakness,
      numbness, etc.)
    Social (social interactions, mobility, family situation, housing,
      medication review)
  Exam
    BP, pulse, respiration, weight   mouth (gums, teeth lesions)
    skin   pelvic
    breast   rectal/prostate
    ear, gross hearing, external canals   mental status (brief screen for
    eye, visual acuity, lens   dementia, paranoia, depression)
    muscular, skeletal (mobility,
      peripheral pulses, feet)

Table 20-2
Continued

Lab	
stool guaiac × 3–6	Hct/Hb
urinalysis	PAP
Immunization	
influenza vaccine*	
tetanus–diphtheria (every	
10 years)	
Patient education	
activities	exercise
nutrition	loss (bereavement)*
accident prevention	

*May be reserved for high-risk patients.

source of medical care are, on the whole, more successful than those set up in a separate agency.

- An outreach program that involves both home and institutional visitation is necessary for an adequate response rate, particularly for those over 75.
- Some form of transportation must be provided for patients with impaired mobility.
- In addition to the physician, the use of nurse practitioners, social workers, and other health care professionals has proved very successful.
- On the other hand, the following factors seem to serve as deterrents. The use of multiphasic screening tests, using automated equipment and measuring large numbers of blood tests, is all too often fruitless in the elder population. The physician who receives such data is often confused since there are usually large numbers of abnormal values. Many of these abnormal values result simply from the fact that most of these tests are continuous variables. The cost and trauma of following up all the abnormalities are often self-defeating. The detection of large numbers of abnormal findings is not equivalent to the detection of actual disease. Finally, the normal range of values for certain tests in the elderly population may differ from adults.
- Many elders cannot tolerate four to five hours of continuous testing nor can they be hurried from one test to another.
- The use of self-administered questionnaires[11] is of distinctly limited value in the elderly population due to frequent physical and mental impairment and elders' underrecognition of problems.

Exercise

The state of the physical body is important to the emotional well-being of the person. The saying "use it or lose it" is especially appropriate to elders. Although exercise will not stop the aging process, it will help to maintain physical capacity and mental well-being. Exercise for elders has a number of outcomes, i.e., limbering, increased heart-lung capacity, strength and endurance, and body awareness. Exercise as an integral part of health maintenance has been underemphasized by health professionals for elders for the following reasons:

- A mistaken belief that the need for exercise diminishes with age
- An exaggeration of the risks involved in exercise
- An overrating of the benefits of light, sporadic work
- An underrating of elders' abilities[12]
- An unfamiliarity with appropriate techniques[13]

It is true that aging produces a decline in physiologic functioning.[12,14] There is a decrease in vital capacity, pulmonary blood flow, aerobic power, physical work capacity, mineralization of bones, lean muscle mass, nerve conduction, velocity, elasticity in all tissues and cardiac output due to a decrease in stroke volume. Unfortunately, the belief that elders should not exert themselves actually induces a more rapid and pronounced decline in function. Inactivity begets loss of function, which reinforces inactivity, accelerating the aging process.

The benefits of exercise, on the other hand, are in direct contrast to the effects due both to inactivity and aging. Exercise can improve muscle tone, posture, range of joint motion, coordination[12,15,16] and

Table 20-3
Approach to Prevention in the Elderly Outlined by Organ System

Listed are suggested screening procedures for *asymptomatic* elderly persons. Specific risks (occupational, genetic, behavioral) or symptoms should result in more extensive evaluation in the areas of risk. In terms of the history, physical examination, and patient education, the areas listed are those that require *special* attention in the elderly.

Sensory
  History: ability to taste and smell food, decreased tearing, pain in
    eyes, vertigo
  Physical exam: Snellen chart and newsprint screen for visual acuity,
    whispered voice hearing check, tuning fork for bone and air conduction,
    tonometry,* audiometry*
Skin and appendages
  History: dryness, breast discharge, or lump
  Physical Exam: careful inspection for conditions such as xerosis,
    actinic keratosis, basal cell, and squamous cell carcinoma, melanoma,
    breast exam
  Laboratory: mammmography*
  Patient education: methods to prevent xerosis, reassurance about
    benign nature of seborrheic keratosis, angioma and senile lentigo,
    checking or instruction of breast self-exam, including encouraging its
    use
Heme—lymph
  Physical Exam: observation for mucus membrane pallor
  Laboratory: hematocrit
  Patient education: nutritional counseling for adequate iron and
    folate intake
Cardiovascular
  History: symptoms suggesting claudication, angina, TIAs, syncope,
    usual exercise level
  Physical exam: blood pressure measurement, inspection of feet for skin
    atrophy, ulceration, loss of hair, palpation for peripheral pulses, pulse rate
  and regularity resting and with mild exercise
  Laboratory: ECG if no previous exam available, triglycerides,*
    cholesterol*
  Patient education: exercise and nutrition counseling, smoking
    cessation
Pulmonary
  History: chronic cough, exercise tolerance, history of tuberculosis,
    and/or result of skin tests
  Physical exam: observation of respiratory rate with mild exercise,
    forced expiration, match test (blowing out lighted match 6 inches from
    non-pursed lips)
  Laboratory: PPD, chest x-rays if no previous exam available
  Patient education: smoking cessation, exercise prescription
Gastrointestinal
  History: appetite, weight loss, swallowing, bowel habits, use of
    laxatives, change in appearance of stool
  Physical exam: inspection of teeth and gums, rectal, protoscopy,
    sigmoidoscopy*
  Laboratory: stool guiac (3–6/year)
  Patient education: nutritional counseling
Endocrine system
  History: (awareness by physician of subtle or atypical presentation
    of hypo- or hyperthyroidism in elderly)

Table 20-3
Continued

Laboratory: urine test for glucose, fasting glucose,* serum thyroxine,* and resin
 T_3 uptake,* calcium*
Genitourinary
 History:
  male—dysuria, hesitancy, dribbling, reduced stream, impotence
  female—dysuria, frequency, sexual dysfunction (dyspareunia,
   etc.), incontinence, vaginal bleeding
 Physical exam: prostate size and consistency
 Laboratory: urinalysis, PAP smear, creatinine/BUN, urine culture*
Musculoskeletal
 History: mobility
 Physical exam: observation of walking, climbing steps, posture and
  fine movements (i.e., picking up and holding a pencil), inspection
  of the feet for bunions, callouses, ulceration, dystrophy, etc.
 Patient counseling: proper foot wear, exercise prescription
Neuropsychiatric
 History: assessment of risk factors for depression/suicide (living
  alone, recent loss of significant other, money or self-function,
  recent hospitalization, lack of social interaction), mental status
  exam, drug usage, socialization, family support, and checking the
  patients' general feeling toward themselves and their aging
 Patient education: discussion of opportunities available to elderly
  in activity centers, senior citizen groups, mental health centers,
  etc., and of the primary care provider role in helping patient work
  through loss and isolation
General
 Immunizations: influenza vaccine,* pneumococcal vaccine,* tetanus–diphtheria
 (if more than 10 years prior immunization)
 Patient education: accident prevention (see Table 20-1)

---

 *Indicates controversial use in general screening and may be of more value in high-risk
elderly.

physical work capacity.[12,17–19] Further, there are increased vital capacity and pulmonary blood flow, stroke volume, and maximal oxygen intake.[12,15,20–22] A decrease in both systolic and diastolic blood pressure has been found.[15,23–26] In addition, exercise may have a protective effect against coronary heart disease, but no direct relationship has been established. Evidence suggests a decreased incidence and severity of myocardial infarction in those who exercise.[27–29] There are other benefits of exercise:

Primary benefits of exercise:
• Improved muscle tone, flexibility, coordination
• Weight control
• Decreased depression, improved body images

Secondary benefits of exercise:
• Reduced low-back pain
• Prevention of accidents
• Increased work capacity

• Social contact
• Improved sleep

Much of the information recounted about exercise as related to physiologic and psychologic parameters has been gathered on young and middle-aged subjects. Several studies have also been done on elders that suggest similar effects from exercise on older age groups.[15] To summarize, exercise can have a beneficial effect in maintaining the independence and functional abilities of individuals in the course of the aging process.

Evaluation for Exercise Prescriptions

An exercise prescription for elders should be to determine the appropriate exercise—including type, intensity, duration, frequency—and not whether the exercise is warranted. Exercise should be part of a therapeutic regimen for all elders, whether well, chronically ill, confined to a wheelchair or bedridden. It is important not to overly stress the physical capacities that may already be compromised by chronic health problems. Exercise may make the difference in maintaining range of motion of joints in an elder who is at risk for loss of ability to maintain independence. Exercise may enhance collateral circulation in the elder with peripheral vascular disease, enabling that person to increase walking distance.

There are many elders whose chronic conditions do not preclude such vigorous exercise as jogging, swimming, or bicycling. For those who are unable to undertake vigorous activity, there are many additional options—such as yoga, T'ai Chi, dance, etc.—that may be suitable. Persons with stable angina, diabetes, arthritis, coronary heart disease, and hypertension may participate in vigorous exercise, beginning gradually and working up to a therapeutic intensity, duration, and frequency. The American College of Sports Medicine (ACSM) has listed the following as absolute contraindications to exercise:[30]

- Congestive heart failure
- Acute myocardial infarction
- Active myocarditis
- Rapidly increasing angina with effort
- Recent embolism
- Systemic or pulmonary dissecting aneurysm
- Acute infections
- Thrombophlebitis
- Ventricular tachycardia or other dangerous dysrhythmias
- Severe aortic stenosis

Evaluation should involve a complete history, including activity patterns, interests, and a physical examination focusing on the organ systems affected by illness. A thorough cardiac and musculoskeletal exam, as well as resting BP, ECG, and heart rate should also be included. In addition, the ACSM recommends that blood chemistries, triglycerides, cholesterol, and a stress test be done.[17]

It may be questioned how productive blood chemistries and a stress test are for exercise prescription for elders. Elders are a high risk group for myocardial infarction. By the age of 65, the majority of the population has at least mild vascular changes, and as many as 30 percent develop myocardial ischemia during exercise.[12] In addition, for many elders, the expense of a stress test is prohibitive.

Exercise Prescription

It is important to be as specific as possible in prescribing exercise. If the health care professional is unfamiliar with a particular practice, he or she would do best to make a referral to a written resource, group, or instructor for further information. The importance of the health care professional's commitment to exercise and health maintenance will be reflected in their ability to prescribe routines for patients. This includes teaching each elder what kind of exercise (range of motion, strengthening, endurance, limbering) there is and how frequently and for how long the exercise should be done.

Exercise should be done while relaxed, at leisure, and with full attention. Relaxation increases bodily awareness and decreases the likelihood of injury due to inattention. (Refer to Chapter 17.) The exercise prescription should emphasize a gradual increase in physical capacity. This approach demands patience but will help the patient avoid injury due to overexercising. Encourage the patient to trust his or her own body's feedback. The person may need to be sensitized to what exercise feels like; these patients may not have used some of their muscles or felt pain and fatigue for years. It does not necessarily feel good to begin to move. Initially, it may remind people of their stiffness and unused ability. Elders need to be able to distinguish between expected discomfort and a warning level of fatigue and/or pain. They should learn when to decrease intensity and when to stop entirely.

Many elders are not limited in their exercise by health problems. For those who are unlimited, exercise should focus on increasing cardiopulmonary function, endurance, limbering, balancing and stretching activities, including brisk walking, jogging, swimming, and bicycling (consider a three-wheel bike to reduce risk of injury). This activity should be rhythmic, sustained, and involve large muscle masses. Running, jumping rope, or weight lifting are among those exercises not recommended. Isometric exercises should be minimized because they rapidly increase heart rate and systolic and diastolic blood pressure. Elders should be taught to stay within their aerobic limits and to allow enough oxygen both to be transported and used by the exercising muscle for as long as the exercise continues.

Again, we stress that the key to exercise prescription in elders is to begin gradually; every program should be graduated. Exercise should be done at least three to four times per week, although some exercise programs may need to be done more frequently than others. Relaxation for 10–15 minutes prior to activity is key to leisurely, attentive exercise. Elders should begin with 10–15 minute activity sessions and build up to a tolerance of at least 30–40 minutes of exercise.

For those persons participating in endurance exercise, the recommended intensity should be 60–75 percent of the maximal heart rate (MHR).[31] MHR can be determined by a stress test or from a chart of norms. An approximation for normal healthy adults can be obtained by subtracting age from 220.[32] All persons participating in endurance exercise should know how to monitor their pulses and adjust the intensity of walking, jogging, cycling, or swimming to reach and maintain at least 60 percent MHR.

As part of the exercise prescription, persons involved in endurance exercise should be instructed to refrain from exercise until two hours after eating a large meal, drinking coffee, tea or alcohol, or smoking cigarettes. Because of a decrease in visual acuity, elders should jog on flat, soft surfaces and, because of decreased hearing, should aovid walking or jogging on streets. They should engage in relaxation processes and warm-up for five minutes before exercise and cool down for the same length of time after exercise. Warm-up activities should put joints through a full range of motion. All of the following joints should be exercised: neck, arm, shoulder, trunk, hip, knee, ankle, and foot.

The cool-down period can consist of slow jogging or walking with arm swings. A lukewarm shower, rather than a cold or hot shower, should be taken after exercise. The intensity of exercise during hot, humid weather and during cold weather should be reduced, since these conditions cause higher pulse rates and blood pressures. Health professionals should advise elders participating in an exercise program of the danger signals and what to do about them.

To encourage exercise in the elderly. In prescribing exercise, the first step is to discover what kind of activity has been enjoyable in the past and to counsel a return to that activity with any necessary modifications. If no activity is identified, there are some excellent resource books from which an exercise program can be designed.[33–35] Often, an exercise program necessitates an educational process change in a number of life-long habits. Members of the individual's support network need to understand and support the changes. The health care team can provide information and referral to exercise resources (gyms, classes, equipment stores, etc.).

The primary care provider should also be part of a support system encouraging exercise. Periodic evaluations should be scheduled. Brief visits two weeks and five weeks (when the dropout rate is greatest) after initiation of the program may be advisable. Visits during this time may convey to the patient that exercise is important to health and will enable the health care provider to evaluate the exercise program. It is often helpful to involve friends and family in the program. Each patient should be given a record sheet to keep track of progress. Levels of fatigue, occurrences of pain, and pain relief measures should be recorded daily by the patient to help the health care provider evaluate the exercise program.

Cost of an exercise program may be a prime consideration of elders. A program that costs little may increase participation in an exercise program. On the other hand, even running shoes may be too expensive for some, so that they may need to be encouraged to walk and to do range of motion and strengthening exercises at no cost.

The booklet, "The Fitness Challenge," prepared by the President's Council of Physical Fitness and Sports and the Administration on Aging, is a guide for patients to use at home.[33]

In addition, *Your Second Life* offers excellent, clearly illustrated exercises, specifically tailored to elders. It combines aerobic, yoga, and other physical enhancement modalities.[34] *Vigor Regained* also offers guidelines for physical fitness and exercise regimes.[35]

NUTRITION

Much attention has been given to promoting sound nutritional practices throughout life that help to minimize the so-called diseases of old age—heart and vascular disease, diabetes and carbohydrate disorders, osteoporosis, and, in some cases, cancer.[36] Attention should be given to nutritional needs that will have the greatest impact on maintaining health and functional ability in elders.

Diet Assessment

Diet assessment is a vital part of an evaluation of elders. The assessment should include a 48-hour diet log, wherein the patient writes down everything consumed. Special attention should be paid to assessing the intake of vegetables, fruits, milk, and milk products, since elders tend to have an inadequate intake of these dietary constituents.[37] Table 20-4 provides a framework in which to assess a number of important additional factors that affect the diets of elders.

The impact of psychological and social factors also needs to be assessed. The nutritional complications brought on by loneliness and depression are awesome. There may be a decreased incentive for preparing meals when there is no one to share them. Depression may cause apathy and neglect of personal and nutritional needs. Forgetfulness or avoidance of meals may thus establish a destructive cycle.

Nutrition Programs for the Elderly

A number of resources are available to assist elders with their nutritional needs. If income is a problem, the elder may be eligible for food stamps. If food preparation is difficult, Meals-on-Wheels will deliver one meal per day on weekdays. The nutrition programs authorized by Title VII of the Older Americans Act also provide at least one hot meal, containing one-third of the RDA, five days a week. These meals are served in a congregate setting, providing companionship and oftentimes other activities to promote the physical, social, and mental well-being of the elder.

Nutrition During Sickness and Injury

Aging does not appear to affect nutritional requirements of healthy elders, except for a decreased need for calories. The recommended dietary allowance established for persons 51 and older reflects this. (See Table 20-5.)

Acute and chronic illness and injury of the elder do alter nutritional requirements. Focusing on nutritional needs during illness and/or injury can avert permanent disability or death.

A major factor to consider when an elder person is ill or injured is the need for increased protein to prevent negative nitrogen balance. The wasting-away syndrome of the debilitated elder person is a very real problem for the practitioner, requiring constant vigilance. Inadequate protein intake at these critical times may be due to:

- The elder person's lack of knowledge about the need for increased protein at a time of illness and/or injury
- The effect of illness and/or medication on protein absorption and/or utilization
- If homebound, inability to prepare adequate meals
- If hospitalized, shortage of staff time and lack of knowledge to encourage dietary protein intake
- Disinterest in food
- Depression
- Inability to afford the additional cost of protein and unawareness of substitutes

In addition to protein, adequate caloric intake is needed. Increasing fat content in the diet may be useful in meeting an increased caloric need. Hyperalimentation or nutritional supplements may also be necessary. Adequate hydration is also essential. Vigorous diet therapy at critical times should always be part of a therapeutic regimen and may mean the difference between recovery from the illness or injury and debilitation.

Vitamin Deficiencies

Vitamin deficiencies have been identified in the elderly populations and may have a major impact on long-term health.[38-40] The significance of these

Table 20-4
Diet Assessment

	1	2	3	4	Intervention
Cost of food					
Shopping					
Transportation					
Food preparation					
Cooking facilities					
Ability to chew foods					
Knowledge of balanced diet					
Emotional status					
Mental status					

Is there someone who helps with meals?

If yes, who?

Are there special cultural or religious considerations involved in food planning, purchase, eating?

1 = no problem; 2 = slight problem; 3 = moderate problem; 4 = major problem.

Table 20-5
Recommended Daily Dietary Allowances, Revised 1979,
Designed for the Maintenance of Good Nutrition of
Practically All Healthy People in the USA

	Males	Females
Age (years)	51+	51+
Weight (kg/lb)	70/154	55/120
Height (cm/in)	178/70	163/64
Protein (g)	56	44
Fat-soluble vitamins		
Vitamin A (μg RE)	1000	800
Vitamin D (μg)	5	5
Vitamin E (mgαTE)	10	8
Water-soluble vitamins		
Vitamin C (mg)	60	60
Thiamin (mg)	1.2	1.0
Riboflavin (mg)	1.4	1.2
Niacin (mg NE)	16	13
Vitamin B_6 (mg)	2.2	2.0
Folacin (μg)	400	400
Vitamin B_{12} (μg)	3.0	3.0
Minerals		
Calcium (mg)	800	800
Phosphorus (mg)	800	800
Magnesium (mg)	350	300
Iron (mg)	10	10
Zinc (mg)	15	15
Iodine (μg)	150	150

Reprinted from Recommended Dietary Allowances, 9th edition (in press). By permission of the National Academy of Sciences, Washington, DC.

deficiencies is not in the rare overt clinical signs of deficiency, but in the relationship to overall functional abilities of the elder.

CALCIUM

A primary concern in the elder is calcium deficiency. The clinical significance of this deficiency is its relationship to osteoporosis, a frequently occurring metabolic bone disease, especially in postmenopausal women. Osteoporosis generally results from a depressed osteoblastic activity with a consequent decrease in the rate of bone deposition. Osteoporosis seems to be related to a complex relationship of a variety of factors, including reduced intake of calcium, vitamin C and vitamin D, estrogen depression, physical inactivity, and possibly fluoride.
The debilitated elders, even those who are temporarily bedridden, are at great risk of intensification of the osteoporotic process, not only because

of inactivity, but also because of poor dietary intake of calcium. Decreased bone density leaves the elder individual vulnerable to vertebral compression, kyphosis, and fractures.[41,42]
Current treatments of osteoporosis with combinations of calcium, vitamin D, estrogen and fluoride are controversial, and, though they may slow the resorption of bone, they do not reverse it. Recent findings suggest that the RDA for calcium (800 mg/d) is sufficient for prevention of calcium depletion in women who have their own or supplemental estrogens, but that postmenopausal requirement may be as high as 1500 mg of calcium per day.[43] It has also been suggested that bone loss can be prevented at any age by adequate calcium intake.[44]

IRON

Iron deficiency is thought to be widespread, especially among sick and low-income elders. Since approximately 10 percent of total dietary iron is absorbed, 10 mg of iron are required daily to replace the estimated 1 mg iron lost. There is some question as to etiology and incidence of iron deficiency anemia in elders.[39,40,45] As a rule, if an elder person is anemic, bleeding should be suspected and ruled out before attributing the anemia to dietary iron deficiency. Dietary iron deficiency is a real concern of the practitioner, especially since a major source of iron is meat, and many elder persons simply cannot afford a diet that will ensure adequate iron supplies. Elders should be directed toward other, less costly sources such as prune juice, beans, spinach, peas, raisins, & fortified cereals.

ASCORBIC ACID

Ascorbic acid may play a role in anemia in that it enhances absorption of iron from the gut. The primary source for ascorbic acid, citrus fruits, is also a frequently omitted dietary constituent.
Pharmacologic doses of ascorbic acid have been proposed to have a therapeutic effect on immunity. Some feel that the potential benefits are worth neither the time nor the risk of taking high doses of ascorbic acid lifelong. Several risks of importance to elder persons have been reported with high doses of vitamin C:

- Potential for scurvy, if stopped
- Falsely negative stool occult blood test
- Destruction of 50–90 percent of the vitamin B_{12} content of a meal by 0.5 g ascorbic acid

- Invalidation of serum uric acid concentration for the assessment of gout
- Increased risk of erythrocyte hemolysis[46]

The first choice should be to encourage adequate natural sources of vitamins including vitamin C.

Clinical Implications of Nutritional Practices

OBESITY

A common nutrition-related problem among elder persons is obesity. There are many etiologies of obesity, including endocrine, genetic, hypothalamic, and addictive behavior disorders, but overeating and underexercise are the primary causes of obesity in elders.

Over half of the diseases and disabilities occurring in elder persons, including hypertension, diabetes, gall bladder disease, gout, and coronary heart disease, are linked to overnutrition.[45]

Several factors associated with the aging process contribute to obesity in elders. There is a loss of lean tissue mass and an increase in adipose tissue. Caloric needs in elders are less than in younger age groups, due to both a decrease in basal metabolic rate and physical activity. The RDA for people 51 years and older suggests reductions of calories to 2400 and 1800 for males and females respectively.[47] The Joint Food and Agriculture Organization–World Health Organizational Committee suggests an additional 10-percent reduction for those over 70.[48]

It is not unusual for elder persons to reveal a pattern of frequnt snacking on high caloric foods with little nutritive value especially in the afternoons and evenings. The reasons for the constant snacking may include boredom, loneliness, anxiety, or habit.

In order to lose one pound per week, caloric intake needs to be 500 cal/day below the number of calories used. This presents a very real problem for weight loss in elder persons since the diet would then require a very high nutrient density diet. This may put a financial strain on elder persons because the usually high nutrient density foods are generally more expensive than a low nutrient density diet. Diet consideration should be given to the less expensive non-meat sources of protein to supplement diets. An excellent publication for these alternative sources is *Laurel's Kitchen*,[49] which provides a basic daily reducing diet having adequate protein (at least 1 g/kg), meeting all nutritional requirements, being inexpensive, and allowing for individual differences.

Emphasis needs to be placed on social and emotional support during a weight loss attempt. In fact, without it, even considering diet and exercise could be fruitless. Groups such as Overeaters Anonymous and Weight Watchers can provide the support and encouragement an older person may need.

There are reasons other than prevention of obesity and possibly coronary heart disease (see Chapter 11) for recommending diets low in fat to elders. High-fat diets are:

- Usually low in fiber
- Associated with lowered carbohydrate tolerance
- Low-density nutrient foods having empty calories that contribute to obesity in the elder person

HIGH-FIBER DIET

Elders frequently complain of constipation, which continues despite chronic use of laxatives. These patients may profit by increasing dietary fiber by as little as 2 g/day.[50] Fiber should be accompanied by adequate fluid intake—estimated at an average of 1.2 liters per day—with 50 percent of the fluid being supplied by water in foods. High-fiber diets have also been useful for treating patients with diverticulosis, diverticulitis, and irritable bowel.

The cheapest source of fiber is raw milled bran, obtainable at health food stores. Bran-containing cereals such as Kellogg's All Bran, Bran Buds, and Nabisco's 100% Bran have the highest crude fiber content of breakfast cereals, but also contain sugar.[50] A 1-ounce serving contains about 2 g of crude fiber, so that a small breakfast serving could provide the required daily amount of fiber. Vegetables and fruits are also high in fiber content and aid the elderly in achieving regular bowel movements and should be recommended as part of a balanced diet. The combination of fiber and fluid is advocated over laxatives, which are costly and tend to cause a "lazy bowel."

The primary care provider should keep in mind when recommending a high-fiber diet that diets high in fiber may lead to sigmoid volvulus, which is a surgical emergency.

VITAMIN USAGE

Many elders take over-the-counter vitamins and vitamins with mineral supplements, and they believe that they are protecting themselves against tired blood, colds, or old age. In spite of what advertisers say, healthy elders who eat well do not need either vitamin or mineral supplements. Given an adequate diet, excess vitamins and minerals will only be excreted.

Evaluation for supplemental vitamin therapy is recommended for persons who are acutely or chronically ill, who have intestinal disorders, who take medications that interfere with absorption, who have an alcohol problem, or who do not eat properly.

SUMMARY

Many preventive measures in elders are simple, straightforward, and represent no invasive procedure. The elder, rather than excluded from preventive measures, should be thought of as the patient who in many ways justifies the most careful efforts of health maintenance. Questioning the patient about his or her social environment, activity status, and dietary habits, in addition to carefully reviewing systems and performing a physical examination, can uncover treatable pathology and potential health problems in many patients. Intervention to correct or minimize these common physical, mental, or social problems in elders will often improve the quality of health.

REFERENCES

1. Rodstein M: Accidents among the aged: Incidence, causes, and prevention. J Chron Dis 17:515–526, 1964
2. Gregg MD, Bregman DJ, O'Brian RJ, Millar JD: Influenza-related mortality. JAMA 239:115–116, 1978
3. Riley ID, Andrews M, Howard R, Tarr PI, et al: Immunization with apolyvalent pneumococal vaccine. Lancet 1:1338, 1977
4. Williamson J, Stokoe IM, Gray S, et al: Old people at home: Their unreported need. Lancet 1:1117–1120, 1964
5. Williams EI: Sociomedical study of patients over 75 in general practice. Bri Med J 1:445–448, 1972
6. Anderson WF, Cowan NR: A consultative health center for older people. Lancet 2:239–240, 1955
7. Wilson JMG: Principles in the practice of screening for disease. WHO Chron 22:473–483, 1968
8. Collen MF, Dales LG, Friedman GD, et al: Multiphasic checkup evaluation study. Prev Med 2:236–246, 1973
9. Rosin AJ, Galinsky D: Health testing in the elderly by the multiphasic method. Geront Clin 17:80–88, 1975
10. Lowther CP, MacLeod RDM, Williams J: Evaluation of early diagnostic services for the elderly. Bri Med J 2:275–277, 1970
11. Chamberlin JOP: Undiagnosed disease in the elderly population. Proc Roy Soc Med 66:888–889, 1973
12. Shephard RJ: Physical Activity and Aging. Chicago, Year Book Medical Publishers, 1978
13. President's Council of Physical Fitness and Sports: Newsletter. Special ed, Washington, DC, May 1973
14. Rockstein M, Chesky JA, Sussman ML: Comparative biology and evolution of aging, in Finch CE, Hayfleck L (eds): Handbook of the Biology of Aging. New York, Van Nostrand Reinhold Co, 1977, pp 3–34.
15. Kasch FW, Wallace JP: Physiology variables during 10 years of endurance training. Med Sci Sports 8:5–8, 1976
16. Shock NW, Norris AH: Neuromuscular coordination as a factor in age changes in muscular exercise, in Brunner D (ed): Medicine and Sport: Physical Activity and Aging. Baltimore, University Press, 1970, vol 4, p 92
17. Cureton TK: The Physiologic Effects of Exercise Programs on Adults. Springfield, Charles C Thomas, 1969
18. Barry AJ, Daly JW, Pruett ED, et al: The effects of physical conditioning on older individuals, I: Work capacity, respiratory function and work electrocardiogram. J Gerontol 21:182–191, 1966
19. DeVries HA: Physiological effects of an exercise training regimen upon men aged 52 to 88. J Gerontol 25:325–336, 1970
20. Pollock ML, Dawson GA, Miller HS Jr, et al: Physiologic response of men 49 to 65 years of age to endurance training. J Am Geriatr Soc 24:97–104, 1976
21. Salten B, Hartley LH, Kilbom A, et al: Physical training in sedentary middle aged and older men. Scand J Clin Lab Invest 24:323–334, 1969
22. Wilmore JH: Alteration in strength, body, composition and anthropomorphic measurements consequent to a 10 week jogging program. Med Sci Sports 6:133–138, 1974
23. Pollock ML, Miller HS Jr, Ribisl PM: Effect of fitness on aging. Phys Sports Med 1978, pp 45–48
24. Sidney KH, Shephard RJ, Harrison JE: Endurance training and body composition of the elderly. Am J Clin Nutr 30:326–333, 1977
25. Stamford BA: Effects of chronic institutionalization on the physical working capacity and trainability of geriatric men. J Gerontal 28:441–446, 1973
26. Stamford BA: Physiologic effects of training upon institutionalized geriatric men. J Gerontol 27:451–455, 1972

27. Paffenburger RS, Laughlin MF, Grimu HS, et al: Work activity of longshoremen as related to death from coronary heart disease and stroke. N Engl J Med 282:1109–1114, 1970

28. Morris JN, Chave SP, Adam C, et al: Vigorous exercise in leisure time and the incidence of coronary heart disease. Lancet 1:333–339, 1973

29. Wood PD, Klein H, Levis S, et al: Plasma lipoprotein concentrations in middle-aged male runners. Circ 49, 50 (suppl 3): 111–115, 1974, (abstr)

30. American College of Sports Medicine: Guidelines for Graded Exercise Testing and Exercise Prescription. Philadelphia, Lea & Febiger, 1975

31. DeVries H: Tips on prescribing exercise regimens for your older patient. Geriatr 34:75–81, 1979

32. Morehouse LE, Gross L: Total Fitness. New York, Simon & Schuster, 1975

33. President's Council on Physical Fitness and Sports, The Administration on Aging: The Fitness Challenge. DHEW Publ No. (OHD) 75-20802, 1975

34. Luce GG: Your Second Life. New York, Delacorte Press, 1979

35. DeVries H: Vigor Regained. Englewood Cliffs, New Jersey, Prentice-Hall, 1974

36. Weir CE: Benefits of human nutrition research: Dietary goals for the United States. Senate Select Committee on Nutrition and Human Needs, 1977

37. Jordon M, Krepes M, Hayes RB, Hammond W: Dietary habits of persons living alone. Geriatr 9:230–232, 1954

38. US Department of Agriculture, Agricultural Research Service: Dietary Levels of Households in the United States, 1965. Report No. 18, 1966

39. Ten-State Survey, Highlights. Nutrition Today, July/August 1972.

40. Department of Health, Education and Welfare: First Health and Nutrition Examination Survey, United States, 1971–72. Dietary intake and biochemical findings. Publ No. (HRA) 74-1219-1, National Center for Health Statistics, January 1974

41. Exton-Smith AN, Millard PH, Payne PH, et al: Pattern of development and loss of bone with age. Lancet 2:1154–1157, 1969

42. Rodstein M: Accidents among the aged: Incidence, causes, and prevention. J Chron Dis 17:515–526, 1964

43. Marx B: Hormones and their effects in the aging body. Science 206:805–806, 1979

44. Lutwak L: Nutritional aspects of osteoporosis. J Am Geriatr Soc 17:115–118, 1969

45. Gershoff SN, Brusis OH, Nino HV, et al: Studies of the elderly in Boston, I: The effects of iron fortification on moderately anemic people. Am J Clin Nutr 30:226–234, 1977

46. Watkin D: Nutrition, health, and aging, in Rechcigl M Jr (ed): Nutrition and the World Food Problem. Karger, Basel, 1979, pp 20–62

47. Recommended dietary allowances. Food and Nutrition Board, National Academy of Sciences, National Research Council, Washington, DC, 8th ed Publ No. 2216, 1974

48. Food and Agricultural Organization/World Health Organization. Energy and protein requirements: Report of a Joint FAO/WHO ad hoc Expert Committee. WHO Tech Petp Ser No. 522: FAP Nutrition Mtgs. Rept Ser 52 WHO: Geneva, 1973

49. Robertson L et al: Laurel's Kitchen. Berkeley, California, Nilgri Press, 1976

50. The high-fiber diet: Its effect on the bowel. Med Letter 17:93–95, 1975

21

Alternative Therapies and Management of Stress and Catastrophic Diseases

James L. Creighton
Ken Dychtwald, Ph.D.

The recognition that emotional state is related to physical health is of particular significance in elder care since most of America's elderly suffer from low levels of mental and physical health.

We have been quite successful at nearly eliminating most infectious and germ-related diseases, but we have done very poorly at initiating and maintaining the kinds of healthy lifestyles, social dynamics, nutritional habits, and exercise activities that would reduce the wear and tear of stress and tension and fortify us against the often debilitating influences of modern living. Doctors and germs alone can no longer be blamed for the ailments of our aging; nor can we expect that lifestyle-related diseases will be eliminated with drugs or after-the-fact symptom-treating intervention. When we look deeply into the physical, psychological, and social issues that generate disease and unhappiness, we realize that the problems of "aging" in America are very much connected to the nature of "how we live" in America.

The Traditional Model of Illness

The barriers to providing effective programs for the elderly are deeply rooted in our traditional concept of illness. In brief, these beliefs are:

1. Illness is the result (or effect) of a specific cause, or agent.
2. Emotional states are "nonphysical," or even "unreal," and therefore irrelevant as a causative factor of illness.
3. Because the causes of illness are physical, effective interventions or therapies are also physical,

such as drugs, surgery, or, in limited cases, manipulation.

It is this set of beliefs, of course, that conditions health professionals to see the complaints of the elderly as a nuisance rather than a potentially key indicator of their overall mental and physical condition. It is also this set of beliefs that is undergoing dramatic reevaluation in light of current research results concerning the links between psychological states and illness.

A Physical Basis for Emotion

Much of the groundwork for the challenge to this prevailing view rests upon the work of Dr. Hans Selye, the distinguished endocrinologist.[1] Selye's research indicates that the body responds to any stress with a set of physical adaptions that allows the body to cope with the stress. The body continues to make these adaptions in response to each stress, but eventually this adaptive capability can be used up. The result is a general system breakdown usually resulting in major illness. Selye's work indicates that the limbic system is central in mediating between emotional states and physiological processes. Since the limbic system is integral to all the activities essential to the self-preservation of the organism, such as the fight-or-flight reaction, it is sensitive to changes in emotional state. The limbic system in turn "communicates" with the hypothalamus leading to pituitary activity and substantial changes in the balance of the endocrine system. The hypothalamic activity may also lead to a suppression of the immune system.

The accumulation of stress effects in the body can itself result in life-threatening physical ailments. While Selye's work does sustain the fundamental premise of modern medicine that illness results from physical processes, it does undermine the three premises cited earlier. His work substantially reduces the importance of the "single cause" of illness and instead places an emphasis on the total state of the organism. It also provides a physiological basis via the mediating influence of the limbic system by which emotional states are translated into physical effects that can have substantial impact on the body. The implications for treatment are that health is a function of the total physical and emotional state of the individual and that remedies must include both.

Stressful Events and Illness

Further confirmation of stress and illness has come from the work of Dr. Thomas Holmes and his associates, Dr. M. Masuda and Dr. R. H. Rahe.[2,3] They studied the relationship of stressful events in people's live (e.g., loss of job, divorce, death of spouse, etc.) and incidence of illness. Results of these studies clearly indicate the correlation between psychological stress and illness. One of the interesting findings made by Holmes et al. was that so-called positive events, such as the birth of a child, marriage, promotion, change in financial condition, could be as stress-producing as "negative events," such as loss of job, death, divorce, etc. Apparently, it is the use of adaptive capability, not its positive/negative qualities, that makes an event stressful.

The literature that demonstrates ties between emotional states and illness is summarized in Pelletier's *Mind as Healer, Mind as Slayer*.[4]

Personality and Illness

Friedman and Rosenman's work demonstrates the relationship between personality and illness in their research on the personality traits of persons with coronary artery disease.[5] They reported two "types" of heart attack patients. The Type A personality is characterized by a constant struggle against other people and time and concentrates solely on status at the expense of personality enhancement. A Type B personality does not fight against life like the Type A. He or she is more likely to value relationships, to explore experiences along the way, to exhibit much less impatience and anxiety. The studies indicated that a Type A individual is ten times more likely to experience a myocardial infarction than a Type B personality.

A more controversial, yet very promising, field of work has been the link between personality characteristics and cancer.[6,7] There is a body of research evidence that suggests cancer to be associated with feelings of helplessness, hopelessness, and powerlessness. This literature is described in some detail in *Getting Well Again* by Simonton, Simonton, and Creighton.[8] In explaining the physical basis for his work, Simonton points to Burnet's "surveillance theory," which suggests that all of us have cancerous cells in our body from time-to-time, either internally generated or in response to an externally induced agent.[9] The body's immune system, however, maintains a constant surveillance and destroys these cells. Cancer occurs only when there is some breakdown in this surveillance. Simonton points to Selye's work, indicating that psychological stress leads to a suppression of the immune system as well as hormonal imbalances which can lead to increased production of abnormal cells—ideal conditions for cancerous growth.

Simonton's work makes an effort to reverse the psychological conditions that may have led to this suppression of the immune system. He works to help the patient regain hope and mobilize the body's defenses against the disease. The dramatic results he has achieved suggest that psychological factors play a role not only in the onset of illness, but can also be mobilized to fight illness as well.

Treatment of the Whole Person

The picture that emerges from research is that it is impossible to separate physical states and psychological states. It is necessary to consider "the whole person." Health is not simply the absence of physical disease, but the presence of a high-level of wellness in physical, emotional, possibly even spiritual, states of the whole person.

There are three significant implications for treatment of the elderly that are derived from this changed conception of health as a function of the whole person:

1. Effective health maintenance of the elderly requires not just an examination of physical condition, but the individual's life-condition. The so-called "complaints" of the elderly are significant indicators of emotional states that may be intimately related to their present or future physical condition.

2. If psychological factors play a role in the onset of disease, they can also play a role in recovery from illness. In effect, if we can have psychosomatic illness, we can also have psychosomatic health. This opens up a whole range of therapies other than drugs or surgery that can play a significant role in physical health.

3. Finally, the recognition that the "whole person" is involved in health, makes "self-help" an essential part of health maintenance. The patient, not just the health professional, can play a critical role in his or her own health by learning to create positive emotional states, by carrying out programs of diet and exercise, and through use of a variety of self-help therapies.

If health is a characteristic of the whole person, then a preventive and multidimensional approach to health care for elders is the way to remedy effectively many of the difficulties that repeatedly and predictably occur during the aging process. A comprehensive approach includes considerations of the social and psychological components of aging, as well as emphasis on all aspects of physical functioning.

Many alternatives to traditional medicine and counseling have begun to find their way into the world of the elderly. Techniques such as biofeedback, relaxation training and stress reduction, yoga, meditation, journal writing, creative art therapies, and various types of personal growth groups for elders have met with strong and positive response, both from elders themselves and from health practitioners.

The Role of the Health Practitioner

The emergence of alternative views and practices call for a shift in the role of the health practitioner. Instead of health being something the health practitioner does "to" the patient, it becomes something the patient creates with the support of the practitioner. The health practitioner must become skilled in assisting the elderly to help themselves, rather than continuing to participate in a relationship in which it is assumed the health practitioner is responsible for the patient's health.

The role of the health practitioner is to mobilize the patient's energy in the direction of health. Yet this shift is not without its pitfalls, for many health practitioners must also learn a new conception of what "helping" means. Many health care practitioners slip into what Dr. Claude Steiner refers to as "the rescue game."[10] The rescuer role, which Steiner describes in his books, *Games Alcoholics Play* and *Scripts People Live,* is a role many health practitioners unconsciously adopt when dealing with people who are weak, helpless, powerless, or unable to take charge of their own lives. The problem is that the rescuer, while appearing to be helping someone, is actually reinforcing their weakness and powerlessness.

The way the game is played would be something like this: the patient (victim) starts out by being absolutely helpless. The victim is unable to eat, get to the bathroom, is victimized by thoughtless or cruel friends, etc. The health practitioner (rescuer) responds to this role by taking care of all the victim's problems. The problem is that by doing this, the rescuer tries to help, but does so by rescuing the victim from self-care.

Either party may then become a persecutor. Frequently, the rescuer will become angry that the victim is doing nothing to help and will begin to criticize or berate the victim for lack of initiative. Often the cycle of feelings moves from pity to anger, eventually to hostility, and finally to guilt for having been hostile. Another pattern is for the victim to sense that the rescuer is contributing to his or her psychological and physical incapacity and become angry and resentful at having been manipulated. The rescuer's efforts to help may also be met with a constant barrage of criticism. The victim has moved to the persecutor role.

Related to the rescuer role is a tendency to reward illness rather than health. Health practitioners are often most loving, supportive, and caring when patients are weak and helpless. They then begin to remove these rewards as soon as the patient starts to regain health. The rewards of love and support are given for sickness, not for health. Some of the behaviors that can initiate a reverse in this pattern and focus on health are:

1. Encourage the patient's efforts of self-care
2. Comment when the patient looks better, thereby focusing on health not illness
3. Spend time with the patient in communication about things other than illness
4. Continue to spend time with the patient as he or she gets well

Another step to building self-health is to acknowledge negative feelings of patients. Often the natural tendency is to try to talk them out of these feelings, reassure or sympathize with them, or occasionally even admonish them. All of these various strategies are based on the assumption that it is not acceptable or "okay" for the person to have these feelings. Yet one fundamental principle of counseling is that if you can accept another person's feelings, this gives a kind of "permission" for him or her to accept them as well. Once accepted, the feeling can bring new insight and can be transformed. This is extremely important with the elderly who face many situations that can engender negative feelings: approaching death, a sense of having no productive role in our society, financial security endangered by inflation, inattention of loved ones, etc. Whether or not they are able to resolve these feelings may be crucial to maintaining a psychological state that can contribute to health. Such feelings are not resolved by avoidance, however. They are resolved by going through the experience of those feelings and coming out on the other side.

AN OVERVIEW OF ALTERNATIVE HEALTH APPROACHS

Complete mastery of many of the alternative health techniques often requires advanced training and experience. Many of the "alternative therapies" can be utilized effectively, however, by primary care clinicians with elders. The primary care clinician learns these techniques by experiencing them, rather than just by developing an intellectual appreciation. The clinician's own experiences can then be passed on to their patients with the practical and personal understanding of their appropriate use. This is a strange concept with an "illness" orientation; there is no need for the practitioner to utilize therapies unless they are sick. In a "wellness" orientation, however, practitioners can find continued benefits in their own lives and can improve their techniques.

Relaxation Techniques

With the growing understanding of the role stress plays in health, there has been an accompanying interest in techniques for relaxation and stress reduction. One important finding of stress research is the realization that many of the activities people call relaxation, e.g., sitting in front of a TV sipping a can of beer, have minimal benefits for stress reduction. There are a variety of techniques, however, that do have demonstrated benefits as stress-reducers. These include biofeedback, autogenic train-

ing, progressive relaxation, yoga, and various forms of physical relaxation exercises.

The breakthrough in recognizing the benefits of these techniques came with the development of biofeedback instrumentation. For many years, researchers have been studying brainwaves and have observed that alpha brainwaves are associated with states of increased relaxation. Dr. Joseph Kamiya of the University of California Medical School was one of the first to note an increased percentage of alpha waves in subjects who had been utilizing a meditative discipline for some time. This suggested that the production of alpha waves was a function of learning, suggesting as well the possibility that it could be directly taught. The teaching methodology that was developed was instrumentation which reported to the subject when alpha brainwave activity was taking place. Research quickly showed that when subjects received accurate information about brainwave activity, they were quickly able to bring it under control. This initial research led to greatly expanded study.[11,12,13]

The startling discovery of biofeedback has been that many people are able to learn to control every internal state for which reliable biofeedback instrumentation can be provided. This includes such diverse internal activities as heart rate, sweat gland activity, dilation of blood vessels, and the firing of individual nerve cells. As a result, biofeedback has proved valuable in treatment of ailments such as hypertension, headaches, Raynaud's syndrome, and many others.

The advent of biofeedback also permitted a study of those psychological states associated with deep relaxation, and allowed the validation of techniques that facilitated these states. This led to the rediscovery of two techniques developed in the early part of this century: Jacobson's Progressive Relaxation[14] and Schultz's Autogenic Training.[15]

Progressive Relaxation is a sophisticated relaxation approach based on a tension–relaxation principle. Individuals are taught to tense specific muscle sets, then relax them. A part of this process is teaching people to become aware of muscular tension and, with this awareness, learn to relax each part of the body systematically. With continued practice the individual is able to achieve the ability to accomplish deep states of relaxation.

Autogenic Training is a form of autohypnosis, which also results in deep states of relaxation. In fact, autogenic training is almost universally employed in the early stages of biofeedback training to help people learn greater states of relaxation. Dr.

C. Norman Shealy, a distinquished neurosurgeon, has also made autogenic training a control element in a nonsurgical approach to pain control.[16]

While both Progressive Relaxation and Autogenic Training can be a highly sophisticated discipline—producing substantially altered emotional states—there are a variety of relatively simple beginning exercises that can be utilized with patients. These are particularly helpful for elders with anxiety, arthritis, chronic pain, etc.

The simplest form of relaxation training is for an individual to sit comfortably with eyes closed and to take a deep breath. He or she fills the lungs with as much air as possible and holds it for a comfortable period, then exhales slowly, letting his or her breath go in a steady sustained flow. This is repeated several times. As the person senses a feeling of "letting go" during each exhalation, he or she permits this feeling to extend through the entire body.

In its basic form, Autogenic Training is also relatively easy to use. Again, an individual sits comfortably in a chair (or lies down unless he or she will fall asleep), and with eyes closed begins the deep breathing exercise described above. While inhaling, the person mentally says, "I am"; while exhaling, he or she mentally says "relaxed." This phrase, "I am . . . relaxed," is repeated five to ten times. Gradually, the sensation of settling in or "centering" will be experienced.

The individual mentally repeats slowly, five to ten times, the phrase "my right hand and arm are heavy and warm," then moves on through the body, from head to toe, using similar phrases appropriate to different body parts. Elders can be instructed to complete these exercises two times a day for ten minutes each. Checking their progress for the first month or so assists them with adapting it as a routine. Most persons experience a sense of relaxation and well-being after the first session.

Meditation

There are a multitude of different types of meditation. Virtually all forms of meditation are processes for gaining high levels of concentration. This is accomplished either by focusing attention down to a single thought, word, or image or by "letting go" of thoughts to the point that the mind becomes free of thought. Both of these are much harder than they sound. If any meditative approach is attempted, a person will quickly experience what has been referred to as "the chatter of the mind."

Stilling this chatter is a primary purpose of meditative practice.

One of the simplest forms of meditation is to repeat a single word or phrase over and over. Transcendental Meditation is based on this simple practice, although the word or phrase that is used is a Sanskrit word—a mantra—that is supposedly endowed with additional spiritual values. Dr. Herbert Benson of Harvard Medical School, however, has successfully demonstrated that equivalent stress-reduction benefits can come from repeating the word "one" over and over, in place of the mantra.[17] When working with patients, it might be just as easy to have them first select a word or phrase that has meaning to them. Then have them sit or lie in a relaxed manner and begin to repeat the word or phrase over and over slowly. Whenever they find their attention drifts away from the word or phrase, they should gently bring their attention back to the word or phrase.

A similar device is to have the individuals focus on their breathing. They might, for example, count both their inhalations and exhalations from 1 to 10, then begin again 1 to 10, for the duration of the meditation. Most people will encounter some difficulties staying focused on their breathing. They are likely to become suddenly aware that they have stopped counting or are now counting "33, 34, 35" instead of stopping at ten. Each time this happens, they should gently bring their attention back to counting from 1 to 10. When they have mastered this with both inhalations and exhalations, have them count only exhalations, and then only inhalations. The final step would be to keep their attention focused solely on their own breathing, with no need to count as a means of sustaining focus.

Obviously, there is no redeeming social purpose just in learning to count breaths or to repeat a word or phrase. The value and related stress-reduction benefits are in learning to develop intense concentration, allowing individuals to drop off all the internal working and reworking of past or present problems, or anxieties about upcoming events.

Visualization

Many of the new therapies that have evolved include the use of visual imagery. The reason for using visual imagery is that it is a powerful means of reprogramming beliefs. Since emotional reactions to life circumstances are based on beliefs about the "meaning" of those life circumstances, to change how one feels requires that he or she change beliefs.

If an elder has a set of beliefs about how an elderly person is "supposed" to behave, and these beliefs are blocking his or her enjoyment of later years, visual imagery can help change these beliefs.

Visual imagery can serve as a reprogramming device by creating such a strong picture of the desired state that it is able to counteract the old belief. This process can be seen in the work of Dr. O. Carl Simonton. Dr. Simonton's early research revealed that a patient's belief about the chances of recovery from cancer was a better predictor of recovery than the severity of the disease itself.[18] If he could change a patient's negative expectancy, he reasoned, he might also influence the course of recovery. Dr. Simonton has his patients visualize three times a day, seeing their disease, seeing the positive effects of whatever treatment they are receiving, seeing their body's immune system mobilized to fight the illness, seeing themselves completely recovered from the disease.

The technique has been extended to other ailments or simply for coping with the problems or stresses of everyday life, or for promoting a higher level of health. It is particularly helpful with patients with cancer, depression, acute illness, and during any rehabilitation of a problem. (See Table 21-1.) By repeating this visual imagery, the patient begins to create a clear belief in recovery. We are not suggesting that the imagery through some form of magic recreates itself at a physical level, but rather that as beliefs change, emotional states change, which in turn produce changes in the physical state.

Work with visual imagery indicates that it is often necessary for people to examine their imagery for underlying beliefs and to revise their imagery to express a more positive belief. Patients' imagery may indicate a clear expectancy that they will not get well or a lack of belief that they will meet the goal. This need to explore the beliefs revealed in imagery was first discovered by the Simontons when a patient of theirs who was visualizing regularly was also steadily declining in health. When questioned about the content of his imagery, the patient reported that the cancer was a big black rat. His treatment (chemotherapy) was a little tiny pill that made the rat sick, but after it got over being sick it was stronger than ever. He had great difficulty seeing himself completely healthy.

By examining the underlying beliefs that are contained in the imagery, the health practitioner can either assist the patient to clarify beliefs that may be contributing to negative emotional states and poor health or help the patient formulate and

Table 21-1
Visual Imagery Technique to Achieve a Desired State of Wellness

The patient is instructed as follows:

1. Lay down, close your eyes, and begin to relax. Take a deep breath, let it out, and relax even more. Continue with deep breaths until the patient is relaxed (two to three minutes).
2. In your mind's eye, see your illness (or problem or pain) however it makes sense to you (two to three minutes).
3. Now see whatever treatment you are receiving as working to remove the illness or improve your level of health. In your mind's eye, see this actually happening (two to three minutes).
4. Now see your body acting to remove the problem, pain, or illness. If you are working on a problem, see a process evolve by which your problem can be resolved (three to four minutes).
5. Now see yourself healthy, completely free of the pain, problem, or illness. See yourself engaging in activities you have put off because of the illness. Really enjoy the feeling of being better (four or five minutes).
6. Continue breathing deeply and when you are ready open your eyes.

reach more positive goals. By involving patients in the imagery process, health practitioners can provide patients with a sense that "they can do something" about their illness, and the process of the patients reassuming responsibility for their own health can be begun.

Exercise, Movement, and Yoga

The state of the physical body is recognized to be as important to emotional states as emotional states are to physical states.

There are now a number of studies in the literature that link regular body movement, like yoga and exercise, to changes not only to transitory emotional states, but also to beneficial long-term personality changes. There is even suggestive evidence that exercise may mobilize the body's defenses in ways that reduce the body' susceptibility to illness.[19]

In general, it is recommended that people exercise daily with a vigorous routine at least three times a week for a period of 30 minutes or longer. The exercise should be appropriate to the physical condition of the elders. If the patient can only get around with a walker, then this might be the exercise chosen. There are times when the exercise program for a bedridden or wheelchair-bound patient can go no further than raising arms and legs. For healthy elders, the level of activity needs to be adjusted upward as appropriate to such forms of exercise as jogging, bicycling, swimming, tennis, vigorous walking, etc. Obviously, if people like the activity, they are also more likely to keep up the exercise regimen.

There are, however, other physical approaches that have beneficial effects in terms of physical relaxation and emotional integration. One is the use of physical relaxation exercises. Most of these appear similar to other more conventional exercises, but use a tension-release principle to release tension systematically. For example, see Table 21-2, which describes simple exercises that can be utilized by elders with relatively limited physical capabilities.

For those who wish to explore the potential of physical movement approaches further, there are the disciplines of yoga and T'ai Chi. Yoga is a highly sophisticated training discipline developed many centuries ago in India. There are a number of different yogic disciplines, but the most widely known in the West is raja yoga, which includes a number of physical exercises, or asanas, designed to achieve physical, mental, and emotional balance. In their basic form, the yogic exercises are not dissimilar from those described in Table 21-2. There is an extensive body of literature on yoga that describes these exercises in considerable detail.[20,21,22]

T'ai Chi is an oriental martial art that in practice is part exercise, part meditation, part dance.[23] It consists of a series of slow graceful movements requiring shifts in balance among all parts of the body. When done by someone practiced in the art, it is flowing, smooth, and graceful. When practiced by a beginner, however, it is immediately clear that this grace is not easily achieved except through intense concentration and a complete integration of all parts of the body. This is a form of movement that needs to be experienced rather than read about.

Touch, Massage, and Bodywork

No practice of quackery has been more scorned by the medical profession than the "laying on of hands" practiced by many faith healers. Dr. Dolores Krieger of New York State University has conducted studies indicating that simple physical touch does appear to have some form of healing effect, although there is no scientific agreement on how this

occurs. Dr. Krieger has conducted numerous training programs for physicians and nurses on the benefits and techniques to achieve healing through touch. Employing a massage routine is particularly important for the bedridden or wheelchair-bound patient at home or in a facility. It can be easily done by family or nursing home staff after prescription by the primary care clinician.

The relaxation benefits of massage are well known, but are often avoided because of its connotations of sexuality and illegitimacy (massage parlors, etc.). In reality, massage can be deeply relaxing and highly integrative when it is not presented in a sexual context. It is often a first introduction to any form of bodywork for the elderly, first as a way of relaxing muscle tension and secondly as a form of caring. There are now numerous training programs in massage and adequate written guides for the beginner.[24,25]

Beyond massage, there is a vast array of new therapies for working with the body designed both to release physical tension and also to encourage emotional release, integration of the personality, and even spiritual development. Among the many forms of bodywork are rolfing,[26] bioenergetics,[27] shiatsu,[28] accupressure,[29] feldenkrais,[30] and tragering.

The essential premise of all bodywork is that body, intellect, and emotions are a unity, or "body–mind." As a result, release of physical tension or other imbalances in physical structure also result in emotional release and emotional restructuring. Several of these disciplines teach practitioners to "read" the body as if it were a map to the personality characteristics of the individual.[31] Some use physical manipulation to release this tension; others use the physical state of the body more as a diagnostic tool, utilizing techniques of emotional release to induce changes in the body. All hold the promise of a medicine of the future that will work simultaneously at mental, emotional and physical levels.

Life Review

An apparently natural process of age is a tendency to reminisce, to review one's life, as if to capture the learning of one's life in a final summation. This natural tendency can be elaborated upon with a variety of techniques to make such a review a process of greatly increased personal growth and consciousness.

Some of the most basic, yet often productive, forms of life review are assignments such as: pre-

Table 21-2
Exercise for Elders With Limited Physical Capabilities

Instruct the patient to exercise the following areas:

Hands: While standing, rotate hands in a circle. They should be loose and relaxed, and should feel like you are flipping your hands in a circular movement. After 10–20 rotations, reverse direction.

Arms: In a standing position, tilt one shoulder slightly so that the arm is hanging straight down from the shoulder. Begin to rotate the arm slowly much as if your hand were rotating the lid of a jar. Begin to rotate your arm rapidly as if it were a wet mop. Rest, close your eyes, and feel the tingling in your arm. Then do the same thing with the other arm.

Back and legs: In a standing position, stretch up as high as you can, as if you were taking something from the ceiling. Then relax in your stomach, bend comfortably at the waist, let your hands drop, and begin bouncing as if you were touching your feet. Don't strive to touch your feet, however. Just bounce up and down from the waist, creating a gentle pull through the lower back and the backs of your legs.

Legs: Stretch out on the floor, then lift one leg up perpendicular to your body. Point your toes towards your head, then away, then towards, several times. Then bend your leg at the knee, and let your foot bounce up and down against the back of your thighs or buttocks. Stretch your leg in the air again, then repeat the process. After completing the sequence the second time, let your leg drop gently to the floor, then repeat the exercise with your other leg.

Lower back: Lying on your back, slide both feet up so they are on the floor near your buttocks, about 18 inches apart. Imagine that someone is pulling your stomach up so that your back is arched. Then relax the arch so that your lower back touches the floor and your hips lift off the floor. Repeat the process several times.

Shoulders: In a sitting position, rotate your shoulders up towards your ears, in back and around to the front again, rotating them in a complete circle. Repeat 5–10 times, then reverse the direction of rotation. Then raise your shoulders as high as you can, as if you were going to touch your ears. Hold that tense position for 1–2 seconds, let the shoulders drop and relax. Repeat this several times.

Neck: In a sitting position, let your head drop back, then roll gently to one side. As it rolls towards the front, let it go completely, then reverse the direction back over the shoulder around the other way in a complete circle. Repeat several times.

Face: Squeeze up your eyes and face as tight as you can, then relax. Open your jaw as wide as it will stretch, hold 1–2 seconds, then relax. Repeat each exercise several times.

pare a list of all the achievements in your life, or write a history of your family. Such exercises can help to shore-up a sagging self-image, or provide a sense of the continuity of life.

INTENSIVE JOURNAL

Dr. Ira Progoff, the former Director of the Institute for Research in Depth Psychology at Drew University Graduate School, has developed a technique he calls the Intensive Journal, which is basically a detailed process for maintaining a journal designed to help people find the interconnectedness of events in their lives and discover the hidden growth process that goes on in us.[32] The subject sits for a period of time in a relaxed state, very similar to forms of meditation in which one lets all thoughts drift away until new images or insights emerge, then writes any new thoughts in the journal. Because life review seems to be a natural process for the elderly, this process holds considerable promise for assisting the elderly in focusing and understanding the meaning of their lives.

DEATH

A significant element in an elder's review of life is the awareness that it is drawing to a close. Friends and loved ones have died, and fewer and fewer remain. This brings with it an acute awareness of one's own mortality. Yet there is a kind of conspiracy of silence regarding death. This may be changing, however, and the person who can be credited with making much of the change possible is Dr. Elizabeth Kubler-Ross.

Dr. Kubler-Ross' extensive studies[33,34] have revealed a definite progression of psychological stages that patients go through when they know they are facing death. These are:

1. Denial and isolation
2. Anger
3. Bargaining
4. Depression
5. Acceptance

She has also discovered that the opportunity to discuss and make meaning out of dying is as essential as finding meaning in any other significant psychological event.

Dr. Kubler-Ross' work has also led to an appreciation that dying is made more painful in our culture by virtue of the fact that people often die in hospitals, which are experienced as strange, antiseptic, and separate from loved ones or any normal life. There is growing appreciation of the need to be concerned with the quality of dying, which includes the environment in which death takes place. The outgrowth of these observations has been the hospice movement.[35] The intent of the hospice movement is to provide the emotional and practical support so that the dying can live out their final days in their own home or in a center designed to provide a feeling of home with large quantities of emotional support and involvement with other people.

DEATH FANTASY

The primary care clinician can assist elders with facing their own death by use of a visualization process, a death fantasy.

Experience working with patients who face a life-threatening illness suggests that death is more frightening when avoided than when confronted directly. Health practitioners can be of great assistance by using processes of visualization to help patients clarify their feelings about death and perhaps to redirect their remaining years in light of this clearer perception of death.

The purpose of this fantasy is not to encourage death, but to encourage patients to look at it squarely and understand their feelings about it. Reports after use of this technique indicate that one of the most frequent patient reactions is that the fantasy of death was not nearly as difficult or painful as had been feared. Also, the life-review aspect of the fantasy is particularly useful in helping patients clarify the changes they would like to make in their lives. By clarifying these changes now, patients are able to change their lives or to say the things they have wanted to say so that they do not spend their last years in lingering regret.[8] The visualization fantasy developed by the Simontons is described in Table 21-3.

Table 21-3
Visualization of the Death Fantasy

1. Sit in a comfortable chair in a quiet room and begin a process of relaxation.
2. When you feel relaxed, imagine being told that you are dying. Experience the feelings and thoughts you have in response to this information. Where do you go? Whom do you talk to? What do you say? Take your time to imagine the scene in detail.
3. Now see yourself moving toward death. Experience whatever physical deterioration takes place. Bring into sharp focus all the details of the process of dying. Be aware of what you will lose by dying. Allow yourself several minutes to experience these feelings and to explore them in detail.
4. See the people around you while you are on your deathbed. Visualize how they will respond to losing you. What are they saying and

(continued on next page)

Table 21-3
Continued

     feeling? Allow yourself ample time to see what is occurring. Imagine the moment of your death.

5. See yourself dead. What happens to your consciousness? Let your consciousness go off to wherever you believe your consciousness goes after death. Stay there quietly for a few moments and experience death.

6. Then let your consciousness go out into the universe until you are in the presence of whatever you believe to be the source of the universe. While in that presence, review your life in detail. Take your time. What have you done that you are pleased with? What would you have done differently? What resentments did you have and do you still have? (Note: Try to review your life and ask yourself these questions no matter what you believe happens to your consciousness after death.)

7. You now have the opportunity to come back to earth in a new body and create a new plan for life. Would you pick the same parents or find new parents? What qualities would they have? Would you have any brothers and sisters? The same ones? What would your life's work be? What is essential for you to accomplish in your new life? What will be important to you in this new life? Think your new prospects over carefully.

8. Appreciate that the process of death and rebirth is continuous in your life. Every time you change your beliefs or feelings, you go through a death and rebirth process. Now that you have experienced it in your mind's eye, you are conscious of this process of death and renewal in your life.

9. Now come back slowly and peacefully to the present and become fully alert.

The Potential of the Wellness Approach

The shift from "treating illness" to "supporting wellness" has important implications for eldercare. It defines the considerable problems of eldercare in ways that invite a multitude of solutions. In addition, it requires their active participation at an age when they are often excluded from meaningful involvement. They are responsible for their own lives. Certainly no one in the field of holistic health has a sense that the techniques described hold all the answers, but the programs do suggest the way to an entirely new form of eldercare.

REFERENCES

1. Selye H: The Stress of Life. New York, McGraw-Hill, 1956
2. Holmes TH, Rahe RH: The social readjustment rating scale. J Psychosom Res 11:213–218, 1967
3. Holmes T, Masuda M: Life changes and illness susceptibility. Paper presented as part of the Symposium on Separation and Depression: Clinical and Research Aspects. Chicago, December 1970
4. Pelletier KR: Mind As Healer, Mind as Slayer. New York, Dell, 1977
5. Friedman M, Rosenman RH: Type A behavior pattern: its association with coronary heart disease. Ann Clin Res 3:300–312, 1971
6. Psychophysiological aspects of cancer. Ann NY Acad Sci 125:773–1055, 1966
7. Second conference on psychophysiological aspects of cancer. Ann NY Acad Sci 164:307–634, 1969
8. Simonton, OC, Matthews-Simonton S, Creighton J: Getting Well Again. Los Angeles, JP Tarcher, 1978
9. Burnet FM: The concept of immunological surveillance. Prog Exp Tumor Res 13:1027, 1970

10. Steiner C: Scripts People Live. New York, Bantam, 1974

11. Green E, Green A: Beyond Biofeedback. New York, Delacorte Press, 1977

12. Brown BB: New Mind, New Body. New York, Harper & Row, 1974

13. Brown BB: Stress and the Art of Biofeedback. New York, Harper & Row, 1977

14. Jacobsen E: Progressive Relaxation, ed 2. Chicago, Chicago Press, 1938

15. Schultz J, Luthe W: Autogenic Training: A Psychophysiologic Approach in Psychotherapy. New York, Grune & Stratton, 1959

16. Shealy CN: The Pain Game. Millbrae, California, Celestial Arts, 1976

17. Benson H, Beary JF, Carol MP: The relaxation response. Psychiatry 37:37–46, 1974

18. Simonton, OC, Simonton S: Belief systems and management of the emotional aspects of malignancy. J Transpers Psychol 7:29–47, 1975

19. Hoffmann S, Pschkis KE, Cantarow A: Exercise, fatigue, and tumor growth. Fed Proc 19:396, 1960 (Abstr)

20. Hittleman R: Introduction to Yoga. New York, Bantam, 1969

21. Iyengar BKS: Light on Yoga. New York, Schocken Books, 1973

22. Vishnude V: The Complete Illustrated Book of Yoga. New York, Pocket Books, 1972

23. Delza S: T'ai Chi Ch'uan: An Ancient Chinese Way of Exercise to Achieve Health and Tranquility. New York, Cornerstone Library, 1972

24. Downing G: The Massage Book. New York, Random House, 1972

25. Yohay LC: Oriental Massage. New York, Award Books, 1973

26. Rolf I: Structural Integration: The Re-Creation of the Balanced Human Body. New York, Viking Press, 1977

27. Lowen A: Bioenergetics. New York, Coward, McCann & Geoghegan, 1975

28. Namikoshi R: Shiatsu Therapy. Tokyo, Japan Publications, 1974

29. Cerney JV: Accupressure. New York, Prentice Hall, 1978

30. Feldendrais M: Awareness Through Movement. New York, Harper & Row, 1972

31. Dychtwald K: Body-Mind. New York, Harcourt & Brace Jovanovich, 1977

32. Progoff I: At a Journal Workshop. New York, Dialogue House Library, 1975

33. Kubler-Ross E: On Death and Dying. New York, MacMillan, 1969

34. Kubler-Ross E: The Final Stage of Growth. New York, Prentice-Hall, 1975

35. Stoddard S: The Hospice Movement. New York, Vintage Books, 1978

22

Approach to Pain Management in Elders

Mary O'Hara-Devereaux, F.N.P., Ph.D.
Len Hughes Andrus, M.D.

The management of pain is a common problem in the care of elders. "Pain perception" and the pathophysiology of pain have been extensively studied. There are specificity, pattern, and biochemical theories of pain, and the most comprehensive explanation of pain is the recently postulated gate-control theory by Melzack and Wall. The "gate" is a neural mechanism in the dorsal bones of the spinal column that can cause an increase or decrease in the flow of impulses from the peripheral to the central nervous system and that modulates pain perception. This theory postulates that emotional states affect the "gate" and influence pain perception.[1] The full usefulness and validity of this theory await further study.

Often the control of chronic pain results less from modifying the physiology of pain production than from the psychological factors that influence the experience of pain. The perception of pain is modified by the attention paid to it, the role of other incoming sensory signals, the continuous–noncontinuous nature of the pain, psychological conditioning, cultural background and many other diverse factors. Extremely important are the meaning that any one patient attaches to the pain and the acceptance of pain. All of these factors play an important role in determining the treatment approach and ultimate success of pain control.

In general, the diagnostic and therapeutic approach to acute and chronic pain in elders is similar to that in all adults. Differences do occur, however.[2] Acute pain, the presenting symptom in young adults for certain problems, is sometimes absent in elders for the same problems. For instance, as many as one half of all myocardial infarcts in elders may occur without pain.[2a] Drug treatment should include the appropriate dosage levels for older persons (see

Chapter 6). Clinicians feel more competent to manage acute pain, but are less comfortable and feel less competent to care for the chronic-pain patient of any age. Often the patient can adapt well to acute pain but becomes anxious and may decompensate with the continuous nature of chronic pain.

Common Pain Problems in Older Persons

The source of chronic pain in elders is frequently chronic disease. There are fewer problems resulting from work-related injuries or accidents, and fewer confusing pain syndromes that seem primarily psychogenic in origin. Headaches are less frequent than in younger age groups. When present, however, they are often symptoms of serious underlying diseases, such as TIA, stroke, and temporal arteritis or even depression or electrolyte disturbances.[3–7] Many painful conditions occur more frequently in elders, such as trigeminal neuralgia and herpes zoster, which occurs in 1–2 percent of elders each year.[8,9] Back pain, resulting from age-associated changes in the spine (including deterioration of intervertebral disks, arthritis, osteoporosis) and from nongenerative changes such as metastatic tumors and Paget's disease, is common.[10–14] Pain in the legs and feet is often a diagnostic and therapeutic problem. The presence of numerous conditions can complicate the diagnosis.[15,16] Hip fractures are extremely common in elders and are a major source of pain and disability. Many painful conditions result from inadequate footcare and from the common conditions of dry skin, poor circulation, and arthritis.[17]

Chest pain is often noncardiac in origin. Herpes

zoster, diseases of the cervical and upper dorsal spine, and psychogenic pain due to anxiety over cardiac disease are common occurrences in treatment of elders.[2] Abdominal emergencies, such as perforation of a peptic ulcer or infarction of the spleen, can manifest as chest pain in elders. It is not uncommon for skeletal conditions in older persons to produce chronic abdominal-wall pain, which may be mistaken for a symptom of intra-abdominal disease.[18]

Other common pain syndromes are due to changes in the oral cavity and problems resulting from pruritis. Good dental care, both curative and preventive, is essential. Pruritis requires careful differential diagnosis, as many internal conditions, such as cholestasis, chronic renal disease, hematologic disorders, neoplasms, and hyperthyroidism, may cause pruritis. Many elders are on a variety of drugs that may cause itching as a side effect. Also of interest is the sensitivity to dyes in black clothing, which is traditionally worn during periods of mourning.[19,20]

The physical aspects of pain are only part of the picture. Elders' pain is often intensified by loneliness. Chronic pain can be managed effectively by clinicians who develop a comprehensive and organized approach.

THE EVALUATION OF CHRONIC PAIN

Chronic pain is that which persists for over six months. By the time pain becomes chronic, it is interwoven with anxiety and depression. The social, psychological, spiritual, and physical aspects must all be recognized and addressed before the pain can be effectively managed. Chronic pain is not an emergency. Too often the clinician hastily resorts to narcotic and non-narcotic pain medications in increasing doses, avoiding the importance of both a thorough history and the patient's involvement in the management of his or her pain. Clinicians are often unnecessarily frustrated by making the complete alleviation of pain their goal, when control is the only realistic possibility. Chronic physical pain is a wearing problem with no time limit, and its relentless nature often has devastating psychological effects. Most chronic pain does come and go and is not ever-present. Explaining to older patients that they cannot be pain-free but that clinical efforts will help control the pain will often assist them in adjusting and tolerating some chronic discomfort.

The foundation of pain control is the reduction of anxiety, the increase of relaxation, and the diversion of attention from the pain. Exploring the patient's fears and his or her attachment of meaning to pain can often alleviate false fears and thereby reduce pain.

It is important for the clinician to share and clarify with elders a perception of their pain. Although less frequent in elders, pain determined to be primarily of psychogenic origin should, in the clinician's conclusions, be explained and discussed with the patient. Only through this kind of meaningful involvement and thoughtful dialogue can pain control, regardless of origin, be accomplished.

All pain problems must be thoroughly investigated, using appropriate consultants (medical, surgical, psychological, etc.). Particularly in elders, persistent pain symptoms require meticulous workups so as not to miss a new or previously undiagnosed underlying problem. Table 22-1 presents some guidelines for the evaluation of chronic pain in elders.

It is important to acknowledge the existence of the pain problem. Regardless of the etiology or prognosis, the chronic-pain patient does experience pain. It is helpful to develop a list of chronic-pain conditions most common in the clinician's practice. These diagnostic labels can be used initially to help organize the clinician's thoughts. Classifying common chronic pain syndromes under such larger headings as neurological disorders, musculoskeletal disorders, ischemic disorders, neoplasms, and psy-

Table 22-1
Guidelines to the Evaluation of Chronic Pain in the Elderly

Acknowledge existence of pain
Identify pain behavior
  Obtain detailed history of pain—diary helpful
  Include how pain affects patient's life
    What pain means to patient
    Does patient have anything to gain—what's the game, what's to gain?
Complete medical workup
  Include physical activity levels
  Include nutritional status
Get complete detailed drug profile
Assess psychological makeup of patient
  Administer MMPI
Explain in honest, simple language an appraisal of pain
Be positive, careful, and respectful—do not frighten patient
Work out a mutually agreed-upon program
  Outline in *writing* for patient

chiatric disorders often provides a place to begin for the bewildered clinician.

It is initially important to identify the patient's "pain behavior." There are several roles that patients frequently play as a chronic-pain patient, including the sick role, the medication-dependent role, the rehabilitation role, and the diagnostic-failure role.[21] Patients often organize their behavior around their pain identity.[22] Identification of the pain behavior is part of the initial workup, as is a detailed history of the pain. It is frequently necessary that careful psychological and sociological interviewing techniques be implemented to uncover pain behavior. Clinicians should seek the aid of a psychological consultant for patients whose pain behavior is less obvious or presents in a more occult form. Included in this evaluation should be details on how the pain affects the patient's life, what the pain means to the patient; such details should identify any secondary gain (attention, financial, medication, need to suffer). It is important during this initial evaluation to interview the patient's family or close friends, as this interview is sometimes a key element in understanding the pain behavior and in gaining insight into the reactions of family and friends to the patient's pain. This interview has important implications for the treatment plan. A diary is an important part of the initial assessment.[21] This should be kept over a one- to two-week period. The diary is sequentially filled out by the patient, describing a week of activity that includes when and for how long pain is present, the severity of the pain, and the relationship of resting, sleeping, and physical activities to pain. Food and medications, including alcohol and smoking, should be recorded, and the patient should assess the effect of the pain on his or her personality. This activity diary will help to define the pain behavior and to discover any association between pain symptoms and food, activities, or relationships. The diary should usually be kept for several weeks to monitor changes in pain as a management program is implemented.

The importance of a medication history cannot be overemphasized. An accurate account of the patient's medication use is essential. This profile is difficult to develop, as patients feel threatened and vulnerable to criticism. It is important for the clinician to be nonjudgmental and supportive of the patient's effort to solve the problem, regardless of how inappropriate the drug use may be.

The level of anxiety and depression that exists with the pain should be assessed. It is helpful to determine the psychological makeup of the patient by using the Minnesota Multiphasic Personality Inventory (MMPI). Determining the extent of the patient's personality problems will be helpful in deciding upon a treatment course and estimating the possibility of success. Most patients with chronic pain score high on depression, and many score high in the hysteria and hypochondriasis scales. These psychological problems are usually the result of pain rather than of a preexisting condition. Patients with abnormal scores in these three areas have good prognosis for participating in and benefiting from a pain program. Chronic pain patients who have elevated scores in paranoia and schizophrenia are difficult to treat. It is often hard for them to gain pain control. Persons with elevations in four to eight personality traits are severely disturbed and unlikely to gain successful pain control. Chronic pain patients who do gain pain control often have MMPIs that return to normal.[23] The MMPI is easy to administer and interpret. Those who do not wish to do personality assessments should identify a psychological consultant in their community who can work with them on an ongoing basis.

Initial evaluation of the patient will take from two to four weeks. The clinician should present to the patient (and the patient's family) his or her evaluation of the pain in a straightforward manner. This should be done in a positive, careful, and respectful manner and should not frighten the patient or family. If a psychogenic factor is to a large degree part of the pain problem, the clinician should discuss this openly and frankly with the patient. The degree to which a pain program can alleviate and relieve the pain is an important part of this discussion. The clinician and the patient should develop a mutually agreed-upon program that will be outlined with the family. The program will be comprehensive in approach with emphasis on modifying pain behavior. It includes improving general health status, discontinuing pain medication, and implementing new measures. The patient's and family's understanding of the treatment program is essential for a successful outcome. An approach to chronic pain management is outlined in Tables 22-1 and 22-2.

Regardless of the underlying medical problem, there are many approaches to pain control. Shealey has made major contributions to pain management; many of his ideas are included in this section.[23] Additionally, Bergman and Werblun recently reviewed chronic pain for *Family Physician*. All pain management programs have a psychological and behavioral modification approach. Other treatment

Table 22-2
Management Approach

Modify pain behavior
- Insist patient stop talking about pain—except to clinician at appropriate times
- Reinforce well behavior—discourage pain pattern Involve family, friends, employees, and community resources
- Develop diversion activity when in pain

Decrease or discontinue or use sparingly all pain medication

Apply simple local measures
- Heat and cold
- Passive exercise
- Massage

Institute relaxation and autogenic training

Maintain general health
- Good nutrition and proper weight
- Vitamin supplement
- Discontinue smoking and alcohol excess
- Exercise program for total body

modalities may be indicated, depending on the patient and the problem. For patients whose pain behavior includes a medication dependence, substitution therapy with methadone can be helpful. Therapeutic plans including nerve stimulation have been effective in certain chronic pain syndromes. It is difficult, however, to predict under what conditions nerve stimulation will work. Transcutaneous nerve stimulation is done by placing battery-powered electrodes with adhesives to sites of predetermined maximal pain relief. Pulsed currents are sent to the nervous system via the "gate relay," producing a counterirritant effect. Through this process the pain "gate" is modified. Transcutaneous nerve stimulation has the most therapeutic success when applied by a clinician experienced in the use of this method. Successful use requires persistance and patience from both patient and clinician. Identifying the sites and regulating the stimulation is a trial and error approach that usually is extremely time consuming.

Local anesthesia nerve blocks have been used with a variety of conditions associated with "trigger points." Some patients with low back pain, postherpetic neuralgia, and cancer have benefited. The use of acupuncture has proved helpful in many chronic-pain conditions. Neurosurgical procedures are generally considered to be a last resort, as many pain symptoms return within a few months to a year after surgery. Patients with severe intractable pain that is unresponsive to other treatments should be referred to a neurosurgeon for consultation.

OPERANT CONDITIONING

By far the most successful management of chronic-pain patients has been attained through operant conditioning. Operant programs are based on the fact that chronic-pain syndromes can be learned behavior. The patient's pain behavior, the operant (the complaint of pain, the physical posture, including rocking behavior and facial expressions) is positively reinforced by sympathy, taking care of the patient, medication, etc. The goals of a behavior modification program are to institute positive reinforcement, increase the patient's physical activity, and decrease medication needs. To achieve an operant program demands involvement of a patient's family and close friends, though, inadvertently, family and close friends often perpetuate the pain behavior and must learn to ignore the pain while rewarding other behavior. This initial and essential part of the program can be very difficult.

A cornerstone of the behavior modification program is an insistance that the patient cease complaining about pain. Only during specific consultations are patients permitted to speak about their pain, and then it is best to limit them to a few simple statements.

Modifying pain behavior includes improving general health. The chronic pain patient often has poor nutrition, is obese or underweight, smokes or consumes alcohol, and has a sedentary lifestyle. The patient must learn to function normally despite the pain. Exercise and increased physical activity are basic to treatment. The patient and his or her family must learn to understand that the pain will not increase if the patient is more active. Improving general health, including physical activity, is an important step for the patient to take towards gaining control of the pain. Rewarding the patient's change in behavior in areas that increase his or her general health is part of operant conditioning (positive reinforcement).

Taking drugs is a major part of the patient's learned behavior and is the most insidious of all the conditioned habits.[23] Drugs never satisfactorily relieve pain and in fact contribute to the patient's problem list. At the least, drugs alter personality and decrease physical activity. As tolerance occurs, higher and higher dosages are necessary, often resulting in drug addiction. It is important that the patient understands at the onset of treatment that drug withdrawal is an integral part of the whole program. There are several approaches that can be used to assist in breaking the drug habit. If the clinician has all the medications packaged in capsules of the same size, shape, and color, or in a syrup (pain cocktail), it will be less difficult to change the dosage and switch drugs without the patient's knowledge. Informed consent must be attained *before* the clinician institutes a drug withdrawal program. All medications should be taken by the patient on a time schedule established by the clinician. It is essential that the clinician, not the patient, be in charge of what, when, and how much pain medication is taken. This will disassociate the patient from experiencing pain and having to experience pain in order to take the drugs. Often clinicians condition patients to experience pain by telling them to take their medication as necessary to relieve pain. This practice reinforces pain behavior. It is a good idea for the clinician to detail a drug reduction program for each chronic-pain patient, this program is then put in the patient's chart and followed. This will allow the clinician to monitor and keep to a schedule. In the beginning, it is important to keep the patient well medicated. From this point of learned comfort, the patient's drugs are gradually reduced.

The pain-control program includes other essential elements, including progressive exercise, massage, application of cold, and relaxation training. Physical exercise and relaxation training are most important in the total pain program. Without them, it is doubtful that pain control can be accomplished. All patients should have a progressive exercise program designed especially for them, which should include aerobic exercises.

Patients not accustomed to exercise can begin very slowly and gradually work up to simple stretching and range-of-motion exercise. It is easy to begin from the head and neck and work downward. Each movement is repeated two or three times, and repetitions are increased gradually. It is often helpful to work with a physical therapist as a consultant to develop individual exercise programs for patients who are quite disabled. Massage is an important part of the program. Total-body massage promotes a general feeling of well-being, relaxation, and decreased pain perception. Local massages to the area of pain can desensitize the patient and usually must be done several times a day to be effective. Family members can learn to give local and total body massage which is an effective and economical way to provide this component of therapy. It not only gets the massage done, but it also brings the family and patient together in a positive and loving way.

Application of heat and cold to painful areas and its relative success are controversial. Shealy feels cold is more effective and quite useful for some localized areas. Ice rubdowns are most effective, although Crygel and Therapac are useful and easier to manage. Care should be taken that cold treatments are not applied so as to burn the patient's skin.[23]

Successful pain-control programs include autogenic training. This is often the most difficult area for the clinician to accept and implement. The perception of Western thinking that the mind and body are separate seems confusing when using the mind-over-body control of autogenics. However, it works. Patients usually accept it readily, and it is easy to teach and learn (see Chapter 21).

Begin autogenic training by thoroughly explaining the philosophy and approach. The clinician should assure patients that he or she does not think their pain is "fake" or all in their head. It is wise to provide patients with a variety of taped exercises, selecting the one(s) that work best. The clinician should first have patients try the exercises out under supervision in the office and then take a tape home and practice with it. Each session should begin with deep breathing and relaxing as the state of relaxation, which the clinician should assist patients to achieve, is essential to the effectiveness of the exercises. In Table 22-3 is a good basic experience for pain control.[23]

It is common in severe pain states for the patient to practice autogenic training many hours a day. Freedom from pain and maintaining an altered state of awareness takes many months of practice. Once achieved, freedom from pain can be carried over into longer and longer periods. The use of verbal and visualization programming is used to alter the patient's behavior and image of him- or herself. Clinicians who are not familiar with autogenic training and visualization should receive training and consultation from knowledgeable resources in their community. There is no reason that every clinician cannot quickly become competent and self-sufficient in this skill. If more desirable, however, a member of the pain-management team can be appointed to acquire skill in this essential component.

Although the authors do not recommend drug therapy for the chronic pain patient, there are times when the total pain-management program will include some medication. In general, patients with chronic pain take too many drugs with only partial relief that often complicates the already complex problem. Chronic pain is not an emergency. Drug

Table 22-3
A Basic Experience for Pain Control

Now relax, close your eyes, take a deep breath and repeat mentally to yourself each
   sentence after I say it:
   My arms and legs are heavy and warm. (Six times)
   My heartbeat is calm and regular. (Six times)
   My body breathes itself. (Six times)
   My abdomen is warm. (Six times)
   My forehead is cool. (Six times)
   My mind is quiet and still. (Three times)
   My mind is quiet and happy. (Three times)
   I am at peace.
   I feel my feet expanding lightly and pleasantly by 1 inch. (Two times)
   My feet are now expanding lightly and pleasantly by 12 inches. (Two times)
   The pleasant 12 inch expansion is spreading throughout all the parts of my legs.
      (Two times)
   My abdomen, buttocks, and back are expanding 12 inches lightly and pleasantly.
      (Two times)
   My chest is expanding 12 inches pleasantly and lightly. (Two times)
   My arms are expanding 12 inches lightly and pleasantly. (Two times)
   My neck and head are joining in the 12 inches of expansion. (Two times)
   My entire body is relaxed, expanded and comfortable. (Six times)
   My mind is quiet and still. (Two times)
   I withdraw my mind from my physical surroundings. (Two times)
   I am free of pain and all other sensations. (Two times)
   My body is safe and comfortable. (Six times)
   My mind is quiet and happy. (Two times)
   I am that I am. (pause Two minutes)
   Each time I practice this exercise my body becomes more and more comfortable.
      And I carry this comfort with me to my normal awareness. As I prepare to
      return to my normal awareness I will bring with me the ideal comfort which I
      have created in my focused concentration. As I open my eyes, I take a deep
      comfortable breath and a big comfortable stretch.

Reprinted from Shealey N: The Pain Game. Millbrae, California, Celestial Arts, 1976, pp
116-117. By permission.

therapy should never be instituted alone as a total management strategy for pain.

When drug therapy is used, it is important to remember the hallmark of drug therapy in elders: start low, go slow. The most common and useful drug for treatment of chronic pain is aspirin, though the side effects—the gastrointestinal problems often associated with long-term aspirin therapy—should be considered. Close medical supervision of a relatively simple drug such as aspirin is important.

Both the minor and major tranquilizers have been used and misused to relieve some types of pain. The principal contribution of these drugs is a decrease in anxiety and attentiveness to the pain. Generally, these drugs should be avoided in elders. The alternative therapies can be just as effective and have neither the dependency problems nor the accompanying decrease in mental alertness and attention that can affect the many daily activities of elders in a hazardous way. Antidepressant drugs have been employed in chronic pain, but they can have adverse effects in elders and should only be used with extreme caution.

The administration of narcotics, except in severe acute or in terminal pain, is largely unwarranted. Low doses of codeine with aspirin are often helpful in a relatively short-term control of pain, but, again, their continuous use is discouraged. Inconsistent, sparing administration of narcotics to patients in terminal pain, under the guise of preventing addiction or avoiding damaging side effects, is totally unwarranted in managing the dying patient. When principles of pain control that are appropriate for those who are not terminally ill are applied to the dying, the result is often inhumane. Relief of pain for dying patients is an important part of their care. The use of major narcotics—heroin, morphine, and Brumpton's cocktails—are indicated with the goal of pain control and patient comfort. For the dying, there is no minimal time interval or maximum dose.

REFERENCES

1. Luce JM, Thompson, TL II, Getto CJ, Byyny RL: New concepts of chronic pain and their implications. Hosp Prac 4:113–123, 1979

2. Pain in the elderly: Patterns change with age. JAMA 241, 1979

2a. Zoob M: Differentiating the causes of chest pain. Geriatrics 33:101, 1978

3. Ziegler DK, Hassanein RS, Couch JR: Characteristics of life headache histories in a nonclinic population. Neurology 27:265–269, 1977

4. Nikiforow R, Hokkanen E: An epidemiological study of headache in an urban and a rural population in northern Finland. Headache 18:137–145, 1978

5. Poser CM: The types of headache that affect the elderly. Geriatrics 31:103–106, 1976

6. Foster JB: Differentiating causes of headache. Geriatrics 32:115–118, 1977

7. Freemon FR: Evaluation and treatment of headache. Geriatrics 33:82–85, 1978

8. Poser CM: Facial pain: Diagnostic dilemma, therapeutic challenge. Geriatrics 30:110–115, 1975

9. Rothman KJ, Monson RR: Epidemiology of trigeminal neuralgia. Chron Dis 26:3–12, 1973

10. Frost HM: Managing the skeletal pain and disability of osteoporosis. Orthop Clin North Am 3:561–570, 1972

11. Cailliet R: Lumbar discogenic disease: Why the elderly are more vulnerable. Geriatrics 30:73–76, 1975

12. Sarkin TL: Backache in the aged. S Afr Med J 51:418–420, 1977

13. Burton C, Nida G, Ray C, et al: Treating low back pain in the elderly. Geriatrics 33:61–65, 1978

14. Stern FH: Coccygodynia among the geriatric population. J Am Geriat Soc 15:100–102, 1967

15. Moylan JA: Diagnosing and treating leg pain due to arteriosclerosis obliterans. Postgrad Med 58:135–138, 141, 1975

16. DeWolfe VG: Iatrogenic and functional leg pain. Geriatrics 38:60–62, 1973

17. Montgomery RM: Relieving painful feet. Geriatrics 29:137–138, 141, 142, 1974

18. Howell TH: Abdominal-wall pain of bony origin: Two clinical entities in geriatric patients. J Am Geriatr Soc 20:312–313, 1972

19. Johnson, SAM: Relieving itching in the geriatric patient. Postgrad Med 58:105–109, 1975

20. Thorne EC: Coping with pruritus—a common geriatric complaint. Geriatrics 33:47–49, 1978

21. Bergman JJ, Werblun MN: Chronic pain: A review for the family physician. J Fam Prac 7:685–693, 1978

22. Sternbach RA: Pain Patients: Traits and Treatment. New York, Academic Press, 1974

23. Shealy CN: The Pain Game. Millbrae, California, Celestial Arts, 1976, pp 95, 116

RECOMMENDED RESOURCES

Bergman JJ, Werblun MN: Chronic pain: A review for the family physician. J Fam Prac 7:685–693, 1978

Degood DE: A behavioral pain-management program: Expanding the psychologist's role in a medical setting. Prof Psych 8:491–502, 1979

Foley KM, Posner JB: Pain, in the American Academy of Neurology Review Book, 1978, pp 199–217

Fordyce WE: An operant conditioning method for managing chronic pain. Postgrad Med 57:123, 1973

Gorsky BH: Chronic pain. Postgrad Med 66:147–154, 1979

Maltbie AA, Cavenar JO Jr, Hammett EB, et al: A diagnostic approach to pain. Psychosomatics 19:359–366, 1978

Melzack R, Wall PD: Pain mechanisms: A new theory. Science 150:971, 1965

Shealy CN: The Pain Game. Millbrae, California, Celestial Arts, 1976

Sternbach RA: Pain Patients. New York, Academic Press, 1974

Szasz T: Pain and Pleasure. New York, Basic Books, 1957

3

COMMUNITY AND MEDICAL RESOURCES

23

Community and Medical Resources

Jack Kleh, M.D.

Eldercare demands a comprehensive approach. It requires that health care professionals become familiar with community resources and options for care. The health care professional often becomes the liaison between the elder, family and friends, and health care sources during critical transitions. The ease and ability with which the health care professional can balance and negotiate community resources to the benefit of the patient is often directly tied to the survival of that individual. The health care team is often called upon to play an advocacy role in negotiating options with elders. Sharing responsibility between the health care team, the family and friends, and the individual produces results that ensure the most independent and successful choices. No longer is there a single person in charge of decision making, with the individual of concern the pawn of the process.

Due to the individual and diverse needs of elders, it may be helpful to think of options along a continuum of care from optimum level to death. This book has addressed in Section 2, Chapters 5–21 the issues involved in prevention, health maintenance, and ambulatory management. This section will focus on the options that are available in the remaining segment of the continuum (see Fig. 23-1). Movement along this continuum does not necessarily follow any set pattern or proceed at any predetermined pace. It is presented solely as a conceptual model from which individuals will create their own map. The health care professional becomes a key resource in the construction of the path to maintain optimum functioning.

CONSIDERATION FOR USE OF RESOURCES

Intelligent use of community services must be based on knowledge, experience of health care providers, and, perhaps more importantly, on information from the recipients of care. The Older Americans Act specifies a number of considerations for the use of community and medical resources. The following would seem most appropriate for the attention of the health care professional:

- Meet basic needs—food, clothing and shelter
- Achieve and maintain functional health
- Provide purpose for living

Experience dictates that a surplus of one cannot entirely compensate for the other. On the other hand, adequacy in all of these makes for successful aging; they impact on each other.

It is obvious, then, that medical care (or health care) can never determine whether or not any of us will age successfully. More significantly, how well our basic needs are met and whether we have a reason for getting up in the morning may well be more important than the best health care. This is why people, communities, and a variety of programs are extremely important to elders. They help meet basic needs, promote health maintenance, and provide the purpose for living.

Direction in Health Care

A balance between the scientific, personal, and social components is always essential at every level

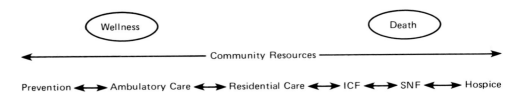

Fig. 23-1. Care options.

of organization in health services for elders. The following four principles are guidelines to orchestrate this balance:

1. Care should be provided to prevent or control disease, relieve suffering, prevent disability, and restore function.
2. Services should be matched to needs. Problems should neither be overlooked or overrated but must be managed according to their significance in the individual's total health picture and way of life.
3. Care providers should be comprehensive, co-ordinated, and have continuity.
4. Management should be participatory with appropriately assigned responsibilities. The patient, his or her family, a variety of disciplines, and even the community must accept responsibilities and participate in the care of the older patient for optimal results.

Models for Treatment

The traditional medical model emphasizes identification of disease and the treatment of disease within clinically acceptable frameworks. The physician has been educated and trained to diagnose and treat disease. The advances in medical knowledge and, more particularly, in technology and therapeutics have sharpened the physician's focus. The patient has become synonymous with his or her disease. This has proven at times detrimental to those aged with multiple diseases; there has been a tendency to fragment, overdiagnose, and overtreat. The health care professional protects the patient from the onslaught of technology and coordinates therapies.

Primary clinicians caring for older patients must realize that their approach is to emphasize the functional evaluation and psychosocial needs and to search for alternatives to institutionalization. Management must include consideration of sensory perception, family and social interrelations, living arrangements, financial resources, and even ethnic and religious considerations. They must make recommendations or even arrangements for a variety of nonmedical services, or at times make trade-offs between scientific and social care needs. This requires a knowledge of resources, as well as the capability to motivate and work with the patient and family to use resources efficiently.

Team Concept

A varied blend of resources and professionals is required to support and augment an elder's optimum living situation effectively. It is the primary care clinician's role to coordinate and direct this multidisciplinary team. Management of this type of approach may necessitate some new models of evaluation of patient progress, blending community and facility-based professionals to form a network of concern for the elder.

Goal Setting

Goal setting is an important part of any treatment plan. In this way, progress can be measured and the plan reevaluated. A goal is neither a dream nor wish but an attainable, reasonable expectation. Setting goals too high only frustrates everyone involved and does not support the reasonable gains that are attained.

Functional evaluation focuses on how well the patient can carry out activities of daily living, how he or she relates to family, friends, and peer groups, and how well he or she can manage the environment. The application of a socially oriented approach using a team model ensures a comprehensive assessment and management plan. A problem list for such a plan may include sensory deprivation, social isolation, inadequate living arrangements, in addition to various disease items. Treatment programs must include efforts to resolve these problems just as drugs or surgery would be recommended for medical problems.

24

How to Keep Elders Alive

James A. Thorson, Ed.D.
Judy Thorson, R.N., M.Ed.

Treating the older person may be one of the major challenges that the medical profession confronts. The practitioner's responsibility to the older client is particularly great since the primary care clinician may become important as a source of affectional support when family, friends, or jobs are lost. Elders accept contact with health care professionals and may be willing to listen to suggestions that are not purely medical in nature. Thus, primary care clinicians have a great opportunity to provide a significant impact on the overall well-being of older persons.

COMPREHENSIVE ASSESSMENT

The starting point of any sound management plan is a comprehensive assessment. Without this, treatment can be fragmented, costly, and iatrogenic. The first step is a life history that concentrates on personal and social conflicts and their resolution; relationships with surviving members and those deceased; patient acceptance of current place in the life cycle; and indications of how this individual is likely to come to terms with aging, illness, and death. Such a life history is not likely to be completed in a single session, but the result of a relationship-building process. Segments of this process can be delegated to team members and all information drawn together and clarified during a final session. Patterns of stress and coping become apparent through this process. Spending an hour or so at the beginning of a relationship can have major benefits for both patient and professional. Patients often benefit from the emotional release of being totally heard. Because of that experience, many patients do not resent it when on occasion clinicians are rushed; they remain secure that clinicians understand. This information is a critical baseline for individuals making life-style changes due to chronic illness or situational developments.

The next step is a functional assessment of the individual's ability to manage in his or her present living situation. The functional assessment combined with a thorough medical evaluation provides the basis for beginning the first phase of the process. The first step in planning is to set reasonable, attainable goals based on the data that have been collected. This is most appropriately done with the elder and any significant support persons in attendance. The primary care clinician's responsibility is then to gather and coordinate the most appropriate mix of services to accomplish the goals.

There are some very important considerations in implementing the plans that are not taken into account in the medical and functional assessments. These factors are related to the psychological strength and adaptability of the individual. Patterns of adjustment will be important factors in the ultimate outcome of any management strategy.

HOW TO KEEP ELDERS ALIVE

In working with elders, stress patterns and coping mechanisms may be key factors in their survival during times of life-style transition. As discussed previously in Chapter 20, there is an emerging body of research that links stress with illness and death. There are some findings that are particularly applicable to eldercare. Seligman's research concluded that "...when we remove the vestiges of control

over the environment of an already physically weakened human being, we may kill him."[1] This perspective is further supported by Wershaw's survey
of nursing home deaths in a major southern city.
He found that of those who die in nursing homes,
44 percent die within the first 30 days after admission.[2] Margaret Blenkner found that ". . .older people admitted to institutions die in excessively high
rates during the first year, and particularly during
the first three months."[3]

PREDICTING REACTIONS TO STRESS

It is exceedingly difficult to predict how much
stress a particular individual might be able to tolerate. Further, although there is no question that at
some point one more straw will break the camel's
back, with humans it is practically impossible to
predict precisely one's reaction to too much stress.
What can be safely predicted is that something
dysfunctional will happen in a person's life if he or
she has been subjected to too many stressful events
in too short a period of time.

In an effort to quantify stress events in a more
scientific manner, Holmes and Rahe[4] developed the
Social Readjustment Rating Scale (SRRS). This
measure has been used to correlate stress with
illness, vulnerability, and death in a number of
research studies.[5-13] Parkes,[14] for example, has cited
data gathered by Young, Benjamin, and Wallis,[15]
who followed a group of 4,486 widowers over the
age of 54 for the first year of bereavement. They
found the group's death rate to be almost 40 percent
higher than other men matched for age during the
first six months; the rate dropped off quickly and,
by the end of the year, was at the same level as that
of married men of the same age. Populations under
stress die at excessively high rates when compared
to similar groups not under stress.[16,17] Blenkner
concluded that institutionalization, particularly involuntary institutionalization, had a disastrous effect
on frail, aged, and otherwise vulnerable populations.[3]

SOCIAL READJUSTMENT RATING SCALE (SRRS) IN PATIENT ASSESSMENT

The SRRS can be used as a quick way to assess a
patient's current stress potential. Life events, both
positive and negative, are ascertained using the

scale found in Table 24-1. This scale is used by
adding the respective values of the occurring items
for each year. The total score represents the number
of Life Change Units (LCU) for the year. Definite
relationships exist between the amount of change

Table 24-1
The Social Readjustment Rating Scale

Life Event	Mean Value
Death of spouse	100*
Divorce	73
Marital separation	65
Jail term	63
Death of close family member	63*
Personal injury or illness	53*
Marriage	50
Fired at work	47
Marital reconciliation	45
Retirement	45*
Change in health of family member	44*
Pregnancy	40
Sex difficulties	39*
Gain of new family member	39
Business readjustment	39
Change in financial state	38*
Death of close friend	37*
Change to different line of work	36
Change in number of arguments with spouse	35*
Mortgage over $10,000	31
Foreclosure of mortgage or loan	30
Change in responsibilities at work	29
Son or daughter leaving home	29*
Trouble with in-laws	29
Outstanding personal achievement	28
Wife beginning or stopping work	26
Beginning or ending school	26
Change in living conditions	25*
Revision of personal habits	24*
Trouble with boss	23
Change in work hours or conditions	20
Change in residence	20*
Change in schools	20
Change in recreation	19*
Change in church activities	19
Change in social activities	18*
Mortgage or loan less than $10,000	17
Change in sleeping habits	16*
Change in number of family get-togethers	15
Change in eating habits	15
Vacation	13
Christmas	12
Minor violations of the law	11

*Those events that are more frequent in the lives of elders.

and risk of illness. Previous studies have shown that 37 percent of people with a total count of 150–199 LCUs will have an associated health change within two years. With 200–299 LCUs, the chance is 51 percent, and, with greater than 300 LCUs, 80 percent of people will have an illness. Furthermore, the more points accumulated the more serious the illness.[18] This framework has a high applicability to elders since many of the life change events are more likely to cluster in old age.

STRESS OF RELOCATION

Applying the information on stress developed by Holmes and Rahe, one can readily see how institutionalization, particularly involuntary institutionalization, forces multiple stresses upon the already vulnerable individual.[19] Elders who are relocated into institutions face disruptions of their entire lives: the sights, sounds, smells, and daily schedule of activities are totally foreign to them and may represent a severe culture shock. Those who cannot adapt quickly to these multiple shocks give up the fight and quietly die.

COPING PATTERNS

Old age may be seen as a time of coping with losses that in most cases are not replaced by corresponding gains or compensations. The pattern of adaptation to these changes will differ with each person, and an individual's success in adapting to the last phase of life commonly can be predicted by his or her pattern of adaptation to previous life changes.

According to Verwoerdt,[20] a pattern of life-long coping is established; this pattern of successful (or unsuccessful) coping strategies determines to a great degree how well an individual will adapt to changes associated with later life. However, certain traits associated with aging—such as a tendency toward less risk-taking behavior, higher fear of failure, and a greater desire to conform—may make the process of adaptation more difficult.

While most people adapt successfully to the changes that come with old age, a minority may exhibit one or more of several dysfunctional patterns of behavior:

- Denial
- Anger
- Withdrawal
- Helplessness

All four of these traits are to one degree or another associated with depression[20]: "Most depressions respond fairly or even quite well to proper treatment. When a depression is characterized by 'emptiness,' apathy, and lack of responsiveness, it is easy to make the mistake of considering the depressed aged patient as being 'senile,' that is, suffering from the effects of irreversible brain changes. This is a serious diagnostic mistake, because, rather than treatment of the depression, the patient may be given only custodial care instead." For a more indepth coverage, see Chapter 5.

MANAGEMENT OF STRESS

Predicting reactions to stress, then, depends on the individual, as well as on his or her personality and social milieu. It appears that the impact of stress is cumulative. Several events of major impact over a short period of time will have a more serious result than the same events spaced over a longer time span. Management of stress in one's life parallels the old saying about not biting off more than you can chew. A new widow would be well advised to wait a year or so to adjust to all the changes that come with widowhood before taking on new life stresses such as changing residence. Postpone stress if possible.

MAINTAIN INDIVIDUAL CONTROL

We have seen from Ferrari's research[19] that people who decide for themselves whether or not to go to the nursing home have a much better survival record. Within the institution, health among populations at risk can be promoted by encouraging individual decision making. Letting patients choose their roommates, what to have for lunch, the color of their rooms, and when to go to bed might seem to be radical notions to health care professionals who are accustomed to the management of others' lives. Most adults make these kinds of everyday decisions for themselves, however, and may react poorly to having this power taken away.

As service providers, too frequently we fail to recognize that we may unwittingly contribute to taking older people's control from them. No matter how confused the person seems to be, or how bad the home situation appears to us, we should think long and hard about "putting" someone in a place against his or her will. It takes a lot of time and patience to discuss all the alternatives with the older person and the family; sometimes it takes a degree of maturity to have our advice rejected and have the patient select what may seem to us to be a poor option. People are generally better off outside of institutions, and placement in an institution should be seen as a last resort. All alternatives must be exhausted before relocation to a nursing home is considered. Home, inadequate as it may be in many cases, is most preferred by the older individual. Resources in the community can be called upon to assist in keeping older persons independent and living at home as long as possible. We should call on social workers with local welfare agencies and councils on aging and on visiting nurses' associations in the attempt to keep people out of institutions. The family itself is often an unrecognized resource; more services are provided for older adults by their families than by all service agencies combined.[21]

ENSURE A CONFIDANT

Eisdorfer[22] suggests that, because of the importance of the confidant relationship, we should make an effort to foster such connections. Two lonely older people may find mutual support from each other and both would benefit when they can give as well as receive. For this reason, the health care professional may be able to match up people who will develop a confidant relationship with each other.

SUMMARY

The practitioner, then, must recognize the social and psychological impact of a particular plan of treatment. We must be particularly cautious about a nursing home placement that, while it may seem like a reasonable alternative to us, may be perceived as devastatingly stressful by the older person. We must be cognizant of the stressful or crisis-producing situations that affect the older people we serve. In some cases, this stress can be ameliorated or at least postponed. We have ample evidence to conclude that pushing old people around kills them. Older adults can be helped to manage stress in their lives, there are alternatives to institutional care, and people can be encouraged to maintain internal control. Our ultimate goal is not only to preserve life but also to add to its quality, and in working toward this goal, we must be aware of the psychological implications of dealing with vulnerable people.

REFERENCES

1. Seligman MEP: Helplessness. San Francisco, WH Freeman, 1975, p 186
2. Wershow HJ: The four percent fallacy: Some further evidence and policy implications. Gerontologist 16:52–55, 1976
3. Blenkner M: Environmental change and the aging individual. Gerontologist 7:101–105, 1967
4. Holmes TH, Rahe RH: The social readjustment rating scale. J Psychosom Res 11:213, 1967
5. Masuad M, Holmes TH: Magnitude estimations of social readjustments. J Psychosom Res 11:219, 1967
6. Ruch LO, Holmes TH: Scaling of life change, comparison of direct and indirect methods. J Psychosom Res 15:221, 1971
7. Wolf HG: Stress and Disease, ed 2. Springfield, Illinois, Charles C Thomas, 1968
8. Rahe RH, Bennett L, Romo M, et al: Subjects' recent life changes in coronary heart disease in Finland. Am J Psychiatry 130:1222, 1973
9. Rahe RH, Romo M, Bennet L, et al: Recent life changes, myocardial infarction, and abrupt coronary death. Arch Intern Med 133:221, 1974
10. Selzer ML, Vinokur A: Life events, subjective stress and traffic accidents. Am J Psychiatry 131:903, 1974
11. Bramwell ST, Masuda M, Wanger NN, et al: Psychosocial factors in athletic injuries. J Human Stress 1:6, 1975
12. Paykel ES: Life stress, depression, and attempted suicide. J Human Stress 2:3, 1976
13. Weyler AR, Masuad M, Holmes TH: Magnitude of life events in seriousness of illness. Psychosom Med 33:115, 1971
14. Parkes CM: The broken heart, in Shneidman E (ed): Death: Current Perspectives. Palo Alto, California, Mayfield, 1975, p 335
15. Young M, Benjamin B, Wallis C: Mortality of widowers. Lancet 2:454, 1963
16. Rees WD, Lutkins SG: Mortality of bereavement. Br Med J 4:13, 1967
17. Parkes CM, Benjamin B, Fitzgerald RG: Broken heart: A statistical study of increased mortality among widowers. Br Med J 1:740, 1969
18. Smith CK, Cullison SW, Polis E, et al: Life change

and illness onset: Importance of concepts for family physicians. J Fam Prac 7:975–981, 1978

19. Ferrari NA: Institutionalization and attitude change in an aged population: A field study and dissidence theory. Unpublished doctoral dissertation, Western Reserve University, 1962

20. Verwoerdt A: Psychiatric aspects of aging, in Boyd R and Oakes C (eds): Foundations of Practical Ger-

ontology. Columbia, University of South Carolina Press, 1973, pp 123–145

21. Tibbitts C: Older Americans in the family context. Aging 9:6–11, 1977

22. Eisdorfer C: The impact of scientific advances on independent living, in Thorson J (ed): Action Now for Older Americans Toward Independent Living. Athens, University of Georgia, 1972, pp 44–51

25

Community-Based Resources

Martha Holstein, M.A.

The health care professional is the key that connects elders to community resources. To keep informed of all the options is challenging and best suited to a team approach.[1]

Just the simple task of taking the time to find out what may exist in the community to help older people retain their independence, and then offering that information to them may be of major significance to their attitudes and sense of commitment to life. If the health care professional can guide them to sources of jobs, housing, income support, or nutrition, he or she may open up a world that may have become restricted.

Where to Begin

Within each community, however small, there are some resources available to elders. The fifty State Agencies on Aging (AOA) can help determine what services there are in any community. Additionally, there are Area Agencies on Aging (AAAs) in approximately 600 American communities, which collect and disseminate information about community services. AAA staff members are also available to speak to groups of health care providers about community resources.

Some resources are available to all older persons, others only to the "needy" among the elderly; some exist in all communities, others are only available in large cities. Each widen the options of older persons in their effort to maintain independence and dignity even into advanced age. By knowing something about these resources, the health care professional can help them in this task.

Self-Help Resources

In the past few years, a number of national and local publications have been produced to guide elders and their families through the maze of resources and services available. They offer numerous addresses and suggestions and can be an excellent starting point for support gathering.[2,3,4]

FINANCIAL RESOURCES

The effects of inadequate financial resources can be fearful and destructive to individual well-being at any age. Old age only exacerbates this condition since there is a declining ability to improve one's income status.

Income in old age comes from several primary sources: Social Security; pensions; savings; dividends; annuities; veteran's benefits; railroad retirement; Supplementary Security Income (SSI); and for an increasing number of older persons, continued employment.

Social Security

Social Security is an entitlement program. If individuals have a work history in covered employment or are married for a lengthy period to someone who does, chances are good that they will be eligible to collect Social Security benefits. To be "fully insured," the worker must be under the program about one-fourth of the time from age 21 (or 1950, whichever is later) until they reach retirement age, become disabled, or die. Consequently,

93 percent of people 65 and over are eligible for Social Security benefits. For those who continue to earn over $4,500 (the 1979 limit) a year, benefits are reduced one dollar for each two dollars earned. Since Social Security rests on a contributory principle, few people feel that there is any stigma attached to deriving benefits from it.[5]

Supplementary Security Income

Unlike Social Security, SSI is a "means-test" program; stringent criteria of financial need determines eligibility. The program began operation in January, 1974 to set a federally mandated income floor, replacing federal–state public assistance programs. Currently, most states supplement these federal payments.

In determining the amount of SSI payment, eligibility workers subtract any income they have from the guaranteed amount and then receive the residual amount. Federal law does not contain any relatives' responsibility clauses, nor does it put a lien on the recipient's home in order to recover the cost of assistance on the person's death. Some states do, however, retain these provisions that many older persons find particularly onerous.

Limited resources ($1,500 in 1977 for an individual), a home, and an automobile do not count as assets in determining eligibility. Life insurance policies with a face value of under $1,500 and household and personal effects with a market value of less than $1,500 also do not count as assets. To apply for SSI, clients should contact any Social Security office.

Nutritional Resources

Obtaining adequate nutrition is a major problem and concern for many elders. Limited income is only one aspect of the nutrition problem. Obesity, poor diet, difficulty in purchase, and preparation, as well as attitudes about eating are involved. There are some very good resources to address each of these concerns.

FOOD STAMPS

The food stamp program subsidizes the purchase of food for a broad category of persons considered to be poor or in need. To obtain information about the food stamp program, call any local (county) welfare department, often called "The Department of Social Services." The practitioner's vital role is to inform elderly clients about programs such as food stamps and to encourage them to overcome any barriers that they may have about receiving such aid.

FOOD CO-OPS, GARDENS, AND GLEANING

Many elders are taking responsibility for combating the high costs of food through the formation of food co-ops, community, backyard, and container gardens. Sometimes a small administrative group helps initiate the program and continues to lend assistance during implementation phases, but any group that has energy and access to a van or a small truck can start a food co-op. For the variety of gardens, availability of land or even space to place containers may be enough. There are groups of elders that have organized specifically to collect or "glean" the fruits and vegetables that are not harvestable or left over at the end of the season. This produce is then made available to individuals or groups who have need of the food.

TITLE VII NUTRITIONAL PROGRAMS

Title VII is a federally funded program that provides meals to elders in group settings—usually senior centers at minimal or no cost—or in-home delivery programs. Meals on Wheels is a service that delivers meals to homebound elders who are unable to prepare their own food. It has allowed many people to stay in their homes who would otherwise be institutionalized.

Employment and Volunteer Activities

A job means more than income to most people; it provides a role, a source of companionship, stimulation. Until 1978, people over 65 had virtually no protection under the law from either mandatory retirement or age discrimination in employment. The Age Discrimination in Employment Act (ADEA) now covers those over 65. Workers in private industry now have protection until aged 70; those in the public sector have lifetime protection.

There are several federally sponsored job programs available to the older worker. The Community Service Employment Program (Title V of the Older Americans Act) provides part-time, public or private, nonprofit employment for low-income older persons. The Comprehensive Employment and Training Act (CETA) provides special treatment for displaced homemakers—women over 35 who have been out of the labor force for a number of years.

In addition, there is a national Displaced Home-makers Network that offers many resources for older women considering a return to the work force. To locate these programs, call the local office of the Department of Labor.

For those who do not work either full time or part time, volunteering can provide a meaningful alternative to paid work. Volunteer activities may also offer training for future paid positions. Many local communities have developed school volunteer programs.

The federal government has created several major national volunteer programs for elders. The Foster Grandparent Program (FGP) provides an hourly stipend to low-income older persons who work with institutionalized children. The Retired Senior Volunteer Program (RSVP) recruits, trains, and places older persons in a broad variety of community service programs.

The federal volunteer agency ACTION has a number of programs that provide volunteer opportunities for the particular capabilities of older adults. These include: Senior Companions, the Service Corps of Retired Executives (SCORE), Active Business Executives (ABE); Volunteers in Service to America (VISTA) and the Peace Corps. There are ACTION agencies available to provide information in every state and in many major cities.

Housing

For elders who have adequate income, housing may not be a major problem. However, all elders, no matter what their income is, have particular concerns for safety, for a barrier-free environment and for housing that offers supports as physical health declines.

The majority of older persons remain homeowners all their lives. The major difficulties they face in maintaining their homes are the ever-increasing tax burden; those minor repairs that may be easy for younger people but that become a serious problem for elders; and the burden of the rapidly increasing costs of energy, particularly of heating oil and coal. To meet one of these difficulties, many state legislators have enacted some form of property tax relief for the lower-income, older homeowner. The county tax collector can be the best informant about various benefits and application procedures.

Many communities have developed special programs to assist with home repairs. The local AAA can provide names of any programs in the com-

munity. Homemaker–choreperson services are an auxilliary service that assists the person in maintaining an independent living arrangement. Cleaning, light cooking, marketing are some of the services provided. Homemaker–choreperson services for low-income individuals are available through Departments of Social Services.

The rising cost of energy may become the most serious problem of all. Weatherization programs have helped some, and there is pending federal legislation designed to assist the elderly in heating their homes.

Each winter, it may be vital for primary care practitioners to be most sensitive to the possibility that cold, unheated houses may cause or contribute to patients' ailments. Many may be unwilling to mention that they could not pay the cost of gas or electricity.

For those seeking alternative living arrangements, many communities offer housing that ranges from separate units for those able to live independently to personal care homes for those who need some assistance with the activities of daily living. There are also residential hotels, mobile home communities, and facilities that include a variety of living arrangements for those who are completely independent or for those who require either temporary or permanent medical care.

For the person with adequate financial resources, selection of appropriate housing may mean a careful analysis of the benefits of relocation or remaining in old surroundings, of choosing a retirement community or living in a multi-age setting. Selection of climate, location of family and friends are all important variables.

For those with less adequate income, appropriate housing may be a serious problem. The two major federal programs that assist the elderly renter are Section 202 Housing and the Section 8 Rent Subsidy Program. Section 202 Housing provides low-interest loans to nonprofit sponsors to build for the elderly. Almost all 202 units are also Section 8, which means that the renter pays a maximum of 25 percent of their monthly income on rent. Unfortunately, there are neither enough Section 202 nor Section 8 units to approach the demand for such housing.

Elders are also eligible for traditional public housing, but in this case they may be competing with families for existing units. Unfortunately public housing is often located in crime-ridden neighborhoods, and the elderly make easy victims.

To obtain information about Section 202, Section

8, or traditional public housing, call the local housing authority (HUD) or the office of community development.

The Farmers Home Administration (FHA) of the U.S. Department of Agriculture sponsors programs for the construction of rural housing for individuals of low and moderate income. These funds can be used to upgrade present housing to include the basic conveniences such as telephones, indoor plumbing, and central heating.[6]

A newly developed housing option is shared-living arrangements, or, in the language of the young, communal living. Some are intergenerational arrangements; others are groupings of older people only. Information on shared housing is still scanty and must be found on a county basis.

Lastly, for those requiring some assistance with daily living, there are board and care (or residential care) homes. These are licensed by county Departments of Social Services and are generally family-run operations. The level of care varies greatly, and on-site inspection is necessary.

Transportation

For many older persons, transportation difficulties may represent the first concrete signs that they are becoming old and will no longer be able to carry out their accustomed way of life.[7] For many Americans, inability to use a car is a major shock in this automobile-dependent society, especially as this loss comes at a time when the replacement of other losses through new activities and the increased availability of leisure time make mobility particularly important.

Walking is one of the most utilized forms of transportation for elders. For many, fatigue, sensory loss, and fears of falling are realistic barriers to walking as a major mode of transportation.

Mass transit presents other possibilities if a community is lucky enough to have any buses, trains, or subways. Those who hold Medicare cards or some other valid form of identification often may receive reduced fares for public transit. There are demand-responsive, personalized transportation systems operating in some communities; taxis offer additional flexibility.[8]

Given the vital role that adequate transportation plays in maintaining the independence of older persons, a check of what is available in the community can be of great assistance to elderly clients. The AAA or the Social Service Department should have information readily available.

Social Needs

SENIOR CENTERS AND RECREATION

One of the oldest means of meeting the need for socialization are senior centers. These may vary from simple drop-in facilities to centers housing a multitude of programs and services. They meet recreational needs and often educational and nutritional ones as well. Senior centers are often the nucleus of highly developed community outreach programs. Some senior centers operate five days or more each week, while others may meet for special programming only one afternoon a week. They are sponsored by a variety of public, church, community, and college groups.

A variety of activities are available through senior centers. Health screening, counseling, tax counseling, legal assistance, college courses, nutritional services, and recreational programs are among the services offered. Park and Recreation Departments, AAA, and colleges are useful referral points.

The many chapters of the National Retired Teachers Association/American Association of Retired Persons (NRTA/AARP) offer a variety of tours, trips, and educational events.

COUNSELING AND SELF-HELP

According to a recently published work, counseling is the process of being "personally useful."[9] It may meet a variety of needs and encounter difficult or chaotic situations. It may be personal in nature or be concerned with particular issues such as housing assistance, legal counseling, tax assistance, or simple guidance in filling out cumbersome Medicare or SSI forms. Decisions made at 40 may no longer be appropriate at 70, but changing decisions may require a new way of perceiving one's self and one's relationship to the world.

Not surprisingly, more and more older couples and individuals are seeking marriage, family, or sex counseling. Retirement roles may place considerable strains on a marriage that may have been shaky, or areas of conflict may appear that business or children effectively hid. Changing attitudes toward sex among the unmarried elderly and the problems created by large numbers of women in the over 65 age group suggest that the need for sex counseling will be increasing. Long-married couples also may need assistance in adapting to changing sexual patterns or desires.

Older couples, forcibly separated as a result of the institutionalization of a mate, benefit from family counseling as do the families and children of institutionalized patients.

Situational crises such as death, job loss, decision to relocate, may result in prolonged cases of depression. Counseling can be effective in these situations. Family service agencies, community mental health centers, and private therapists provide help to older persons. Peer counseling—such as a widow-to-widow program—provides another source of support.

The Friendly Visitor programs around the country again help the homebound or institutionalized older person to find friendship and someone to talk to on the many interminably long days. Church groups or service clubs, as well as Telephone Reassurance services, often initiate these programs. Some provide a regular, daily phone call to people who live alone. If no one responds at the set time, then appropriate emergency measures are initiated.

For more independent and basically well elders, there are newly emerging clinics and self-help groups. Health screening, health and nutrition education, exercise programs, yoga, and meditation are just a few activities of these groups. SAGE (Senior Actualization and Growth Experience)* in Oakland, California is one of the most exciting and successful of these projects.[10] Since its inception in 1974, SAGE has been attempting to generate positive images of aging by demonstrating that people over 60 can grow and transcend the often negative expectations of our culture.

Staffed by 20 psychologists, physicians, and breathing, movement and art therapists, SAGE work is electric in technique. It draws from Western therapeutic practices such as cocounseling, biofeedback, autogenic and relaxation training, and psychodrama, as well as Eastern self-developmental disciplines such as yoga, meditation and T'ai Chi. The SAGE approach is holistic in practice since it focuses on the individual as a whole person working simultaneously with the mind, body, and spirit.

The SAGE Project continues to grow and expand each year and to date has already successfully extended its resources into nursing homes, community centers, hospitals, universities, medical centers, growth centers, and health clinics nationwide.

An offshoot of the SAGE Project is the Association for Humanistic Gerontology (AHG), which is located in Berkeley and was founded in 1977 in response to the need for positive images of aging and prev-

entative services for the elderly.* AHG serves simultaneously as a professional association, an international resource sharing network, and as an information clearing house. AHG publishes a quarterly newsmagazine that lists workshops, lectures, training seminars, conferences, publications, and bibliographic material.

Senior Organizations

For those who enjoy and value participation in organizational activity, old age may finally permit time to become fully involved. The variety is legion; there probably is an organization to meet most basic needs for friendship and companionship.

NRTA/AARP

NRTA/AARP is the largest such organization in the country, with a membership of several million older persons. They are involved in legislative analysis of policies that affect elders. Membership brings two magazines, participation in trips and tours, and the opportunity to meet regularly in chapters across the country.**

NATIONAL COUNCIL OF SENIOR CITIZENS

One of the oldest of the senior activist organizations, NCSC has been involved in the fight for Medicare, for Social Security reform, and is now in the struggle for National Health Insurance.†

GRAY PANTHERS

Organized in the mid-1970s by the charismatic Maggie Kuhn, the Gray Panthers represent the most radical component of the aging activists. The Panthers' theme is "youth and age in action," but they welcome members of all ages. Housing, health care, and redistribution of wealth are some major concerns of the Panthers. Each Panthers network chapter selects its conveners and issues. The main office in Philadelphia publishes a useful newsletter and can help locate a chapter in areas where one exists.‡

---

*Address: SAGE, 114 Montecito Avenue, Oakland, California 94610.

*Address: AHG, 1711 Solono Avenue, Berkeley, California 94705.
**Address: NRTA/AARP, 1909 K Street, NW, Washington, DC 20006.
†Address: NCSC, 1511 K Street, NW, Washington, DC 20005.
‡Address: Gray Panthers, 3700 Chestnut Street, Philadelphia, Pennsylvania 19104.

ORGANIZATIONS FOR PROFESSIONALS

The National Council on Aging (NCOA), Gerontological Society, and the Western Gerontological Society (WGS) are good resources for professionals who serve elders.*

There are several national organizations particularly concerned with minority elders. These are: Asociacion Nacional Pro Personas Mayores (Los Angeles), the National Caucus on the Black Aged (Washington, D.C.), the National Indian Council on Aging (Albuquerque), and the Pacific Asian Coalition (Seattle).†

Legal Services

Although the special area of providing legal assistance to elders is relatively new, it has become one of the mandated services of the 1978 amendments to the Older Americans Act. Special legal issues for elders involve SSI income eligibility, retroactive denials of Medicare benefits, denial of disability payments, discrimination in employment, lawsuits on behalf of nursing home patients. Nursing home residents each have a federal patient's bill of rights from which major claims have arisen. Wills, estates, guardianship and conservatorship continue to be important areas of legal concern.

The private bar frequently provides either pro bono or reduced-rate services to older persons. Private attorneys or the AAAs can recommend legal service programs that may be of great help to clients.

CONCLUSION

There is a wide range of services and programs that exist in communities throughout the United States to reinforce and support the goal of the Older American Act, and probably of each older American to stay independent and living at home for as long as possible. It may take some looking and some time to identify what precisely exists in any given community so that the information can be made available for elder clients, but the potential results—their health, well-being, and joy in life—make it all worthwhile.

---

*Addresses: NCOA, 1828 L Street, NW, Suite 504, Washington, DC 20036; Gerontological Society, 1835 K Street, Suite 305, Washington DC 20006; WGS, 785 Market Street, Room 616, San Francisco, California 94103.

†Addresses: Asociacion Nacional Pro Personas Mayores, 1730 W. Olympic Blvd., Suite 401, Los Angeles, California 90015; National Caucus on the Black Aged, 1730 M Street, NW, Suite 811, Washington, DC 20036; National Indian Council on Aging, PO Box 2088, Albuquerque, New Mexico 87103; The National Pacific/Asian Resource Center on Aging, Alaska Building, Suite 423, 618 Second Avenue, Seattle, Washington 98104.

REFERENCES

1. Pfeiffer E: Mental health and aging: Prevention, innovation, intervention. Unpublished speech presented at the Western Gerontological Society Training Institute, October 5, 1979

2. Silverstone B, Hyman HK: You and Your Aging Parent. New York, Pantheon Books, 1976

3. Galton L: Don't Give Up On an Aging Parent. New York, Crown Publishers, 1975

4. Percy CH: Growing Old in the Country of the Young: With a Practical Resource Guide for the Aged and Their Families. New York, McGraw-Hill Book Co, 1974

5. Ball R: Social Security, Today and Tomorrow. New York, Columbia University Press, 1978, p 365

6. Atchley R, Miller SJ: Housing and households of the rural aged, in Byerts, T, Howell S, Pastalan L (eds): Environmental Context of Aging. New York, Garland STPM Press, 1979, p 77

7. Golant SM: Interurban transportation needs and problems of the elderly, in Lawton PM, Newcomer RJ, et al (eds): Community planning for an aging society. Strousberg, Pennsylvania, Dowden, Hutchinson & Ross, Inc, 1976, p 283

8. Transportation for the elderly: The state of the art. United States Department of Health, Education and Welfare. January, 1975, p 25

9. Herr JJ, Weakland JH: Counseling Elders and Their Families. New York, Springer Publishing Company, 1979, p 6

10. Luce GG: Your Second Life. New York, Delacorte Press, 1979

26

Approaching Institutionalization

Georgia Barrow, Ph.D.

The goal of maintaining the elder independently in the community cannot always be met. Continued health declines may force the elder to ask, "Is a change in my living environment necessary?" Along with friends and relatives, the health care professionals are typically called upon in the decision-making process. Most elders go into long-term facilities, not from their own homes, but from a hospital. The decision to institutionalize is not always clear cut. It should be made cautiously and as systematically as possible. The physical and mental health of the patient, as well as the existing community resources, which could be used in keeping the elder at home are factors to be considered.

Geriatric Assessment Centers

Sometimes an assessment center or geriatric evaluation unit is located in the area, and patients can be referred for comprehensive evaluation. In most centers, patients receive an initial comprehensive evaluation by an internist, neurologist, psychiatrist, and social worker and a functional appraisal in a therapeutic milieu. Short-term treatments may be given. Both the family and the health care professionals are made aware of the diagnosis and can discuss recommendations made by the staff. Such geriatric assessment centers are not always available, and the clinician then assumes more of a role in helping to decide on an appropriate living environment.[1]

UNNECESSARY INSTITUTIONALIZATION

Many elders have been institutionalized because the home care services needed to keep them functioning independently in their community were not available or were not tapped. It has been estimated that as many as 25 percent of all aged in long-term care facilities would not have to be there if appropriate home care and community services had been available and utilized.[2]

Evaluation of an older person for long-term care cannot be made simply on the basis of presence or absence of diseases. It is the *ability to function* that counts most. Some elders are severely limited by chronic conditions such as arthritis; others are not. One elder may have a long list of ailments, yet be able to function quite well. Others may be disabled by one chronic condition. The elderly person who cannot function independently at home and cannot get outside help is the one who may need long-term care.

The personality of the elder plays a part in determining whether institutionalization is appropriate. In some instances, two patients may have the same physical capacity for independent living; yet one seems to need nursing home care because of anxieties and fears. Some individuals need a highly structured and secure environment while others do not want it. A source of resistance to nursing homes by some is the fear of loss of control over one's life. Hostility and resistance to the idea of a nursing home may seem to negate the benefits. What the elderly body seems to need is not always something the mind can tolerate. The decision-making process is then very difficult.

PLAN AHEAD

Whether older patients are going to need nursing home care can sometimes be anticipated some months before they actually enter the facility. The limitations in behavior brought on by chronic illness or age may be progressive and irreversible. This means there is usually time to prepare the individual and the family, make a thoughtful and careful selection of homes, and ease the transition from one living arrangement to another.

Unfortunately, too few people are willing to entertain the possibility of a nursing home and simply wait for circumstances to force a quick, hurried decision filled with emotional trauma for all concerned. Statistics indicate that the typical nursing home patient enters the facility from a general hospital rather than from a private home. This usually signifies that nursing home care has become a necessity rather than a choice. Families often burden themselves for long periods of time trying to care for an aged parent who would receive care that was as good, perhaps better, in a nursing home. Feelings of guilt, duty, loyalty, and even shame often are associated with any attempt to consider nursing home care prior to critical need.

Involving the Elder

It is possible for the family and the physician to anticipate the eventual need and involve the elder in the decision-making process. All concerned can discuss the advantages and disadvantages and together can make inquiries, as well as visit potential facilities. In addition, a grandparent may not always be happy to be in the midst of bustling young people or to be the cause of unusual alterations or deviations in a family routine. These problems can be talked about in an atmosphere of love and concern for one another. Otherwise an aged person may feel "dumped" in a nursing home if it is done suddenly following a medical crisis without any previous discussion or plan.

OPTIONS FOR CARE

An understanding of the kinds of care available is a step in making the best possible placement.

Day Care

In some communities, adult day care is available. Many older people need services on a daily or weekly basis. Day care centers provide services on an out-patient basis. Older people may come to a center for health care, meals, and social activity, or practitioners from the center may, on occasion, deliver services to them. These centers allow people to enjoy the advantages of both institutional care and home living. Day care facilities may meet the medical rehabilitative and social needs of individuals.

Total Care Facilities

Nursing homes provide different categories of care depending on the personal needs of the individual. As a consequence, there are three kinds of nursing home facilities in operation, all of which are designed to serve the needs of elders.

SKILLED NURSING FACILITY (SNF)

These homes provide nursing service on a 24-hour basis for patients with chronic illness or who are convalescing from illness. Registered nurses interpret orders from physicians, supervise patient care, and licensed practical nurses provide direct patient care. Individuals who require continuous daily medications, injections, catheterizations, cardiac or orthopedic care are typical patients in a SNF.

INTERMEDIATE CARE FACILITY (ICF)

The emphasis in these nursing homes is less on intensive nursing care and more on personal care service. The typical patient in an ICF is not in medical distress or crisis but needs help with functions such as walking, dressing, bathing, eating, or getting in or out of bed. While a registered nurse may be available as a consultant, patient supervision is done by licensed practical nurses, and patient care is administered by aides.

RESIDENTIAL CARE FACILITY

These homes are for people who are functionally able to be independent and want a safe, hygienic, and sheltered environment in which to live. Emphasis here is on meeting social and recreational needs rather than medical needs, and providing personal services such as housekeeping and dietary requirements.

Skilled Nursing Facilities and Intermediate Care Facilities are the most commonly utilized and represent what is generally meant by the term "nursing home." The California Association of Health Facilities[3] has developed a profile of the typical patient in SNF and ICF homes. The most typical patient is female, white, widowed, aged 79, and has lived in the facility 2.6 years. Most of the patients in SNF and ICF homes came there from another institution, usually a general, medical hospital rather than from their own homes. The typical patient has multiple health problems with an average of three diagnoses upon admission. In addition to physical impairments, there are usually problems of behavioral management such as mental disorientation (confusion), impulse control (anger), and emotional affect level (depression). Approximately 72 percent of these patients need help dressing, one-half require assistance in eating; two-thirds require help with toileting; and about 94 percent need assistance with bathing.[3]

The Hospice

The hospice is a part of the concept of continuous care. It provides personal attention to the needs of the dying patient and tries to meet physical, spiritual, and psychological needs. Some hospice programs have only an office for counseling to which patients and their families come in to discuss openly the fears, anxieties, and sorrow that death brings. Other hospice programs have more extensive services and facilities. They have hospital wings or other facilities where the terminally ill come periodically or live. Doctors and nurses who work in a hospice have special preparation in assisting individuals to die pain-free and with dignity, whether in the home or the hospital.

FINANCIAL RESOURCES: PAYING THE BILL

Medicare and Medicaid

Medicare and Medicaid are nationwide programs that help many older persons with medical bills. Nearly all persons 65 and older are eligible for Medicare. Needy, low-income elderly persons may also be eligible for Medicaid. Medicare is a federal program that is the same all over the country; Medicaid is a federal–state partnership under which benefits vary from state to state.

Medicare, handled by the Social Security Administration, has two parts. Part A, called Hospital Insurances, covers a portion (about 66 percent) of short-term hospital bills. Most people on Social Security pay no premiums for Part A. Part B consists of optional major medical insurance for which the individual pays a fee ($8.70 per month as

of July 1, 1979). Part B helps pay for necessary doctor's services and outpatient services for physical and speech problems.

The hospital care an elder receives must be "reasonable and necessary for an illness or injury" to qualify for Medicare payments. Therefore, each participating hospital and SNF has a Utilization Review Committee of at least two physicians to determine this for each patient. Medicare was established by congress to pay only a restricted portion of a citizen's medical expenses resulting from only the most serious illnesses. Therefore, the most common health needs of the elderly (routine checkups, drugs, false teeth, etc.) are not covered. In addition, there is both a dollar limit and a time limit on what is covered. For example, Part A does not pay the first $100 or so ($160 in 1979) in any benefit period. This is known as the hospital insurance deductible. It means that the patient must pay the deductible in each benefit period that he or she is hospitalized. If one is still in the hospital after 60 days, that person must pay from the sixty-first through the ninetieth day. Part A pays for standard hospital services, but it does not pay for such items as personal conveniences, private duty nurses, or a private room. Again, there are some restrictions and limitations. Typically, one must pay $40 a day for the third month of an extended stay. Beginning in 1979, participants also had to pay $80 a day for a limited number of "reserve days" after the ninetieth day of a stay.

If an aged person needs part-time skilled health care at home, Medicare can help pay for it, provided the services are by an agency participating in Medicare. Medicare can also pay for physical and speech therapy. It does not pay for full-time nursing care at home, but it does pay for "visits." Thus, if a nurse comes twice a day, that is counted as two visits. Medicare pays for up to 100 visits per year. It neither pays for meals delivered to the home nor for homemaker and personal services such as cleaning, cooking, bathing, or dressing.

For the low-income elderly, Medicaid helps pay for a wide variety of hospital or other services. Medicaid often pays for services not covered by Medicare such as eye glasses, dental care, prescribed drugs, and long-term nursing home care.

Costs of care can vary in SNFs and ICFs from $600–1,200 a month with an average somewhere between $800–1,000 a month.[4] These recent figures are very tentative because the health care industry is especially subject to inflation. There are a variety of ways that nursing home care may be financed.

Medicare will only pay partial costs in a SNF. The patient must have spent three consecutive days in a hospital and be admitted to the SNF within 14 days of discharge from the hospital. A physician must certify that extended care with daily nursing is needed for the same or a related illness for which the patient was originally hospitalized. Medicare will cover only 100 days of care in a SNF for one documented illness. Consequently, a limited amount of nursing home care can be financed in this way since the average length of an individual's stay in a nursing home is two to three years. In addition, Medicare does not provide for those under 65 or for those who do not qualify as disabled, according to the guidelines of the Social Security Administration.

Low-income persons may get help from Medicaid in covering nursing home costs. Medicaid will cover an individual's partial costs in either a SNF or an ICF. Utilization of Medicaid and eligibility requirements differ somewhat in the various states, but generally the provisions for prolonged care are more flexible and generous than those provided by Medicare. In California, the Medicaid program is called Medical.

Private Health Insurance

The policies of many comprehensive health insurance plans of a private nature (e.g., Blue Cross) will pay some portion of nursing home care for some limited period of benefit for specified conditions. These policies should be carefully reviewed for allowed financial conditions.

Religious and Fraternal Organizations

These groups often provide financial assistance to members either directly or in homes owned and operated by the church or fraternal group. These homes often have long waiting lists, and it would be wise to determine eligibility well in advance of need.

Paying the Bill Alone

This usually means using personal funds or funds provided by the family, and it might include pen-

sions, savings, revenues from stocks, bonds or other investments, or the proceeds from the sale of an individual's home. The American Health Care Association (1978) estimates that about 30 percent of all nursing home patients pay their bills entirely out of their own pockets.[4]

REVIEWING OPTIONS

Nursing homes in general have a bad reputation. But the question remains whether all homes are as bad as some imagine them to be, or whether a bad nursing home is relatively rare. This question is quite difficult to answer because no one knows what conditions exist in all the homes, and standards for measuring good and bad vary. Butler and Lewis state that there are good nursing homes. But the remainder " . . . run the gamut from filthy and unsafe to clean but cheerless and depressing. The worst are firetraps, with unhealthy living conditions and neglect of patient care. Others are stylized motel like, antiseptically clean horrors."[5] There is a clearly stated patient's bill of rights for SNFs to assist in designing their operations.[6]

Finding a Home for the Aged

There are many nursing homes that provide a good quality of care for the aged, but they are not necessarily the newest, cleanest, or fanciest. Many of the better homes have long waiting lists, so early planning is helpful in eventual successful placement.

Immediate resources that can be used to begin the search for the right nursing home include: (1) physician, clergyman, relatives, and friends; (2) state and local Office of Aging; (3) county Medical Society; (4) state and local Departments of Health and Departments of Social Services; (5) hospital social service departments; (6) Gray Panthers[6]; and (7) Social Security office.

See Table 26-1 for guidelines in comparing several homes. As stated earlier, there will more than likely be some trade-offs involved in the decision-making process. Availability may be the most important criteria. It is often necessary to place elders hundreds of miles from their homes due to scarcity of beds. Preplanning is the most direct insurance against this occurrence.

Table 26-1
Guidelines for Comparing Nursing Homes

I. What to notice about the general atmosphere.
    A. Are visitors welcome?
        1. Are you encouraged to tour freely?
        2. Do staff members answer questions willingly?
    B. Is the home clean and odor-free?
    C. Is the staff pleasant, friendly, cheerful, affectionate?
    D. Are lounges available for socializing?

II. Is attention paid to the patients' morale?
    A. Are they called patronizingly by their first names or addressed with dignity as "Mr.," "Mrs.," "Miss" _____?
    B. Are they dressed in nightclothes or street clothes?
    C. Do many of them appear oversedated?
    D. Are they allowed to have some of their own possessions?
    E. Are they given sufficient privacy?
        1. Are married couples kept together?
        2. Are "sweethearts" given a place to visit with each other in complete privacy?
    F. Is good grooming encouraged?
        1. Beautician and barber available?

III. What licensing to look for:
    A. State Nursing Home License
    B. Nursing Home Administrator License
    C. Joint Committee on Accreditation of Hospital Certificate
    D. American Association of Homes for the Aging
    E. American Nursing Home Association

IV. Location:
    A. Is it convenient for visiting?
    B. Is the neighborhood safe for ambulatory residents?
    C. Is there an outdoor garden with benches?

V. Safety considerations:
    A. Does the home meet federal and state fire codes?
        1. Ask to see the latest inspection report.
        2. Are regular fire drills scheduled?
    B. Is the home accident-proof?
        1. Good lighting?
        2. Hand rails and grab bars in halls and bathrooms?
        3. No obstructions in corridors?
        4. No scatter rugs or easily tipped chairs?
        5. Stairway doors kept closed?

VI. Living arrangements:
    A. Are the bedrooms comfortable and spacious?
    B. Is the furniture appropriate?
        1. Enough drawer and closet space?
        2. Doors and drawers easy to open?
        3. Can residents furnish their rooms with personal items?
    C. Can closets and drawers be locked?
    D. Is there enough space between beds, through doorways, and in corridors for wheelchairs?
    E. Are there enough elevators for the number of patients?

VII. Food services:
    A. Is there a qualified dietician in charge?

(continued on next page)

Table 26-1

Continued

      1.   Are special therapeutic diets followed?

      2.   Are individual food preferences considered?

B.   Are you welcome to inspect the kitchen?

C.   Are menus posted?

      1.   Do the menus reflect what is actually served?

D.   Are dining rooms cheerful?

      1.   Are patients encouraged to eat in the dining room rather that at the bedside?

E.   Are bedridden patients fed when necessary?

F.   Are snacks available between meals and at bedtime?

      1.   Are snacks scheduled too close to meals in order to accomodate staff shifts?

      2.   Is there too long a period between supper and breakfast the the next morning?

VIII. Medical services:

A.   Is there a medical director qualified in geriatric medicine?

B.   Are patients allowed to have private doctors?

C.   If there are staff physicians, what are their qualifications?

      1.   Is a doctor available 24 hours a day?

      2.   How often is each patient seen by a doctor?

D.   Does each patient get a complete physical examination before or upon admission?

E.   Does the home have a hospital affiliation or a transfer agreement with a hospital?

F.   Does each patient have an individual treatment plan?

G.   Is a psychiatrist available?

H.   Is provision made for dental, eye, and foot care, as well as for other specialized services?

I.   Are there adequate medical records?

IX. Nursing services:

A.   Is the nursing director fully qualified?

B.   Is there a registered nurse on duty at all times?

C.   Are licensed practical nurses graduates of approved schools?

D.   Is there adequate nursing staff for the number of patients?

E.   Is there an inservice training program for nurse's aides and orderlies?

X. Rehabilitation services:

A.   Is there a registered physiotherapist on staff?

      1.   Good equipment?

      2.   How often are patients scheduled?

B.   Is there a registered occupational therapist on staff?

      1.   Is functional therapy prescribed in addition to diversionary activities?

C.   Is a speech therapist available for poststroke patients?

D.   Is the staff trained in reality orientation, remotivation, and bladder training for the mentally impaired?

XI. Group activities:

A.   Is the activities director professionally trained?

B.   Are a variety of programs offered?

      1.   Ask to see a calendar of activities.

C.   Are there trips to theaters, concerts, and museums for those who go out?

D.   Are wheelchair patients transported to group activities?

E.   Is there a library for patients?

Table 26-1

Continued

 F. Is there an opportunity to take adult education courses or participate in discussion groups?

XII. Social services:

 A. Is a professional social worker involved in admission procedures?

  1. Are both the applicant and family interviewed?

  2. Are alternatives to institutionalization explored?

 B. Is a professional, trained social worker available to discuss personal problems and help with adjustment of patient and family?

 C. Are social and psychological needs of patients included in treatment plans?

 D. Is a professional, trained social worker available for consultation to the staff?

  1. On social and psychological problems of patients?

  2. On roommate choices and tablemates?

XIII. Religious observances

 A. Is there a chapel on the grounds?

 B. Are religious services held regularly for those who wish to attend?

 C. If the home is run under sectarian auspices, are clergy of other faiths permitted to see patients when requested?

XIV. Citizen participation:

 A. Is the patient's bill of rights prominently displayed and understood?

 B. Is there a resident council?

  1. How often does it meet?

  2. Does it have access to the administrator and department heads?

 C. Is there a family organization?

  1. How often does it meet?

  2. Does it have access to the administrator and department heads?

 D. Do the patients vote in local, state and federal elections?

  1. Are they taken to the polls?

  2. Do they apply for absentee ballots?

XV. Financial questions:

 A. What are the basic costs?

  1. Are itemized bills available?

  2. Are there any extra charges?

 B. Is the home eligible for Medicare and Medicaid reimbursement?

  1. Is a staff member available to assist in making applications for these funds?

  2. Is assistance available for questions about veterans' pensions? Union benefits?

 C. What provision is made for patients' spending money?

REFERENCES

1. Kleh J: When to institutionalize the elderly, in Reichel W (ed): The Geriatric Patient. New York, Hospital Practice Publishing Co, 1970

2. Special Senate Committee on Aging: Congregate Housing for Older Adults. Washington, DC, US Govt Printing Office, 1975

3. California Association of Health Facilities: Facts about California Nursing Homes. Sacramento, California, 1977

4. American Health Care Association: The Nursing Home Dilemma. Washington, DC, 1978

5. Butler RN, Lewis MI: Aging and Mental Health, ed 2. St Louis, CV Mosby Co, 1977

6. Horn L, Griesel E: Nursing Homes: Citizens Action Guide. Boston, Beacon Press, 1977

Author Index

Subject Index